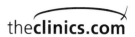

PEDIATRIC CLINICS
OF NORTH AMERICA

Complementary and Alternative Medicine

GUEST EDITORS
Lawrence D. Rosen, MD, FAAP
David S. Riley, MD

December 2007 • Volume 54 • Number 6

SAUNDERS

An Imprint of Elsevier, Inc.
PHILADELPHIA   LONDON   TORONTO   MONTREAL   SYDNEY   TOKYO

W.B. SAUNDERS COMPANY
A Division of Elsevier Inc.

1600 John F. Kennedy Boulevard • Suite 1800 • Philadelphia, Pennsylvania 19103

http://www.theclinics.com

THE PEDIATRIC CLINICS OF NORTH AMERICA	Volume 54, Number 6
December 2007	ISSN 0031-3955
Editor: Carla Holloway	ISBN-13: 978-1-4160-5323-1
	ISBN-10: 1-4160-5323-9

The ideas and opinions expressed in *The Pediatric Clinics of North America* do not necessarily reflect those of the Publisher. The Publisher does not assume any responsibility for any injury and/or damage to persons or property arising out of or related to any use of the material contained in this periodical. The reader is advised to check the appropriate medical literature and the product information currently provided by the manufacturer of each drug to be administered to verify the dosage, the method and duration of administration, or contraindications. It is the responsibility of the treating physician or other health care professional, relying on independent experience and knowledge of the patient, to determine drug dosages and the best treatment for the patient. Mention of any product in this issue should not be construed as endorsement by the contributors, editors, or the Publisher of the product or manufacturers' claims.

The Pediatric Clinics of North America (ISSN 0031-3955) is published bi-monthly by Elsevier Inc. 360 Park Avenue South, New York, NY 10010-1710. Months of publication are February, April, June, August, October, and December. Business and Editorial Offices: 1600 John F. Kennedy Blvd., Suite 1800, Philadelphia, PA 19103-2899. Customer Service Office: 6277 Sea Harbor Drive, Orlando, FL 32887-4800. Periodicals postage paid at New York, NY and additional mailing offices. Subscription prices are $149.00 per year (US individuals), $315.00 per year (US institutions), $202.00 per year (Canadian individuals), $411.00 per year (Canadian institutions), $226.00 per year (international individuals), $411.00 per year (international institutions), $72.00 per year (US students), $119.00 per year (Canadian students), and $119.00 per year (foreign students). To receive students/resident rare, orders must be accompanied by name of affiliated institution, date of term, and the signature of program/residency coordinator on institution letterhead. Orders will be billed at individual rate until proof of status is received. Foreign air speed delivery is included in all Clinics subscription prices. All prices are subject to change without notice. POSTMASTER: Send address changes to *The Pediatric Clinics of North America*, Elsevier Periodicals Customer Service, 6277 Sea Harbor Drive, Orlando, FL 32887-4800. **Customer Service: 1-800-654-2452 (US). From outside of the US, call 1-407-345-4000.** E-mail: hhspcs@harcourt.com.

The Pediatric Clinics of North America is also published in Spanish by McGraw-Hill Inter-americana Editores S.A., Mexico City, Mexico; in Portuguese by Riechmann and Affonso Editores, Rua Comandante Coelho 1085, CEP 21250, Rio de Janeiro, Brazil; and in Greek by Althayia SA, Athens, Greece.

The Pediatric Clinics of North America is covered in *Index Medicus, Excerpta Medica, Current Contents, Current Contents/Clinical Medicine, Science Citation Index, ASCA, ISI/BIOMED,* and *BIOSIS.*

Printed in the United States of America.

GOAL STATEMENT
The goal of the *Pediatric Clinics of North America* is to keep practicing physicians and residents up to date with current clinical practice in pediatrics by providing timely articles reviewing the state-of-the-art in patient care.

ACCREDITATION
The *Pediatric Clinics of North America* is planned and implemented in accordance with the Essential Areas and Policies of the Accreditation Council for Continuing Medical Education (ACCME) through the joint sponsorship of the University Of Virginia School Of Medicine and Elsevier. The University Of Virginia School of Medicine is accredited by the ACCME to provide continuing medical education for physicians.

The University of Virginia School of Medicine designates this educational activity for a maximum of 15 *AMA PRA Category 1 Credits™*. Physicians should only claim credit commensurate with the extent of their participation in the activity.

The American Medical Association has determined that physicians not licensed in the US who participate in this CME activity are eligible for 15 *AMA PRA Category 1 Credits™*.

Credit can be earned by reading the text material, taking the CME examination online at http://www.theclinics.com/home/cme, and completing the evaluation. After taking the test, you will be required to review any and all incorrect answers. Following completion of the test and evaluation, your credit will be awarded and you may print your certificate.

FACULTY DISCLOSURE/CONFLICT OF INTEREST
The University of Virginia School of Medicine, as an ACCME accredited provider, endorses and strives to comply with the Accreditation Council for Continuing Medical Education (ACCME) Standards of Commercial Support, Commonwealth of Virginia statutes, University of Virginia policies and procedures, and associated federal and private regulations and guidelines on the need for disclosure and monitoring of proprietary and financial interests that may affect the scientific integrity and balance of content delivered in continuing medical education activities under our auspices.

The University of Virginia School of Medicine requires that all CME activities accredited through this institution be developed independently and be scientifically rigorous, balanced and objective in the presentation/discussion of its content, theories and practices.

All authors/editors participating in an accredited CME activity are expected to disclose to the readers relevant financial relationships with commercial entities occurring within the past 12 months (such as grants or research support, employee, consultant, stock holder, member of speakers bureau, etc.). The University of Virginia School of Medicine will employ appropriate mechanisms to resolve potential conflicts of interest to maintain the standards of fair and balanced education to the reader. Questions about specific strategies can be directed to the Office of Continuing Medical Education, University of Virginia School of Medicine, Charlottesville, Virginia.

The authors/editors listed below have identified no financial or professional relationships for themselves or their spouse/partner:
Gerard A. Banez, PhD; Shay Beider, MPH, LMT; Brian Berman, MD; Cora Collette Breuner, MD, MPH; Andreas Cohrssen, MD; Timothy P. Culbert, MD, FAAP; Jeffrey I. Gold, PhD; Carla Holloway (Acquisitions Editor); Kara M. Kelly, MD; Kathi J. Kemper, MD, MPH; Benjamin Kligler, MD, MPH; Anjana Kundu, MBBS, MD; Nicole E. Mahrer, BA; John D. Mark, MD; Hilary H. McClafferty, MD, FAAP; Sanford Newmark, MD; David S. Riley, MD (Guest Editor); Lawrence D. Rosen, MD, FAAP (Guest Editor); Susan F. Sencer, MD; Scott Shannon, MD; Sunita Vohra, MD, MSc; and Wendy Weber, ND, MPH.

The authors/editors listed below identified the following professional or financial affiliations for themselves or their spouse/partner:
Michael H. Cohen, JD, MBA serves as the principal attorney for the Law Offices of Michael H. Cohen.
Paula Gardiner, MD, MPH is a consultant for the Council for Responsible Nutrition.
Patrick Hanaway, MD is employed by Genova Diagnostics.

Disclosure of Discussion of Non-FDA Approved Uses for Pharmaceutical and/or Medical Devices:
The University of Virginia School of Medicine, as an ACCME provider, requires that all authors identify and disclose any "off label" uses for pharmaceutical and medical device products. The University of Virginia School of Medicine recommends that each physician fully review all the available data on new products or procedures prior to clinical use.

TO ENROLL
To enroll in the *Pediatric Clinics of North America* Continuing Medical Education program, call customer service at 1-800-654-2452 or visit us online at www.theclinics.com/home/cme. The CME program is available to subscribers for an additional fee of $195.00.

GUEST EDITORS

LAWRENCE D. ROSEN, MD, FAAP, Chair, Integrative Pediatrics Council; Clinical Assistant Professor, New Jersey Medical School; and Chief, Pediatric Integrative Medicine, Department of Pediatrics, Hackensack University Medical Center, Hackensack, New Jersey

DAVID S. RILEY, MD, Clinical Associate Professor, University of New Mexico Medical School, Department of Internal Medicine, Santa Fe, New Mexico; and Editor-in-Chief, EXPLORE—The Journal of Science and Healing, Philadelphia, Pennsylvania

CONTRIBUTORS

GERARD A. BANEZ, PhD, Director, Behavioral Pediatrics Treatment Service; and Postdoctoral Fellowship in Pediatric Psychology, Cleveland Clinic Children's Hospital, Cleveland, Ohio

SHAY BEIDER, MPH, LMT, Founder and Executive Director, Integrative Touch for Kids, Beverly Hills, California

BRIAN BERMAN, MD, Professor, Family and Community Medicine; Director, Program in Complementary Medicine; and Director, Center for Integrative Medicine, University of Maryland School of Medicine, Kernan Hospital Mansion, Baltimore, Maryland

CORA COLLETTE BREUNER, MD, MPH, Associate Professor, Department of Pediatrics, University of Washington, Adolescent Medicine Section, Children's Hospital and Medical Center, Seattle, Washington

ANDREAS COHRSSEN, MD, Assistant Professor of Family and Social Medicine, Albert Einstein College of Medicine, Bronx; and Program Director, Beth Israel Residency Program in Urban Family Practice, New York, New York

MICHAEL H. COHEN, JD, MBA, Law Offices of Michael H. Cohen, Cambridge, Massachusetts

TIMOTHY P. CULBERT, MD, Medical Director, Integrative Medicine Program, Children's Hospitals and Clinics of Minnesota; and Assistant Professor of Clinical Pediatrics, University of Minnesota Medical School, Minneapolis, Minnesota

PAULA GARDINER, MD, MPH, Assistant Professor, Department of Family Medicine, Boston University Medical School, Boston, Massachusetts

JEFFREY I. GOLD, PhD, Pain Management and Palliative Care Program, Department of Anesthesiology Critical Care Medicine, Children's Hospital Los Angeles; and Keck School of Medicine, University of Southern California, Los Angeles, California

PATRICK HANAWAY, MD, Chief Medical Officer, Genova Diagnostics, Asheville, North Carolina

KARA M. KELLY, MD, Associate Professor of Clinical Pediatrics, Division of Pediatric Oncology, Columbia University Medical Center, Morgan Stanley Children's Hospital of New York Presbyterian, New York, New York

KATHI J. KEMPER, MD, MPH, Caryl J. Guth Chair for Holistic and Integrative Medicine; and Professor, Pediatrics and Public Health Sciences, Wake Forest University School of Medicine, Winston-Salem, North Carolina

BENJAMIN KLIGLER, MD, MPH, Associate Professor of Family and Social Medicine, Albert Einstein College of Medicine, Bronx; and Research Director, Continuum Center for Health and Healing, New York, New York

ANJANA KUNDU, MBBS, MD, Assistant Professor, Department of Anesthesiology and Pain Medicine; and Director, Complementary and Integrative Medicine Program, Children's Hospital and Regional Medical Center, University of Washington School of Medicine, Seattle, Washington

NICOLE E. MAHRER, BA, Research Assistant, Department of Anesthesiology Critical Care Medicine, Children's Hospital Los Angeles, Los Angeles, California

JOHN D. MARK, MD, Clinical Associate Professor of Pediatrics, Pediatric Pulmonary Medicine, Lucile Packard Children's Hospital, Stanford University Medical Center, Palo Alto, California

HILARY H. McCLAFFERTY, MD, FAAP, Director, The Center for Children's Integrative Medicine, Chapel Hill, North Carolina

SANFORD NEWMARK, MD, Director, Center for Pediatric Integrative Medicine; and Faculty and Medical Editor, Program in Integrative Medicine, University of Arizona, Tucson, Arizona

DAVID S. RILEY, MD, Clinical Associate Professor, University of New Mexico Medical School, Department of Internal Medicine, Santa Fe, New Mexico; and Editor-in-Chief, EXPLORE—The Journal of Science and Healing, Philadelphia, Pennsylvania

LAWRENCE D. ROSEN, MD, FAAP, Chair, Integrative Pediatrics Council; Clinical Assistant Professor, New Jersey Medical School; and Chief, Pediatric Integrative Medicine, Department of Pediatrics, Hackensack University Medical Center, Hackensack, New Jersey

SUSAN F. SENCER, MD, Medical Director, Department of Pediatric Oncology, Children's Hospitals and Clinics of Minnesota, Minneapolis, Minnesota

SCOTT SHANNON, MD, Northern Colorado Center for Holistic Medicine, Fort Collins, Colorado

SUNITA VOHRA, MD, MSc, Director, Complementary and Alternative Research and Education (CARE) Program, Stollery Children's Hospital; and Associate Professor, Department of Pediatrics, Faculty of Medicine, University of Alberta, Edmonton, Alberta, Canada

WENDY WEBER, ND, MPH, Research Associate Professor, School of Naturopathic Medicine, Bastyr University, Kenmore, Washington

CONTENTS

Ethics of Complementary and Alternative Medicine Use in Children 875

Sunita Vohra and Michael H. Cohen

Complementary and alternative medicine (CAM) has enjoyed tremendous public interest in North America in recent years. CAM is used most often by those who have serious, chronic, or recurrent illness, sometimes for symptom control and sometimes to combat the primary disease. Others use CAM to promote wellness or as a prophylaxis. CAM therapies are increasingly being offered in conventional medical settings and at various other centers and institutes. The relevant ethical commitments or values that must be considered are social commitment to public welfare, nonmalefi-cence, respect for patient autonomy/consumer choice, recognition of medical pluralism, and public accountability. This article explores the major ethical principles involved in pediatric CAM use and how they affect clinical care and research.

Acupuncture for Pediatric Pain and Symptom Management 885

Anjana Kundu and Brian Berman

Over 2 million people in the United States are estimated to use acupuncture annually, primarily for musculoskeletal complaints and pain management, evidence that the integration of acupuncture into Western health care is increasing. Despite the increase in the quality of trials demonstrating the efficacy and safety of acupuncture in medicine, the pediatric acupuncture literature lacks the quantity and quality of the same body of evidence. Contributing to this paucity of evidence may be the acceptability of acupuncture in pediatric patients. There is an urgent need for high-quality randomized controlled trials on the use of acupuncture in the pediatric population. This review aims to highlight the evidence for use of acupuncture in pain and symptom management.

Complementary and Alternative Medicine Therapies to Promote Healthy Moods 901

Kathi J. Kemper and Scott Shannon

Pediatric mood disorders (unipolar depression and bipolar disorder) are serious, common, persistent, and recurrent medical conditions. Depression is the second leading cause of illness and disability among young people worldwide. A healthy lifestyle and healthy environment are the cornerstones for promoting positive moods. In addition, several complementary therapies, including nutritional supplements, herbs, mind-body therapies, massage, and acupuncture can be helpful. The focus of this article is the fundamental lifestyle approaches and complementary therapies that enhance mental health in young people. Various resources are available to clinicians to help patients and families promote mental health.

Constipation and encopresis (fecal soiling) are common childhood disorders that may lead to significant functional impairment. The etiology and course of constipation and encopresis are increasingly conceptualized from a broad biopsychosocial perspective, and therefore a holistic approach to assessment and treatment is indicated. Many children experience symptoms of chronic constipation and/or encopresis that are only partially responsive to conventional medical therapy. Complementary/alternative therapies can often help in the treatment of constipation/encopresis and are well accepted by patients and families.

The gastrointestinal flora plays a complex and important role in the development of healthy immunologic and digestive function in children. Probiotics are safe in healthy children and effective in reducing the risk of antibiotic-associated diarrhea and the duration of acute infectious diarrhea. Probiotics may also be effective in preventing community-acquired diarrheal infections, in reducing the risk of necrotizing enterocolitis in premature infants, and in the prevention and treatment of atopic dermatitis. The exact strain or combination of strains most effective for common clinical indications has yet to be determined, but the exact strain used seems less important than whether an adequate dose is used (typically 5 to 10 billion CFUs per day or higher). Clinicians should familiarize themselves with the products available because there is a wide range in their quality.

Integrative medicine blends conventional medicine with carefully evaluated complementary therapies and considers all elements of a patient's lifestyle (physical, mental, spiritual). Integrative medicine therapies and philosophies have characteristics similar to those of successful treatment programs for pediatric obesity. This article defines pediatric obesity and explores those similarities in more detail. It also updates the practitioner on selected integrative approaches as they relate to prevention and treatment of pediatric obesity.

and methodology, with long-term follow-up, for examining the longitudinal effects of pediatric MT.

Evidence on the science of complementary and alternative medicine (CAM) in children with cancer is slowly evolving. Most parents of children with cancer want their children to receive state-of-the-art therapy, which generally includes chemotherapy, radiation, and surgery. Increasingly, they also want the concomitant use of CAM therapies to help effect a cure or to alleviate symptoms. The ideal model of integrative pediatric oncology offers safe and effective CAM therapies in a pediatric hospital or medical center setting which participates in the clinical trials network of a pediatric oncology cooperative group setting.

FORTHCOMING ISSUES

RECENT ISSUES

ELSEVIER
SAUNDERS

PEDIATRIC CLINICS
OF NORTH AMERICA

Pediatr Clin N Am 54 (2007) xv–xviii

Preface

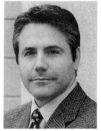 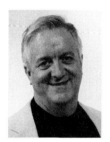

Lawrence D. Rosen, MD, FAAP   David S. Riley, MD
Guest Editors

Complementary and alternative medicine (CAM) is defined by the National Center for Complementary and Alternative Medicine as "a group of diverse medical and health care systems, practices, and products that are not presently considered to be part of conventional medicine" [1]. This is changing. Patient interest and use of CAM continues to grow, the pool of licensed healthcare providers specializing in CAM is increasing, and the interest in CAM research and therapies continues to expand in conventional medical centers.

The increasing prevalence of CAM use in adults has been widely publicized [2,3], whereas the use of such therapies in children has been underreported [4]. In fact, CAM use in pediatric populations has been increasing over the past decade, in both well and chronically ill children, according to numerous publications [5–18]. Safety and efficacy issues in the pediatric population for conventional therapies have been front and center for some time, as there has been increasing recognition that extrapolation from adult treatments is often not justified. These same questions are important in the pediatric usage of CAM. What is safe and what is not? What works and what does not? What sort of evidence-based practice guidelines do we need and how should they be developed? What is the role for the categories of evidence [19] used by the World Health Organization (WHO) (Table 1)?

Recent surveys indicate that pediatricians want evidence-based guidance on how to safely and effectively integrate CAM therapies in their practices [20,21]. Educational efforts to address this need include the inclusion of more CAM topics at the American Academy of Pediatrics (AAP) National

doi:10.1016/j.pcl.2007.09.003   *pediatric.theclinics.com*

Table 1
World Health Organization categories of evidence

Category	Source of evidence
Ia	Systematic review of randomized controlled trials
Ib	At least one randomized controlled trial
IIa	At least one well-designed quasi-experimental trial
IIb	At least one other type of well-designed quasi-experimental study
III	Well-designed nonexperimental descriptive studies (eg, comparative, correlation, or case control studies)
IV	Expert committee reports or opinions, and clinical experience of respected authorities

Convention and Exhibition [22], and the growth of the international Pediatric Integrative Medicine Conference, Pangea [23]. In this spirit, this issue is the first in the history of the *Pediatric Clinics of North America* dedicated to reviewing the principles and practices of CAM use.

The growing practice of pediatric integrative medicine, which advocates for an examined integration of conventional and CAM therapies in the holistic care of children, is evidenced by the burgeoning number of professional groups supporting pediatric CAM education [24]. These include the AAP Provisional Section on Complementary, Holistic, and Integrative Medicine (PSOCHIM) [25], the Ambulatory Pediatric Association's Special Interest Group in Integrative Pediatrics [26], and the Integrative Pediatrics Council [27]. Many of the leaders of this movement serve as authors in this remarkable issue dedicated to pediatric integrative medicine. Articles included in this issue review current hot topics such as integrative approaches to obesity, mood disorders, autism and asthma, the ethics of CAM use in children, and how to integrate therapies such as acupuncture, herbals, massage, and mind-body medicine. These subjects should be relevant for all primary care practitioners and specialists who care for children. We thank our colleagues for their contributions to this important work.

Lawrence D. Rosen, MD, FAAP
Integrative Pediatrics Council
Pediatric Integrative Medicine
Department of Pediatrics
Hackensack University Medical Center
Hackensack, NJ 07601, USA

E-mail address: lrosen@integrativepeds.org

David S. Riley, MD
University of New Mexico Medical School
Santa Fe, NM 87508, USA
EXPLORE–The Journal of Science and Healing

E-mail address: dsriley@integrativemed.org

References

[1] What is CAM? NCCAM CAM Basics. Available at: http://nccam.nih.gov/health/ whatiscam/. Accessed September 4, 2007.

[2] Eisenberg DM, Kessler RC, Foster C, et al. Unconventional medicine in the United States: prevalence, costs, and patterns of use. N Engl J Med 1993;328:246–52.

[3] Eisenberg DM, Davis RB, Ettner SL, et al. Trends in alternative medicine use in the United States, 1990–1997: results of a follow-up national survey. JAMA 1998;280:1569–75.

[4] Rosen LD. Complementary and alternative medicine use in children is underestimated. Arch Pediatr Adolesc Med 2004;158:291.

[5] Spigelblatt L, Laine-Ammara G, Pless IB, et al. The use of alternative medicine by children. Pediatrics 1994;94:811–4.

[6] Braganza S, Ozuah PO, Sharif I. The use of complementary therapies in inner-city asthmatic children. J Asthma 2003;40:823–7.

[7] Braun CA, Bearinger LH, Halcon LL, et al. Adolescent use of complementary therapies. J Adolesc Health 2003;37:76e.1–76e.9.

[8] Day AS, Whitten KE, Bohane TD. Use of complementary and alternative medicines by children and adolescents with inflammatory bowel disease. J Paediatr Child Health 2003;40: 681–4.

[9] Harrington JW, Rosen L, Garnecho A, et al. Parental perceptions and use of complementary and alternative medicine practices for children with autistic spectrum disorders in private practice. J Dev Behav Pediatr 2006;27:S156–61.

[10] Loman DG. The use of complementary and alternative health care practices among children. J Pediatr Health Care 2003;17:58–63.

[11] Losier A, Taylor B, Fernandez CV, et al. Use of alternative therapies by patients presenting to a pediatric emergency department. J Emerg Med 2005;28:267–71.

[12] Ottolini MC, Hamburger EK, Loprieato JO, et al. Complementary and alternative medicine use among children in the Washington, D.C. area. Ambul Pediatr 2001;1:122–5.

[13] Pitetti R, Singh S, Hornyak D, et al. Complementary and alternative medicine use in children. Pediatr Emerg Care 2001;17:165–9.

[14] Reznick M, Ozuah PO, Franco K, et al. Use of complementary therapy by adolescents with asthma. Arch Pediatr Adolesc Med 2002;156:1042–4.

[15] Sanders H, Davis MF, Duncan B, et al. Use of complementary and alternative medical therapies among children with special health care needs in southern Arizona. Pediatrics 2003; 111:584–7.

[16] Sawni A, Ragothaman R, Thomas RL, et al. The use of complementary/alternative therapies among children attending an urban pediatric emergency department. Clin Pediatr (Phila) 2007;46:36–41.

[17] Sawni-Sikand A, Schubiner H, Thomas RL. Use of complementary/alternative therapies among children in primary care pediatrics. Ambul Pediatr 2002;2:99–103.

[18] Sinha D, Efron D. Complementary and alternative medicine use in children with attention deficit hyperactivity disorder. J Paediatr Child Health 2005;41:23–6.

[19] WHO Division of Traditional Medicine. General guidelines for methodologies on research and evaluation of traditional medicine. Geneva (Switzerland): World Health Organization; 2000.

[20] Sikand A, Laken M. Pediatricians' experience with and attitudes toward complementary/ alternative medicine. Arch Pediatr Adolesc Med 1998;152:1059–64.

[21] Periodic Survey of Fellows #49, American Academy of Pediatrics Division of Health Policy Research: Complementary and Alternative Medicine (CAM) Therapies in Pediatric Practices, October 2002. Available at: http://www.aap.org/research/periodicsurvey/ps49bexs. htm. Accessed September 4, 2007.

[22] American Academy of Pediatrics National Conference and Exhibition. Available at: http:// www.aap.org/nce. Accessed September 4, 2007.

[23] Pangea: a conference for the future of pediatric wellness. Available at: http://www.pangeaconference.com. Accessed September 4, 2007.

[24] Rosen LD. Integrative pediatrics: past, present, and future. Explore 2006;2:455–6.

[25] American Academy of Pediatrics Provisional Section on Complementary, Holistic and Integrative Medicine. Available at: http://www.aap.org/sections/CHIM. Accessed September 4, 2007.

[26] Ambulatory Pediatrics Association Special Interest Group in Integrative Pediatrics. Available at: http://www.ambpeds.org/Site/sp_int_groups/sig_comp_alt_peds.htm. Accessed September 4, 2007.

[27] The Integrative Pediatrics Council. Available at: http://www.integrativepeds.org. Accessed September 4, 2007.

ELSEVIER
SAUNDERS

Pediatr Clin N Am 54 (2007) xix

PEDIATRIC CLINICS
OF NORTH AMERICA

Dedication

This issue is dedicated to our children and to children everywhere. We appreciate the support of our friends, families, and colleagues who are working with us to advocate for the optimal health and wellness of this and future generations.

Lawrence D. Rosen, MD, FAAP
David S. Riley, MD

0031-3955/07/$ - see front matter © 2007 Elsevier Inc. All rights reserved.
doi:10.1016/j.pcl.2007.09.004

Primary Care from Infancy to Adolescence

Lawrence D. Rosen, MD, FAAP[a],*,
Cora Collette Breuner, MD, MPH[b]

[a]*Department of Pediatrics, Division of Pediatric Integrative Medicine,
Hackensack University Medical Center, Hackensack, NJ 07601, USA*
[b]*Department of Pediatrics, University of Washington, Adolescent Medicine Section,
Children's Hospital and Medical Center, Seattle, WA 98105, USA*

What is primary care? And who is this primary care practitioner/pediatrician or "PCP" to whom we so often refer? How limited or wide is our role? Primary care, in the world of medicine, is conventionally defined as "the activity of a health care provider who acts as a first point of consultation for all patients" [1]. Historically, many types of health care practitioners have served as primary care providers for children, including pediatricians, family practice doctors, nurses, and alternative health care practitioners. In truth, the primary care of a child is shared by many: pediatricians or other health care practitioners, the child's family and community, and the child herself. The scope of primary care includes a focus on prevention and well care, and implies a comprehensive, collaborative, and coordinated approach exemplified by the medical home model developed by the American Academy of Pediatrics (AAP) [2]. The medical home model is holistic in the sense that it views the health of a child as intricately connected to the child's environment—her family, her community, and the world around her. And holistic pediatrics—the concept of nurturing the whole child toward optimal wellness—is simply "good medicine," as noted by Dr. Kathi Kemper [3] in her Presidential Address to the Ambulatory Pediatric Association.

Integrative pediatrics, a holistic practice that includes an examined integration of complementary and alternative medicine (CAM) and conventional therapies, is ideally suited for primary care. In addition to supporting medical home tenets, integrative pediatrics emphasizes a collaborative and individualized approach to working with families and other health care

* Corresponding author.
E-mail address: lrosen@integrativepeds.org (L.D. Rosen).

0031-3955/07/$ - see front matter © 2007 Elsevier Inc. All rights reserved.
doi:10.1016/j.pcl.2007.09.007
                                                              pediatric.theclinics.com

practitioners, including open discussions about CAM therapies, environmental health concerns, nutrition, immunization, and parenting practices. The appeal of integrative pediatrics for pediatric primary care is indeed growing, as evidenced by the increased use of CAM therapies for well children and those who have special health care needs [4–7]. Adolescent use of CAM in particular is rising [8,9], and primary care practitioners need to engage teens in discussions about safety and efficacy concerns, as they would with any therapies. Pediatricians are in fact more interested than ever in learning about CAM therapies so that they can more effectively communicate and connect with their patients and families [10]. To increase awareness and knowledge of commonly used CAM therapies in primary care practice, we describe three cases that illustrate the potential for evidence-based integrative care from infancy through adolescence.

Infancy

Ideally, primary care is grounded in the concept of prevention and emphasizes regular well care visits to provide anticipatory guidance for families. We meet with families most frequently in the first months of a child's life to assess growth and development and also to establish a relationship so that together we can create a foundation for optimal health for each and every child. In the scope of daily practice, however, primary care pediatricians encounter various common conditions requiring an acute intervention. These acute problems offer us opportunities not simply to treat the presenting problem but to modulate the course of an infant's health for the future.

Case I

A 6-week-old baby, new to your practice, is brought in by his parents for a well visit. The family is interested in more holistic care and has heard in the community that you are open minded to "natural approaches." The baby was full term and has been generally healthy; he is breastfed with occasional supplemental bottles of a cow's milk–based formula. The parents are concerned about how fussy their baby has become over the past month, and are wondering if you can help them.

Colic

The typical baby cries an average of 2.25 hours per day [11]; others are excessively irritable and are said to have colic. Surveys indicate that more than one quarter of infants are diagnosed with colic [12], making the condition one of the most common reasons for infant visits to primary care practitioners today. Dr. Morris Wessel [13], who studied infant crying behavior as part of the Yale Rooming-In Project, defined colic as paroxysmal fussing in infancy for more than 3 hours per day, at least 3 days per week, for at least 3 weeks' duration. Colic is currently best understood as an extreme variant of infant irritability, perhaps related to neural regulation differences. Pediatrician Harvey Karp [14] speculates that some babies have a more difficult time adjusting to what he terms the "fourth trimester," a 3-month period of time in which infants must cope with potentially overwhelming sensory stimuli. Just like adults, babies vary in how well they integrate external stimuli, and colic may well represent an adjustment disorder, the far end of an infant irritability syndrome, or perhaps an early sensory integration disorder. Most parents who have colicky babies believe that there is some component of abdominal pain; in fact, the gastrointestinal tract may be involved in colic through neuro-gut-immune pathways. Atopic disorders (discussed in more detail later) have been associated with colic, perhaps through an immunomodulatory mechanism involving gastroesophageal reflux [15]. Of greatest concern, a recently published 10-year prospective study challenges the commonly held view that there are no long-term health-related issues in children who had colic in infancy [16]. In this prospective study of 100 children, there was an association noted between infantile colic and later recurrent abdominal pain, atopic disease, and sleep disorders. This association does not prove causation, but suggests that processes involved in the development of colic may also predispose children to subsequent health concerns. Larger prospective studies are needed for confirmation, but the theoretic impetus for colic intervention is strengthened by the trial's findings.

Complementary and alternative medicine therapies for colic

It is often difficult to distinguish conventional from CAM approaches for managing colic because culture and geography play such a large role in what is considered conventional. Surveys of CAM use in culturally diverse populations indicate that colic is a common reason for use of herbal and nutritional therapies [17,18]. The largest systematic review to date of treatments for colic found little evidence to support many routinely advocated therapies, including simethicone, while noting that several nutritional and botanically based approaches were safe and effective [19]. Individualizing a treatment plan is extremely important in the management of colic because some approaches work well for some families and not at all for others. Common CAM approaches for colic include the use of mind–body therapies, infant massage, botanically based therapies, nutritional modulation, and probiotics.

Mind–body medicine

Mind–body medicine, according the National Center for Complementary and Alternative Medicine (NCCAM), "focuses on the interactions among the brain, mind, body, and behavior, and on the powerful ways in which emotional, mental, social, spiritual, and behavioral factors can directly affect health" [20]. Stress can indeed modulate neurologic responses, supporting the need to promote parental stress-coping mechanisms in the face of excessive infant irritability. In a chicken–egg analogy, it is likely that parental stress and infant colic exacerbate each other. There are established links between maternal mood states, including postpartum depression, and the development of colic in infants [21]. Reducing parenting stress is a proven method of helping families cope with irritable infants, and there are many strategies to do so. A study by Keefe and colleagues [22] used a home-based nursing intervention for stress reduction, but teaching families other mind–body therapies may be equally helpful. Other parenting interventions, included parent-to-parent guidance, have been demonstrated to reduce crying time in colicky babies [23,24]. Despite the lack of randomized controlled trials proving efficacy or cost effectiveness in colic management, practices such as guided imagery, self-hypnosis, mindfulness-based stress reduction, or yoga might be equally helpful in reducing parental distress.

Infant massage

Infant massage is a specific therapeutic massage technique developed for soothing babies and for facilitating bonding between parent and child. A Cochrane Database Systematic Review of infant massage acknowledged "evidence of benefits on mother–infant interaction, sleeping and crying, and on hormones influencing stress levels" [25]. Infant massage is effective in reducing excessive crying in even the most vulnerable of infants, including premature babies and cocaine-exposed neonates [26,27]. Self-care is an important part of the healing power for many CAM modalities, including massage, and families can learn infant massage techniques for safe and effective use at home. This positive effect for soothing infants seems to be superior to simple vibration devices [28] and may be enhanced by the use of essential oils, such as sesame seed oil [29]. Whether this latter effect is related to the oil as aromatherapy or simply adds to the physical massage technique, or both, is unknown.

Botanically based therapies

Botanically based therapies for colic have been used historically in many cultures. One of the more widely known in recent times, gripe water, dates back to the 1800s, when it was developed by William Woodward, a British pharmacy apprentice [30]. Woodward's formula, a mixture of dill seed oil, sodium bicarbonate, and alcohol, among other substances, derived from a solution used at the time to treat babies who had "fen fever," related to malaria. Babies soothed by the concoction reportedly found relief from gastrointestinal troubles ("watery gripes"). Over the years, the gripe water formula has changed and commercially available solutions may contain any number of botanicals, though alcohol has been removed from many of these products. One must ask families specifically about the use of gripe water and other herbal blends for colic treatment to determine which herbs are being ingested.

One natural health product database lists five separate products labeled as gripe water, all with different constituents [31]. Herbs most commonly found in these preparations include dill (*Anethum graveolens*), fennel (*Foeniculum vulgare*), ginger (*Zingiber officinale*), and German chamomile (*Matricaria recutita*). There have been several published studies of herbal remedies for colic. Weizman and colleagues [32] evaluated an herbal tea preparation containing chamomile, vervain, licorice, fennel, and lemon balm. In this trial, 68 colicky infants aged 2 to 8 weeks were randomized to receive either tea or placebo for 7 days. Infants were allowed drink up to 5 ounces up to three times per day, but the average actual intake per baby was approximately 3 ounces per day. Significantly more babies in the treatment group (57%) improved than in the placebo group (26%). No significant adverse effects were reported. Unfortunately, many unknown variables in the study design make it difficult to base recommendations on the results. The amounts and types of each herb and the exact nature of the placebo are unspecified and may have had an impact on resolution of colic. Alexandrovich and colleagues [33] examined the effect on colic of an emulsion of fennel seed oil in a randomized controlled trial of 125 infants. The babies were allowed 5 to 20 mL of either fennel seed oil emulsion or placebo up to four times per day for 1 week, but actually ingested an average of two to three doses per day, for a total of less than 2 ounces per day. Colic was eliminated in 65% of the treatment group versus 23.7% of the placebo group. There were no reported adverse effects in this trial. Savino and colleagues [34] compared a standardized extract of three herbs (chamomile, fennel, and lemon balm) with a placebo in 93 breastfed colicky infants. Each infant received a standardized dose of extract or placebo at 2 mL/kg/d twice daily before breastfeeding for a 7-day trial period. A significant reduction in crying time was observed in 85.4% of patients receiving the treatment extract and in 48.9% of infants receiving the placebo. Interestingly, crying time was still reduced 2 weeks after the end of the trial in the intervention group. There were no reported adverse side effects in either group.

Nutritional modulation

Modulating the diets of babies, whether breastfed or formula-fed, is often attempted to reduce infant fussiness. Although breastfeeding exclusively does not seem to prevent colic [35], nursing mothers may have success in reducing infant irritability by altering their nutritional intake. Hill and colleagues [36] found that elimination from maternal diet of common allergenic foods (cow's milk, soy, wheat, eggs, peanuts, tree nuts, and fish) was associated with a reduction in colic in breastfed infants. Cruciferous vegetables (eg, broccoli, cauliflower) and chocolate in the maternal diet have been linked to colic in breastfed babies [37,38]. Some food constituents, like essential fatty acids, may actually be desirable in higher amounts; although not directly connected to colic, maternal docosahexaenoic acid levels have been associated with positive infant sleep patterning [39].

Certain formulas have been shown to reduce colic symptoms, although no prospective studies evaluating prevention of colic have been published. Extensively hydrolyzed casein and whey formulas are more effective than nonhydrolyzed cow's milk formulas in reducing crying times in colicky babies [40,41]. Studies do not support either soy or partially hydrolyzed formulas as options for colic reduction [42,43].

Probiotics and prebiotics

Probiotics are "viable, defined microorganisms in sufficient numbers, which alter the microflora (by implantation or colonization) in a compartment of the host and by that exert beneficial health effects in this host" [44]. Prebiotics are biologic substances that increase the growth and activity of probiotic organisms. There are differences in the types and number of probiotic microorganisms colonizing the intestinal tracts of infants who have colic versus those who do not [45,46].

Savino and colleagues [47] have evaluated the effect of probiotics and prebiotics on colic. In one trial, they compared a probiotic (*Lactobacillus reuteri*) with simethicone in a randomized controlled trial in 90 exclusively breastfed colicky infants. Simethicone, a conventional nonprescription medication, has been previously shown to be ineffective for colic treatment [19]. After the 1-month trial, 95% of the probiotic treatment group responded (no longer met Wessel criteria for colic) versus only 7% of the simethicone group. The second study randomized 267 formula-fed infants to one of two arms [48]. The treatment group was fed a novel partially hydrolyzed whey protein formula supplemented with prebiotic oligosaccharides and the control group received the standard formula (without prebiotics) and simethicone. The treatment group, after both 1 and 2 weeks, had a significant reduction in crying episodes when compared with the control group.

Case I, continued

The parents return for a visit several weeks later. They have been using chamomile tea and gripe water with some success, and find that the infant massage lessons they took are helping to calm their baby also. Although he is less fussy, he is now spitting up most of his feedings, although his mother is trying to avoid dairy and other common food allergens in her diet; they are still occasionally supplementing with an "easier-to-digest" cow's milk formula. Furthermore, he is covered by a patchy, dry, red rash and has noticeable nasal congestion with a frequent nighttime cough.

Atopic disorders

Atopic disorders, including asthma and food allergies, are widely considered to be increasing in prevalence at epidemic rates [49]. In primary care pediatric practice, we are seeing many more infants suffering from early atopic signs (dermatitis, gastroesophageal reflux, chronic rhinorrhea, and recurrent wheezing). Some infants who have colic develop signs and symptoms of atopy, including eczema, chronic rhinitis, and gastroesophageal reflux. Research supports the finding that atopy may be responsible for symptoms of colic [15], although infants who have colic do not necessarily develop atopy at higher rates than other babies later in life [50]. The atopic march, as it has come to be known, represents the natural tendency of children who have early signs of allergic reaction to environmental stimuli (eg, atopic dermatitis) to progress to more severe manifestations of allergic disease (eg, asthma) [51].

What predisposes certain infants to develop atopic symptoms? Although it has long been appreciated that some are at higher risk for atopic disorders based on family history, we are only now recognizing how complicated the nature–nurture equation might be. Even single nucleotide polymorphisms (SNPs, or very small DNA shifts) may not only account for the presence or absence of atopy in a given person but may also affect the severity of disease, the likelihood of other atopic conditions developing, and the success of various therapies [52]. A baby who has a given genomic predisposition, under certain environmental conditions, manifests immune dysregulation, resulting in an imbalance between Th1-dominant and Th2-dominant responses [53]. Th2 dominance leads to immune dysregulation marked by a proliferation of inflammatory cellular mediators (eg, cytokines, interleukins, leukotrienes). Inflammation involves excess mucous production and other clinically observable phenomena we call allergies.

The "hygiene hypothesis" is a popular current theory to explain why we are experiencing a surge in atopic disease prevalence [54]. According to this theory, our environments are now too clean—we are not exposed to as many antigens (bacterial, fungal, viral) as previous generations. With a reduction in infectious exposure, certain individuals over time may produce altered gastrointestinal, immunologically active microorganisms, leading to a Th2 immune shift [55]. Numerous studies also have supported a correlation between early life antibiotic exposure and atopy (particularly wheezing) in children [56–61]. Other environmental factors, too, have been implicated in triggering allergic responses. These include immune and endocrine disrupting agents in air, water, food, and industrial products [62–64].

Complementary and alternative medicine therapies for atopy

Many families turn to CAM therapies for their children suffering atopic disorders [65–69]. Among the most well studied for prevention and treatment of infant atopy are nutritional modulation and probiotics.

Nutritional modulation

For those infants at risk, exposure to certain foods in and ex utero may contribute to the development of atopy. We focus on the following key areas: maternal pre- and postnatal antigen avoidance, breastfeeding, choice of infant formula supplementation, timing of solid food introduction, and fatty acid intake (in breastfeeding mothers and in infants).

General antigen avoidance (milk, soy, eggs, tree nuts, peanuts, shellfish) for the population as a whole is not supported by current data [70]. In families at highest risk (parents or siblings who have significant atopic history), avoidance of most highly allergenic foods, especially peanuts and tree nuts, should be considered during pregnancy and during duration of breastfeeding. The AAP advises avoiding peanuts and tree nuts for nursing mothers for maximal atopy prevention [71]. If avoiding specific food groups, one must take great care to ensure proper compensatory intake of vitamins, minerals, and amino acids.

The AAP also supports breastfeeding as a means to reduce allergic disorders. Exclusive breastfeeding for 4 to 6 months is associated with a lower risk for developing atopic dermatitis, food allergy, allergic rhinitis, and asthma [72–75]. If exclusive breastfeeding is not possible, the AAP recommends hydrolyzed protein formulas for high-risk babies [71]. A Cochrane Database Systematic Review supports this recommendation [76]. These formulas may contain extensively or partially hydrolyzed cow's milk proteins (casein or whey), and there is debate about whether they are equivalently effective in preventing atopic expression [77]. Most experts currently recommend extensively hydrolyzed products, but cost and availability issues are factors. The AAP recommends against using soy formulas for atopic prevention in high-risk infants [71]; again, this recommendation is supported by a Cochrane Database Systematic Review [78].

There is no clear consensus guideline for treating infants who develop atopic symptoms, even in the absence of family history. Common practice includes advising exclusive breastfeeding with maternal antigen avoidance, or, if not possible, using extensively hydrolyzed formulas.

When is the optimal time to introduce solid foods to infants for the general population and those at high risk? Prevention of atopy seems to be the key focus in published trials. With increasing prevalence of allergic disorders, some experts are advocating for delaying solid food introduction in all babies until 6 months, with the introduction of highly allergenic foods as follows: dairy products at 12 months, eggs at 24 months, and peanuts, tree nuts, and shellfish at 36 months [79]. These guidelines are supported by other major United States and European groups, but only for infants at high risk [71]. Early solid feeding (before 4 months of age), particularly of gluten-containing products, is associated with atopic disease and celiac disease [80,81]. There have also been several encouraging studies looking at the treatment of atopic disorders with nutritional modulation (avoiding specific food allergens) [82–84].

Recent studies have examined the role of essential fatty acids in preventing and reducing allergic disease. Atopy can be prevented when mothers ingest higher amounts of omega-3 polyunsaturated fatty acids (PUFAs) [85]. It also seems that babies who ingest breast milk relatively rich in omega-3 are less likely to develop allergic symptoms [86,87]. This effect is most evident in those babies at highest risk genetically. The results of directly feeding infants PUFAs are not as clear. Some studies of dietary modification with omega-3 PUFAs in children at high risk demonstrated reduction in atopy [88,89], and another study showed improvement with supplementation of evening primrose oil, an omega-6 PUFA [90]. Perhaps it is the balance of the two that is most important, and one must also take into account pre-existing dietary deficiencies and genomic factors. More research is clearly needed in this realm before universal recommendations can be made.

Probiotics

Randomized controlled trials have demonstrated that probiotics (*Lactobacillus* GG) given prenatally to women and then postnatally to either breastfeeding mothers or directly to formula-fed infants can reduce the incidence of atopic dermatitis by half in those infants at high risk for up to 4 years postnatally [91,92]. Prebiotics have also been shown to prevent eczema in a vulnerable infant population [93]. Several randomized controlled trials have pointed toward a positive effect of probiotics and prebiotics on the course of atopic dermatitis [94–97], although one publication reported no such effect [98]. More research is needed to determine the ideal doses and types of pre- and probiotics for atopy prevention and treatment.

Adolescence

Adolescence is a time full of changes and a particularly challenging period of life not only for the patients and their families but also for the primary care practitioner. In adolescence there is a recapitulation of many of the stages of infantile emotional development, including the oral, anal, and genital, where the fires of conflict are rekindled. During early adolescence (11–13 years) teens are preoccupied with body image and peer group identity. Middle adolescence (14–16 years) is characterized by desire for separation from the family and development of individual identity. In late adolescence (16–20 years), the young adult begins to foster long-term relationships and plan for his or her future. The physical and psychosocial transitions of adolescence are challenging in healthy teens and even more so in those who have chronic illnesses requiring frequent medical interventions and hospitalizations. It is important to recognize that the psychosocial issues faced by an adolescent can be different from a child or older adult, although the medical treatment may be similar. The tasks of adolescence include winning the acceptance of peers, achieving independence from families, developing the capacity to love a person of the opposite or same sex, and achieving an effective ego (a sense of self; an individuality inclusive of sexual and vocational identities) and an effective superego (eg, a conscience, a value system, a sense of right and wrong).

Integrative care—complementary and alternative medicine and adolescents

Holistic care in the adolescent population is exciting territory that resonates with many avenues for improving outcomes in this population. An integrative approach can be helpful in discussing pregnancy prevention, sexually transmitted diseases, the effects of smoking, the need for immunizations, substance use, and health education regarding improved efforts at compliance in those who have specific health care needs.

CAM has a large range of use in children and adolescents and is more common in certain geographic areas of North America and in those young people who have chronic illnesses [99–106]. CAM use is considerably higher in specific groups of children and adolescents, such as in those who have cystic fibrosis, cancer, or arthritis, and in those undergoing surgery [103–108]. Other frequent users of CAM in adolescence include homeless youth, who have a 70% use rate [107]. Why teens and their families turn to CAM in the face of chronic illness is a subject of much conjecture but may be because conventional medical approaches may only target specific aspects of the illness. The integrative and alternative interventions may support the child and the family as the illness becomes more physically and psychologically pervasive.

Case study II

D' Andree is a 12-year-old who has been on stimulant medication twice daily for his attention-deficit/hyperactivity disorder (ADHD). His teacher thinks he is not focused enough and needs more medication. Mom is concerned about his weight and self esteem. He eats voraciously when the medication wears off and has been battling obesity for many of his school years. His mom has been seeing a nutritionist for her own weight issues and has used some nutritional supplements and herbals with good results. It turns out that D'Andree already had been taking some herbs and supplements. He tells you he has been drinking two or three cans of energy drink daily to "lower my appetite." He also thinks it is helping him pay better attention at school. Mom and D'Andree come to the follow-up appointment with a bag of many different herbs and supplements, including yerba mate, guaraná, green tea, ginseng, and hoodia, recommended by the nutritionist, and they are wondering whether you think they might help him.

Herbal therapies and nutritional supplements

Among adolescents, it is common to find the use of herbal therapies for several conditions: weight loss, depression and anxiety, upper respiratory tract infections, and the enhancement of athletic performance. Outlined here is a brief review of a few commonly used herbal therapies pertinent to the above case.

Caffeine is the only stimulating supplement that can be easily and abundantly consumed and even purchased by children and adolescents. Caffeine is found in pain relievers, diuretics, cold remedies, weight control products, and sport supplements. A U.S. Department of Agriculture survey showed that for children (6 to 9 years old), the mean daily caffeine intake was 20 mg compared with adults in whom the average is 200 mg per day [108]. A survey of 8- to 11-year-olds in Massachusetts found the average daily caffeine intake was 18.9 mg, or 0.6 mg/kg, and that greater than 50% of the caffeine consumed was from carbonated beverages [109].

Caffeine, a member of the methylxanthine drug class, increases norepinephrine and epinephrine secretion and blocks central adenosine receptors. It increases the heart rate and basal metabolic rate, promotes secretion of acid in the stomach, is a diuretic, and acts as a vasoconstrictor and vasodilator. Caffeine enhances alertness and gives a person a jolt by peaking in the blood plasma within 30 minutes after ingestion. The half-life of caffeine varies from several hours to days; the average in adults is 3 to 7 hours. In one clinical study, school-aged boys who consumed caffeine showed a greater increase in motor activity and in rate of speech and decrease in reaction time compared with adults. There was also improvement in attention with less nervousness and jitteriness and fewer omission errors on a continuous performance test [110]. For ADHD, caffeine has been shown to have mixed results [111]. Studies have demonstrated that caffeine is not more effective than placebo and is less effective than stimulant medication in treating ADHD symptoms [112].

Caffeine withdrawal symptoms in the child or adolescent can occur after only 2 weeks of daily caffeine use and include irritability, depression, anxiety, fatigue, and headache. In one study, during caffeine withdrawal children had a worse performance reaction time on a task requiring sustained attention; this deterioration may persist for a week [113]. Importantly, caffeine can interact with stimulant, analgesic, and other over-the-counter medications. Its use is not recommended in those who take prescribed stimulant medications. Caffeine has been believed to cause decreased bone mineral density because of its propensity to increase urinary calcium excretion in adults. In a study in adolescent women, however, dietary caffeine consumed by American white, adolescent girls was not correlated with a decrease in total bone mineral gain or hip bone density at age 18 [114]. This remains an ongoing area of concern and there is a need for further research.

Ephedra, also known by its Chinese name *Ma huang*, is a naturally occurring substance derived from plants. Its principal active ingredient is ephedrine. Although it was not recommended in the above case study many teens know about its propensity to assist in weight loss. Ephedra products have been used to suppress appetite, enhance sports performance, and increase energy. Ephedra acts by increasing the levels of norepinephrine, epinephrine, and dopamine, and stimulating alpha and beta adrenoreceptors. This stimulation leads to anorectic and thermogenic effects by speeding up metabolism, which leads to increased alertness, less fatigue, and a decreased perceived need for sleep. Ultimately there is increased anxiety, jitteriness, and insomnia. In a meta- analysis of 52 controlled trials and 65 case reports, ephedrine and ephedra were shown to promote modest short-term weight loss (~0.9 kg/mo compared with placebo) [115].

It is well known that ephedra has the potential to cause serious side effects that have led to several reported deaths. In 2004, the FDA banned the sale of dietary supplements containing ephedra because of reported serious adverse effects; although the ban has been contested legally, the medical concerns remain. Based on known side effects and minimal benefit, this product should not be recommended for use. Combining caffeine and ephedra may lead to psychiatric symptoms, such as euphoria, neurotic behavior, agitation, depressed mood, giddiness, and extreme irritability. Other side effects may include elevated blood pressure, palpitations, tachycardia, chest pain, coronary vasospasm, and possibly cardiomyopathy.

Guaraná (*Paullinia cupana*) is a small shrub native to Venezuela and northern Brazil, known for the high stimulant content of the fruit. The dried paste made from the crushed seeds of guaraná is used to enhance athletic performance, as an appetite suppressant, and as an aphrodisiac. Guaraná seeds contain the caffeine-like product guaranine, along with theobromine, theophylline, xanthine, and other xanthine derivatives. There are several energy drinks containing guaraná equivalent to 3.6% to 5.8% caffeine (compared with 1% to 2% in coffee). One study of overweight adults reported that the combination of guaraná, yerba mate (see later discussion), and damiana (*Turnera diffusa*, a purported aphrodisiac) significantly delayed gastric emptying, causing prolonged perceived gastric fullness with an associated weight loss over 45 days [116]. The side effects are similar to those of ephedra and caffeine.

Yerba mate (*Ilex paraguariensis*), a member of the holly family, is a widely cultivated medium-sized evergreen tree native to South American countries. Yerba mate tea leaves are used as a diuretic, for weight loss, and for fatigue and depression. The primary active chemical constituents are caffeine (0.3%–2.0%), theobromine, theophylline, saponins, tannins, and chlorogenic acid. Yerba mate may cause insomnia, gastric irritation, nervousness, diuresis, and arrhythmias. Side effects are similar to those herbs that contain caffeine [117].

Hoodia gordonii is a succulent from the Kalahari Desert in southern Africa. Bushmen from the area have been using hoodia for centuries to help ward off hunger during long trips in the desert. A steroidal glycoside termed P57AS3 (P57) has been isolated from *H gordonii* and may increase the content of ATP causing a decrease in hunger [118]. Preliminary data suggest that overweight men who consume P57 have significantly lower calorie intake than those taking a placebo. No side effects have been reported to date [119].

Green tea (*Camellia sinensis*) is a popular drink among adolescents and has been advertised as a weight loss aid and a treatment for fatigue, gastrointestinal disorders, and headaches. It can be found everywhere, including in grocery stores, in energy drinks, and at ever-present fancy chain coffee shops. Green tea leaves are steamed and heated, rather than rolled and exposed to air as in black tea, to remove the enzyme that promotes oxidation. The caffeine in green tea is believed to be milder than that in black tea because of its combination with catechin in the steaming process. The active ingredients include caffeine, 2-amino-5-(N-ethylcarboxyamido)-pentanoic acid, catechins, and polyphenolic compounds. In vitro studies show green tea to be antibacterial, antimutagenic, and anticarcinogenic [120]. Thermogenesis, fat oxidation, or both may be affected by green tea; a cup may contain 22 to 46 mg of caffeine [121].

Side effects of green tea include those similar to caffeine and include withdrawal after 2 weeks of consumption if ingestion is abruptly discontinued. As with any caffeine product, excessive green tea consumption should be avoided in pregnant or breastfeeding women, in those who have cardiac arrhythmias, hypertension, gastrointestinal ulcers, anxiety, or renal disease, and in those taking antifungal medications or aminophylline. There is a precautionary use in infants and young children. A retrospective trial noted that microcytic anemia can occur in infants consuming daily green tea [122].

Ginseng (*Panax ginseng*) has been used for more than 2000 years to strengthen mental and physical capacity. Recently, ginseng has become popular as an "adaptogenic" (stress-protective) agent. Ginseng is believed to have effects on nitric oxide synthesis in endothelial tissue of lung, heart, and kidney. In addition, effects on serotonin and dopamine may also be responsible for its actions. Other effects may be related to activity on the hypothalamic-pituitary-adrenal system. To date, seven trials investigating ginseng's effects on physical performance in young, active volunteers during cycle ergometer exercises have been reported. Four studies found no significant difference between ginseng and placebo, whereas three studies found a significant decrease in heart rate and increase in maximal oxygen uptake with ginseng [123]. Adverse effects may include nervousness, insomnia, and gastrointestinal disturbance associated with prolonged use. Because of the estrogen-like effect, ginseng has been reported to cause mastalgia and vaginal bleeding in women. Importantly, ginseng may interact with oral anticoagulants, antiplatelet agents, corticosteroids, and hypoglycemic agents [124].

Case III

Alicia is a 17-year-old referred to the clinic by her naturopathic physician with a history of a 15-pound weight loss over the past 6 months. Her weight has decreased from 100 to 85 pounds; her height is 5 ft 1 in, putting her at 80% of her ideal body weight. She has had no menses for 3 months. Alicia's parents and her naturopathic physician are concerned about her increasing anxiety and insomnia. The family would like to avoid conventional medications at all costs and ask you about alternative therapies to help Alicia. They were wondering about interventions such as meditation, yoga, and massage. They describe Alicia as extremely anxious. She obsesses about her grades and relationships with friends and has considerable difficulty falling asleep.

Eating disorders represent a devastating condition that primarily affects adolescent women. Although the lifetime prevalence rates according to the Diagnostic and Statistical Manual of Mental Disorders, 4th Edition, Text Revised are listed as 1% to 3%, more recent research suggests it is much higher, with a range of 3% to 6% in young women [125]. Adolescents who have eating disorders experience various symptoms, including food preoccupation, anxiety, and depression. They may also face low body weight, loss of menses, biochemical imbalances in the brain, family difficulties, financial hardship, poor adaptation, disruption of academic progress, prolonged care in hospital settings, and ultimately death. Conventional treatments for these eating disorders include psychopharmacologic interventions, nutritional interventions, and psychologic treatments. CAM therapies integrated in the management of eating disorders often include mind–body therapies (eg, meditation and yoga), natural health products, and therapeutic massage.

Mind–body therapies

The use of relaxation psychotherapies for the treatment of physical and mental ailments is an old practice. Historically, various relaxation psychotherapies have been used to alleviate symptoms associated with psychologic and medical conditions, including stuttering, cancer treatment, insomnia, diabetic care, affective disorders, irritable bowel syndrome, and eating disorders [126]. One important benefit has been the reduction of problematic symptomatology (eg, anxiety, sleep disorders) by way of relatively low-risk and cost effective methods of care.

The use of *meditation* in the treatment of eating disorders originates from various sources. Mindfulness meditation can be defined as "intentional self-regulation of attention from moment to moment [127]. It is neither contemplation nor rumination, as in thinking about a conceptual theme." In mindfulness meditation, the individual observes thoughts and experiences from a detached perspective thus allowing thoughts and experiences to come into awareness, be noticed, and dissipate from consciousness. Mindfulness meditation has been used in the treatment of pain amplification disorders, depression, and various other chronic conditions. Success with this approach has spurred researchers to examine the impact of mindfulness meditation on individuals who have eating disorders.

A meditation intervention for the treatment of binge eating disorder was studied and results indicated that the number of binges dropped significantly over the course of treatment, with nine participants binging less than once a week and five participants bingeing less than once or twice a week post-treatment. Participants who spent time using eating meditation were subsequently able to change their bingeing behaviors with an increased sense of eating control, sense of mindfulness, and awareness of hunger cues and satiety cues [128]. Results were comparable to cognitive-behavioral therapy (CBT) interventions, which suggest that meditation may be an alternative to CBT in cases in which CBT is not feasible because of financial or geographic concerns [129].

Another mind–body therapy integrated in the treatment of eating disorders is *yoga*. Because yoga is viewed as form of exercise by some practitioners, the use of yoga to treat eating disorders is controversial. Most clinics advise against strenuous exercise because of the possibility of increasing weight loss. There are known negative effects of long-term abstinence from exercise, however, such as decreased bone mass and an increased risk for atherosclerosis. In a study examining the positive effects of yoga, eating disorder patients who completed yoga trended toward experiencing an improved quality of life and did not lose weight compared with those who did not receive yoga [130]. Although these results suggest a preliminary positive use for yoga, controlled clinical trials are needed to support these results.

The use of yoga to treat anxiety is mostly theoretic. Although several articles have attempted to examine the impact of yoga on anxiety or other affective states, the lack of controlled clinical trials or adequate statistical analysis makes it difficult to interpret the results. In a multifaceted treatment approach for individuals who have eating disorders yoga may help reduce severe physical discomfort and feelings of guilt after eating [131]. In another study, yoga was noted to decrease food preoccupation in adolescents who had eating disorders [132]. Scheduling yoga sessions before and after meals helps reduce many typical anxiety responses that occur in patients who have eating disorders and alleviates some of the problems of after-meal supervision.

Natural health products

Kava is an important cultural product in the South Pacific, particularly in the Fiji Islands, where it is used as a ceremonial drink. It is also used for its calming effects. More recently, it has been used as a natural alternative to sedatives and anxiolytics.

It is believed to work by inhibiting γ-aminobutyric acid (GABA) receptor binding. A Cochrane Systematic Review found that kava does have an antianxiety effect compared with placebo [133]. Adverse effects include kava dermopathy, a yellowing and flaking of the skin associated with excessive use of kava, which resolves with discontinuation of the herb. There is a potential risk for liver injury associated with the use of kava-containing dietary supplements, although some speculate the liver toxicity is reversible on discontinuation of the herb [134].

Valerian has been used for centuries as a sedative agent and sleep aid. Valerian root has effects on GABA receptors, leading to its sedative effects. Several human trials confirm a mild sedative effect. Few studies exist regarding the anxiolytic effects of valerian root in vivo. A Cochrane Systematic Review concluded that "there is insufficient evidence to draw any conclusions about the efficacy or safety of valerian" [135]. Side effects include headache, excitability, uneasiness, and cardiac disturbances.

Chamomile has been used for gastrointestinal discomfort, peptic ulcer disease, infantile colic, and mild anxiety. Chamomile may act by binding to central benzodiazepine receptors [136]. Several small human trials have noted chamomile to have hypnotic-sedative properties. None of these trials have been randomized or controlled, however. The FDA regards chamomile as safe when used as a spice, seasoning, or flavoring agent. Although several cases of allergic reactions to chamomile have been reported, no significant toxicity or herb–drug interactions have been noted.

Melatonin is a hormone produced nocturnally by the pineal gland and functions as a biologic and circadian cue to promote sleep. Melatonin also has a direct radical scavenging and antioxidant action. It has been used to successfully alleviate jet lag [137]. Reports are conflicting for those who have chronic sleep disorders, however. A retrospective study in adolescents who had delayed sleep phase syndrome revealed that those treated with 3 to 5 mg/d of melatonin for an average of 6 months reported quicker sleep onset, longer sleep duration, and a decrease in school difficulties. No adverse effects of melatonin were noted [138].

Therapeutic massage

It is important to briefly mention therapeutic massage as a CAM therapy commonly used by patients who have eating disorders. In a small placebo controlled study, massage therapy was shown to decrease body dissatisfaction. Massage may help those who have eating disorders by decreasing levels of cortisol and increasing levels of serotonin and dopamine [139]. Risk for adverse effects is theoretically low, but more research is necessary before routine recommendations can be made.

Summary

The integration of CAM therapies into primary care pediatric practice is well illustrated by these case discussions. From infancy to adolescence, CAM therapies are being used more frequently in the pediatric population, and primary care pediatricians are in an ideal position to work with families to explore all safe and effective remedies. Evidence supporting the use of CAM therapies for common conditions, such as colic, atopy, ADHD, eating disorders, and anxiety, has steadily increased in volume and improved in quality. Although we clearly need additional research examining the safety and efficacy of all therapies for these common childhood conditions, evidence to date supports the judicious use of specific CAM therapies. Primary care practitioners should routinely discuss the use of CAM therapies with their patients and their families.

References

[1] Primary care. Available at: http://en.wikipedia.org/wiki/Primary_care. Accessed August 23, 2007.
[2] American Academy of Pediatrics. AAP medical home initiatives for children with special needs project advisory committee: the medical home. Pediatrics 2002;110(1):184–6.
[3] Kemper KJ. Holistic pediatrics = good medicine. Pediatrics 2000;105(1 Pt 3):214–8.

[4] Loman DG. The use of complementary and alternative health care practices among children. J Pediatr Health Care 2003;17:58–63.

[5] Sanders H, Davis MF, Duncan B, et al. Use of complementary and alternative medical therapies among children with special health care needs in southern Arizona. Pediatrics 2003; 111:584–7.

[6] Sawni-Sikand A, Schubiner H, Thomas RL. Use of complementary/alternative therapies among children in primary care pediatrics. Ambul Pediatr 2002;2:99–103.

[7] Spigelblatt L, Laine-Ammara G, Pless IB, et al. The use of alternative medicine by children. Pediatrics 1994;94:811–4.

[8] Braun CA, Bearinger LH, Halcon LL, et al. Adolescent use of complementary therapies. J Adolesc Health 2005;37:76E1–9.

[9] Wilson KM, Klein JD. Adolescents' use of complementary and alternative medicineAmbul Pediatr 2002;2:104–10.

[10] American Academy of Pediatrics Division of Health Policy Research. Periodic survey of fellows #49: complementary and alternative medicine (CAM) therapies in pediatric practices. 2001. Available at: http://www.aap.org/research/periodicsurvey/ps49bexs.htm. Accessed August 22, 2007.

[11] Brazelton TB. Crying in infancy. Pediatrics 1962;29:579–88.

[12] Fireman L. Colic. Pediatr Rev 2006;27:357–8.

[13] Wessel MA, Cobb JC, Jackson EB, et al. Paroxysmal fussing in infancy, sometimes called "colic". Pediatrics 1954;14:421–35.

[14] Karp H. The "fourth trimester": a framework and strategy for understanding and resolving colic. Contemp Pediatr 2004;21:94–116.

[15] Heine RG. Gastroesophageal reflux disease, colic and constipation in infants with food allergy. Curr Opin Allergy Clin Immunol 2006;6:220–5.

[16] Savino F, Castagno E, Bretto R, et al. A prospective 10-year study on children who had severe infantile colic. Acta Paediatr Suppl 2005;94:129–32.

[17] Lohse B, Stotts JL, Priebe JR. Survey of herbal use by Kansas and Wisconsin WIC participants reveals moderate, appropriate use and identifies herbal education needs. J Am Diet Assoc 2006;106:227–37.

[18] Smitherman LC, Janisse J, Mathur A. The use of folk remedies among children in an urban black community: remedies for fever, colic, and teething. Pediatrics 2005;115: E297–304.

[19] Garrison MM, Christakis DA. A systematic review of treatments for infant colic. Pediatrics 2000;106:184–90.

[20] Mind-body medicine: an overview (NCCAM). Available at: http://nccam.nih.gov/health/backgrounds/mindbody.htm#intro. Accessed September 25, 2007.

[21] Akman I, Kuscu K, Ozdemir N, et al. Mothers' postpartum psychological adjustment and infantile colic. Arch Dis Child 2006;91:417–9.

[22] Keefe MR, Kajrlsen KA, Lobo ML, et al. Reducing parenting stress in families with irritable infants. Nurs Res 2006;55:198–205.

[23] Dihigo SK. New strategies for the treatment of colic: modifying the parent/infant interaction. J Pediatr Health Care 1998;12:256–62.

[24] Wolke D, Gray P, Meyer R. Excessive infant crying: a controlled study of mothers helping mothers. Pediatrics 1994;94:322–32.

[25] Underdown A, Barlow J, Chung V, et al. Massage intervention for promoting mental and physical health in infants aged under six months. Cochrane Database Syst Rev 2006;4: CD005038.

[26] Field T. Massage therapy for infants and children. J Dev Behav Pediatr 1995;16:105–11.

[27] Wheeden A. Massage effects on cocaine-exposed preterm neonates. J Dev Behav Pediatr 1993;14(5):318–22.

[28] Huhtala V, Lehtonen L, Heinonen R, et al. Infant massage compared with crib vibrator in the treatment of colicky infants. Pediatrics 2000;105:E84–9.

[29] Agarwal KN, Gupta A, Pushkarna R, et al. Effects of massage and use of oil on growth, blood flow and sleep pattern in infants. Indian J Med Res 2000;112:212–7.

[30] Blumental I. The gripe water story. J R Soc Med 2000;93:172–4.

[31] Natural medicines comprehensive database. Available at: http://www.naturaldatabase.com. Accessed August 23, 2007.

[32] Weizman Z, Alkrinawi S, Goldfarb D, et al. Efficacy of herbal tea preparation in infantile colic. J Pediatr 1993;122:650–2.

[33] Alexandrovich I, Rakovitskaya O, Kolmo E, et al. The effect of fennel (Foeniculum vulgare) seed oil emulsion in infantile colic: a randomized, placebo-controlled study. Altern Ther Health Med 2003;9:58–61.

[34] Savino F, Cresi F, Castagno E, et al. A randomized double-blind placebo-controlled trial of a standardized extract of Matricariae recutita, Foeniculum vulgare and Melissa officinalis (ColiMil) in the treatment of breastfed colicky infants. Phytother Res 2005;19:335–40.

[35] Clifford TJ, Campbell MK, Speechly KN, et al. Infant colic: empirical evidence of the absence of an association with source of early infant nutrition. Arch Pediatr Adolesc Med 2002;156:1123–8.

[36] Hill DJ, et al. Effect of a low-allergen maternal diet on colic among breastfed infants: a randomized, controlled trial. Pediatrics 2005;116:E709–15.

[37] Lust KD, Brown JE, Thomas W. Maternal intake of cruciferous vegetables and other foods and colic symptoms in exclusively breast-fed infants. J Am Diet Assoc 1996;96:46–8.

[38] Cambria S, et al. Hyperexcitability syndrome in a newborn infant of chocoholic mother. Am J Perinatol 2006;23:421–2.

[39] Cheruku SR, Montgomery-Downs HE, Farkas SL, et al. Higher maternal plasma docosahexanoic acid during pregnancy is associated with more mature neonatal sleep-state patterning. Am J Clin Nutr 2002;76:608–13.

[40] Jakobsson I, Lothe L, Ley D, et al. Effectiveness of casein hydrolysate feedings in infants with colic. Acta Paediatr 2000;89:18–21.

[41] Lucassen PLBJ, Assendelft WJ, Gubbels JW, et al. Infantile colic: crying time reduction with a whey hydrolysate: a double-blind, randomized, placebo-controlled trial. Pediatrics 2000;106:1349–54.

[42] American Academy of Pediatrics, Committee on Nutrition. American Academy of Pediatrics, Committee on Nutrition. Soy protein-based formulas: recommendations for use in infant feeding. Pediatrics 1998;101:148–53.

[43] American Academy of Pediatrics, Committee on Nutrition: Hypoallergenic infant formulas. Pediatrics 2000;106:346–9.

[44] Schrezenmeir J, de Vrese M. Probiotics, prebiotics, and synbiotics—approaching a definition. Am J Clin Nutr 2001;73:361S–4S.

[45] Savino F, Cresi F, Pautasso S, et al. Intestinal microflora in breastfed colicky and non-colicky infants. Acta Paediatr 2004;93:825–9.

[46] Savino F, Bailo E, Oggero E, et al. Bacterial counts of intestinal Lactobacillus species in infants with colic. Pediatr Allergy Immunol 2005;16:72–5.

[47] Savino F, Pelle E, Palumeri E, et al. Lactobacillus reuteri (American Type Culture Collection Strain 55730) versus simethicone in the treatment of infantile colic: a prospective randomized study. Pediatrics 2007;119:E124–30.

[48] Savino F, Palumeri E, Castagno E, et al. Reduction of crying episodes owing to infantile colic: a randomized controlled study on the efficacy of a new infant formula. Eur J Clin Nutr 2006;60:1304–10.

[49] Asher MI, Montefort S, Bjorksten B, et al. Worldwide time trends in the prevalence of symptoms of asthma, allergic rhinoconjunctivitis, and eczema in childhood: ISAAC Phases One and Three repeat multicountry cross-sectional surveys. Lancet 2006;368:733–43.

[50] Castro-Rodriguez JA, Stern DA, Halonen M, et al. Relation between infantile colic and asthma/atopy: a prospective study in an unselected population. Pediatrics 2001;108(4): 878–82.

[51] Spergel JM, Palier AS. Atopic dermatitis and the atopic march. J Allergy Clin Immunol 2003;112S:118–27.

[52] Negoro T, Orihara K, Irahara T, et al. Influence of SNPs in cytokine-related genes on the severity of food allergy and atopic eczema in children. Pediatr Allergy Immunol 2006;17: 583–90.

[53] Kidd P. Th1/Th2 balance: the hypothesis, its limitations, and implications for health and disease. Altern Med Rev 2003;8:223–46.

[54] Noverr MC, Huffnagle GB. The "microflora hypothesis" of allergic diseases. Clin Exp Allergy 2005;35:1511–20.

[55] Duramad P, Harley K, Lipsett M, et al. Early environmental exposures and intracellular Th1/Th2 cytokine profiles in 24-month-old children living in an agricultural area. Environ Health Perspect 2006;114:1916–22.

[56] Johnson CC, Ownby DR, Alford SH, et al. Antibiotic exposure in early infancy and risk for childhood atopy. J Allergy Clin Immunol 2005;115:1218–24.

[57] Marra F, Lynd L, Coombes M, et al. Does antibiotic exposure during infancy lead to development of asthma? A systematic review and metaanalysis. Chest 2006;129: 610–8.

[58] Noverr MC, Noggle RM, Toews GB, et al. Role of antibiotics and fungal microbiota in driving pulmonary allergic responses. Infect Immun 2004;72:4996–5003.

[59] Thomas M, Custovic A, Woodcock A, et al. Atopic wheezing and early life antibiotic exposure: a nested case-control study. Pediatr Allergy Immunol 2006;17:184–8.

[60] Kummeling I, Stelma FF, Dagnelie PC, et al. Early life exposure to antibiotics and the subsequent development of eczema, wheeze, and allergic sensitization in the first 2 years of life: the KOALA Birth Cohort Study. Pediatrics 2007;119(1):E225–31.

[61] Kozyrskyj AL, Ernst P, Becker AB. Increased risk of childhood asthma from antibiotic use in early life. Chest 2007;131(6):1753–9.

[62] Bornehag CG, Sundell J, Weschler CJ, et al. The association between asthma and allergic symptoms in children and phthalates in house dust: a nested case-control study. Environ Health Perspect 2004;112:1393–7.

[63] Chalubinski M, Kowalski ML. Endocrine disrupters—potential modulators of the immune system and allergic response. Allergy 2006;61:1326–35.

[64] Sherriff A, Farrow A, Golding J, et al. Frequent use of chemical household products is associated with persistent wheezing in pre-school age children. Thorax 2005;60:45–9.

[65] Bielroy L. Complementary and alternative interventions in asthma, allergy, and immunology. Ann Allergy Immunol 2004;93(Suppl 1):S45–54.

[66] Braganza S, Ozuah PO, Sharif I. The use of complementary therapies in inner-city asthmatic children. J Asthma 2003;40:823–7.

[67] Johnston GA, Bilbao RM, Graham-Brown RA. The use of complementary medicine in children with atopic dermatitis in secondary care in Leicester. Br J Dermatol 2003;149: 566–71.

[68] Reznick M, Ozuah PO, Franco K, et al. Use of complementary therapy by adolescents with asthma. Arch Pediatr Adolesc Med 2002;156:1042–4.

[69] Ko J, Lee JI, Munoz-Furlong A, et al. Use of complementary and alternative medicine by food-allergic patients. Ann Allergy Asthma Immunol 2006;97:365–9.

[70] Kramer MS, Kakuma R. Maternal antigen avoidance during pregnancy or lactation, or both, for preventing or treating atopic disease in the child. Cochrane Database Syst Rev 2006;3:CD000133.

[71] Zeiger RS. Food allergen avoidance in the prevention of food allergy in infants and children. Pediatrics 2003;111:1662–71.

[72] Friedman NJ, Zieger RS. The role of breast-feeding in the development of allergies and asthma. J Allergy Clin Immunol 2005;115:1238–48.

[73] Kull I, Bohme M, Wahlgren CF, et al. Breast-feeding reduces the risk for childhood eczema. J Allergy Clin Immunol 2005;116:657–61.

[74] Kull I, Almquist C, Lilja G, et al. Breast-feeding reduces the risk of asthma during the first 4 years of life. J Allergy Clin Immunol 2005;114:755–60.

[75] Kull I, Wickman M, Lilja G, et al. Breast feeding and allergic disease in infants—a prospective birth cohort study. Arch Dis Child 2002;87:478–81.

[76] Osborn DA, Sinn J. Formulas containing hydrolysed protein for prevention of allergy and food intolerance in infants. Cochrane Database Syst Rev 2006;4:CD003664.

[77] Hays T, Wood RA. A systematic review of the role of hydrolyzed infant formulas in allergy prevention. Arch Pediatr Adolesc Med 2005;159:810–6.

[78] Osborn DA, Sinn J. Soy formula for prevention of allergy and food intolerance in infants. Cochrane Databse Syst Rev 2006;4:CD003741.

[79] Fiocchi A, Assa'ad A, Bahna S, et al. Food allergy and the introduction of solid foods to infants: a consensus document. Adverse Reactions to Foods Committee, American College of Allergy, Asthma and Immunology. Ann Allergy Asthma Immunol 2006;97:10–20.

[80] Tarini BA, Carroll AE, Sox CM, et al. Systematic review of the relationship between early introduction of solid foods to infants and the development of allergic disease. Arch Pediatr Adolesc Med 2006;160:502–7.

[81] Norris JM, Barriga K, Hoffenberg EJ, et al. Risk of celiac disease autoimmunity and timing of gluten introduction in the diet of infants at increased risk of disease. JAMA 2005;293: 2343–51.

[82] Fiocchi A, Bouygue GR, Martelli A, et al. Dietary treatment of childhood atopic eczema/ dermatitis syndrome (AEDS). Allergy 2004;59(Suppl 78):78–85.

[83] Johnston GA, Bilbao RM, Graham-Brown RA. The use of dietary manipulation by parents of children with atopic dermatitis. Br J Dermatol 2004;150:1186–9.

[84] Lothian JB, Grey V, Lands LC. Effect of whey protein to modulate immune response in children with atopic asthma. Int J Food Sci Nutr 2006;57:204–11.

[85] Denburg JA, Hatfield HM, Cyr MM, et al. Fish oil supplementation in pregnancy modifies neonatal progenitors at birth in infants at risk of atopy. Pediatr Res 2005;57:276–81.

[86] Wijga AH, van Houwelingen AC, Kerkhof M, et al. Breast milk fatty acids and allergic disease in preschool children: the prevention and incidence of asthma and mite allergy birth cohort study. J Allergy Clin Immunol 2006;117:440–7.

[87] Oddy WH, Pal S, Kusel MM, et al. Atopy, eczema and breast milk fatty acids in a high-risk cohort of children followed from birth to 5 yr. Pediatr Allergy Immunol 2006;17:4–10.

[88] Peat JK, Mihrshahi S, Kemp AS, et al. Three-year outcomes of dietary fatty acid modification and house dust mite reduction in the childhood asthma prevention study. J Allergy Clin Immunol 2004;114:807–13.

[89] Mihrshahi S, Peat JK, Webb K, et al. Effect of omega-3 fatty acid concentrations in plasma on symptoms of asthma at 18 months of age. Pediatr Allergy Immunol 2004;15:517–22.

[90] Biagi PL, Bordoni A, Masi M, et al. A long-term study on the use of evening primrose oil (Efamol) in atopic children. Drugs Exp Clin Res 1988;14:285–90.

[91] Kalliomaki M, Salminen S, Poussa T, et al. Probiotics in primary prevention of atopic disease: a randomised placebo-controlled trial. Lancet 2001;357:1076–9.

[92] Kalliomaki M, Salminen S, Poussa T, et al. Probiotics and prevention of atopic disease: 4-year follow-up of randomised placebo-controlled trial. Lancet 2003;361:1869–71.

[93] Moro G, Arslanoglu S, Stahl B, et al. A mixture of prebiotic oligosaccharides reduces the incidence of atopic dermatitis during the first six months of age. Arch Dis Child 2006;91: 814–9.

[94] Rosenfeldt V, Benfeldt E, Nielsen SD, et al. Effect of probiotic Lactobacillus strains in children with atopic dermatitis. J Allergy Clin Immunol 2003;111:389–95.

[95] Weston S, Halbert A, Richmond P, et al. Effects of probiotics on atopic dermatitis: a randomized controlled trial. Arch Dis Child 2005;90:892–7.

[96] Viljanen M, Savilahti E, Haahtela T, et al. Probiotics in the treatment of atopic eczema/dermatitis syndrome in infants: a double-blind placebo-controlled trial. Allergy 2005;60: 494–500.

[97] Passeron T, Lacour JP, Fontas E, et al. Prebiotics and synbiotics: two promising approaches for the treatment of atopic dermatitis in children above 2 years. Allergy 2006;61:431–7.

[98] Brouwer ML, Wolt-Plompen SA, Dubois AE, et al. No effects of probiotics on atopic dermatitis in infancy: a randomized placebo-controlled trial. Clin Exp Allergy 2006;36: 899–906.

[99] Lee ACC, Kemper KJ. Homeopathy and naturopathy. Arch Pediatr Adolesc Med 2000; 154:78–80.

[100] Stem RC, Canda ER, Doershuk CF. Use of non-medical treatment by cystic fibrosis patients. J Adolesc Health 1992;13:612–5.

[101] Sawyer MG, Gannoni AF, Toogood IR, et al. The use of alternative therapies by children with cancer. Med J Aust 1994;169:320–2.

[102] Southwood TR, Malleson PN, Roberts-Thomson PJ, et al. Unconventional remedies used by patients with juvenile arthritis. Pediatrics 1995;85:150–1554.

[103] Neuhouser ML, Patterson RE, Schwartz SM, et al. Use of alternative medicine by children with cancer in Washington state. Prev Med 2001;33(5):347–54.

[104] Friedman T, Slayton WB, Allen LS, et al. Use of alternative therapies for children with cancer. Pediatrics 1997;100(6):E1.

[105] Faw C, Ballentine R, Ballentine L, et al. Unproved cancer remedies. A survey of use in pediatric outpatients. JAMA 1977;238:1536–8.

[106] Paramore LC. Use of alternative therapies: estimates from the Robert Wood Johnson Foundation national access to care survey, US Cancer Pain Relief Committee. J Pain Symptom Manage 1997;13:83–9.

[107] Breuner CC, Barry P, Kemper KJ. Alternative medicine use by homeless youth. Arch Pediatr Adolesc Med 1998;152(11):1071–5.

[108] Ahuja J. Caffeine and theobromine intakes of children: results from CSF II 1994–96, 1998. Family Economics and Nutrition Review 2001;13(2):47–52. Available at: http://www.barc. usda.gov/bhnrc/foodsurvey/pdf/fenrv13n2p47.pdf. Accessed August 23, 2007.

[109] Ellison RC. Caffeine intake and salivary levels in children. Presented at the 7th International Caffeine Workshop. Santorini, Greece, June 1993.

[110] Rapoport JL, Berg CJ, Ismond DR, et al. Behavioral effects of caffeine in children. Relationship between dietary choice and effects of caffeine challenge [Clinical Trial. Controlled Clinical Trial. Journal Article]. Arch Gen Psychiatry 1984;41(11):1073–9.

[111] Stein MA, Krasowski M, Leventhal BL, et al. Behavioral and cognitive effects of methylxanthines. A meta-analysis of theophylline and caffeine. Arch Pediatr Adolesc Med 1996; 150(3):284–8.

[112] Huestis RD, Arnold LE, Smeltzer DJ. Caffeine versus methylphenidate and d-amphetamine in minimal brain dysfunction: a double-blind comparison. Am J Psychiatry 1975; 132(8):868–70.

[113] Bernstein GA, Carroll ME, Dean NW, et al. Caffeine withdrawal in normal school aged children. J Am Acad Child Adolesc Psychiatry 1998;37(8):858–65.

[114] Lloyd T, Rollings NJ, Kieselhorst K, et al. Dietary caffeine intake is not correlated with adolescent bone gain. J Am Coll Nutr 1998;17(5):454–7.

[115] Shekelle PG, Hardy ML, Morton SC, et al. Efficacy and safety of ephedra and ephedrine for weight loss and athletic performance: a meta-analysis. JAMA 2003;289(12):1537–45.

[116] Andersen T, Fogh J. Weight loss and delayed gastric emptying following a South American herbal preparation in overweight patients. J Hum Nutr Diet 2001;14(3):243–50.

[117] Mate monograph, natural medicines comprehensive database. Avaialble at: www. naturaldatabase.com. Accessed August 23, 2007.

[118] Avula B, Wang YH, Pawar RS, et al. Determination of the appetite suppressant P57 in Hoodia gordonii plant extracts and dietary supplements by liquid chromatography/electrospray ionization mass spectrometry (LC-MSD-TOF) and LC-UV methods. J AOAC Int 2006;89(3):606–11.

[119] Hoodia cactus plant and P57 research. Available at: http://www.cellhealthmakeover.com/hoodia-p57.html. Accessed September 27, 2007.

[120] Mukhtar H, Wang ZY, Katiyar SK, et al. Tea components: antimutagenic and anticarcinogenic effects. Prev Med 1992;21:351–60.

[121] Dulloo AG, Duret C, Rohrer D, et al. Efficacy of a green tea extract rich in catechin polyphenols and caffeine in increasing 24-h energy expenditure and fat oxidation in humans. Am J Clin Nutr 1999;70(6):1040–5.

[122] Merhav H, Amitai Y, Palti H, et al. Tea drinking and microcytic anemia in infants. Am J Clin Nutr 1985;41(6):1210–3.

[123] Vogler BK, Pittler MH, Ernst E. The efficacy of ginseng. A systematic review of randomised clinical trials. Eur J Clin Pharmacol 1999;55(8):567–75.

[124] Ginseng. Natural medicines comprehensive database website. Available at: www.naturaldatabase.com. Accessed September 27, 2007.

[125] Beumont P, Touyz S. What kind of illness is anorexia nervosa? Eur Child Adolesc Psychiatry 2003;12(Suppl 1):I20–4.

[126] Barabasz M. Efficacy of hypnotherapy in the treatment of eating disorders. Int J Clin Exp Hypn 2007;55(3):318–35.

[127] Miller JJ, Fletcher K, Kabat Zinn J. Three year follow up and clinical implications of a mindfulness meditation based states reduction intervention in the treatment of anxiety disorders. Gen Hosp Psychiatry 1995;17(3):192–200.

[128] Kristeller JL, Hallett B. An exploratory study of a meditation-based intervention for binge eating disorder. J Health Psychol 1999;4(3):357–63.

[129] Garfinkel PE, Dorian BJ. Factors that may influence future approaches to the eating disorders. Eat Weight Disord 1997;2(1):1–16.

[130] Thien V, Thomas A, Markin D, et al. Pilot study of a graded exercise program for the treatment of anorexia nervosa. Int J Eat Disord 2000;28(1):101–6.

[131] Giles G. Anorexia nervosa and bulimia: an activity-oriented approach. Am J Occup Ther 1985;39(8):510–7.

[132] Carei T, Breuner CC, Fyfe-Johnson A. The evaluation of yoga in the treatment of eating disorders. J Adolesc Health 2007;40(2):S31–2.

[133] Pittler MH, Ernst E. Kava extract for treating anxiety. Cochrane Database Syst Rev 2003;1:CD003383.

[134] Clough AR, Bailie RS, Currie B. Liver function test abnormalities in users of aqueous kava extracts. J Toxicol Clin Toxicol 2003;41(6):821–9.

[135] Miyasaka LS, Atallah AN, Soares BG. Valerian for anxiety disorders. Cochrane Database Syst Rev 2006;4:CD004515.

[136] Viola H, Wasowski C, Levi de Stein M, et al. Apigenin, a component of Matricaria recutita flowers, is a central benzodiazepine receptors-ligand with anxiolytic effects. Planta Med 1995;61(3):213–6.

[137] Herxheimer A, Petrie KJ. Melatonin for the prevention and treatment of jet lag. Cochrane Database Syst Rev 2002;2:CD001520.

[138] Szeinberg A, Borodkin K, Dagan Y. Melatonin treatment in adolescents with delayed sleep phase syndrome. Clin Pediatr (Phila) 2006;45(9):809–18.

[139] Hart S, Field T, Hernandez-Reif M, et al. Anorexia nervosa symptoms are reduced by massage therapy. Eat Disord 2001;9:289–99.

ELSEVIER
SAUNDERS

PEDIATRIC CLINICS
OF NORTH AMERICA

Pediatr Clin N Am 54 (2007) 859–874

Herbs to Homeopathy—Medicinal Products for Children

Paula Gardiner, MD[a],*, David S. Riley, MD[b]

[a]Department of Family Medicine, Boston University Medical Center, 1 Boston Medical
Center Place, Dowling 5 South, Boston, MA 02118, USA
[b]University of New Mexico Medical School, Santa Fe, NM 87508, USA

Medicinal products in pediatric integrative medicine range from non-pharmaceutical herbs, dietary supplements, and vitamins regulated as foods to homeopathy regulated as a drug or "pharmaceutical" therapy. These products are designed for a wide range of applications, from treating specific conditions to supporting a healthy life, and the evidence supporting their use ranges from historical patterns of prescribing to randomized, controlled trials. Issues of safety and efficacy are impacted by a variety of factors. Even if a medicinal product has a single ingredient, how that ingredient is regulated or manufactured and its indications of use will help define its categorization. Iron, for example, might be sold as a dietary supplement or a homeopathic preparation or be present in a food. To complicate matters further, single products are commonly combined into multi-ingredient preparations with varying methods of manufacturing and more than one route of administration. How can clinicians make recommendations for products in the marketplace when research supporting an intervention has been conducted on only a single ingredient?

The categories of herbs, dietary supplements, and homeopathy often overlap. Herbal products are regulated as dietary supplements under the Dietary Supplement Health and Education Act of 1994 (DSHEA); but when these same products are diluted and prepared according to the Homeopathic Pharmacopoeia of the United States they become pharmaceutical products according to federal regulations. For example, chamomile and calendula, both medicinal plants, may be classified as either dietary supplements or homeopathic drugs by the Food and Drug Administration (FDA). Chamomile and calendula are used as herbal preparations for colic and burns,

---

* Corresponding author.
E-mail address: Paula.gardiner@bmc.org (P. Gardiner).

respectively, and when prepared homeopathically are also used at lower concentrations for the same and other indications. The concentration at which an herbal product or dietary supplement transitions to its homeopathic counterpart is often confusing.

Regulation of dietary supplements

Dietary supplements, regulated under the DSHEA, are products designed to "supplement the diet" and include herbal and other botanical products, vitamins, minerals, amino acids, and other dietary substances for use." The DSHEA allows dietary supplements that were on the market before 1994 to be marketed without the approval of efficacy and safety that the FDA requires for prescription medications. Manufacturers are permitted to claim that the product affects the structure or function of the body, as long as there is no claim of effectiveness in the prevention or treatment of a specific disease and provided there is a disclaimer informing the user that the FDA has not evaluated the product for any claim.

In June of 2007, the FDA finalized its good manufacturing practices regulations for dietary supplements. These regulations will be useful to professionals and consumers alike. They will help standardize the lot-to-lot quality of dietary supplements throughout the manufacturing, packaging, labeling, and storing processes. The final rule includes requirements for establishing quality-control procedures, designing and constructing manufacturing plants, and testing ingredients and the finished product.

Regulation of homeopathy

Homeopathic remedies, on the other hand, have been regulated as drugs since the 1938 Food Drug and Cosmetic Act that defines the term "drug" to mean "articles recognized in ... the official Homeopathic Pharmacopeia of the United States ... and articles intended for use in the diagnosis, cure, mitigation, treatment, or the prevention of disease in man .... Whether or not they are official homeopathic remedies, those products offered for the cure, mitigation, prevention, or treatment of disease conditions are regarded as drugs within the meaning of Section 201(g)(l) of the Act. Homeopathic drugs must comply with the labeling provisions of Sections 502 and 503 of the [Food, Drug, and Cosmetic] Act and Part 201 Title 21 of the Code of Federal Regulations (CFR)...."

What do these regulations mean to pediatricians, their patients, and the patients' families? The two primary concerns, as in all of medicine, are safety and effectiveness. For both homeopathic drugs and dietary supplements, clinicians often depend on the evidence available from clinical trials in adults and animals studies. As one ventures into the realm of the complex herbal mixtures that are used in Chinese herbal medicines and Ayurvedic practice, where international herbal pharmacopoeias may differ in growing and harvesting conditions, and manufacturing practices may differ from Western standards, identifying the plant itself and determining its safety become challenging. Both determining and measuring effectiveness are complicated as one balances the evidence from patterns of historical usage and personal experience and the small pool of randomized, controlled trials against traditional medical practices that are hundreds or thousands of years old. Establishing a rigorous evidence profile is challenging when intellectual property rights do not exist and the economic engine of patent law is not available.

Trends in pediatric use of dietary supplements

Many children and adolescents use dietary supplements and homeopathy. The prevalence of use of these products depends on population characteristics (healthy versus sick), the age of the child or adolescent, race/ethnicity, and other factors such as methods of data collection (interviews versus surveys) and the extent of the survey (national versus regional).

Recent national surveys indicate that more than 20% to 40% of all young children and 20% to 30% of adolescents in the United States have used dietary supplements [1–6]. Vitamins and minerals are the dietary supplements most commonly used by children and adolescents.

Regional surveys of the general pediatric population show varying prevalences. Among parents who report using complementary and alternative medicine (CAM), 40% to 45% gave their child an herbal product, and 34% to 50% used vitamin supplementation [7–9]. In a survey of parents in a primary care practice in Washington, DC, more than 50% of pediatric CAM users reported specific vitamin supplementation, more than 40% used herbal therapies, and 25% used other nutritional supplements or elimination diets [8].

Outpatient clinical surveys have reported that children and adolescents who have medical conditions are more likely to use dietary supplements. Chronic pediatric conditions for which dietary supplements are commonly used include attention deficit hyperactivity disorder (ADHD), asthma, atopic dermatitis, allergic rhinitis, cancer, inflammatory bowel disease, headache, and cystic fibrosis [10–22]. For example, in a cross-sectional survey of 117 parents of children seen in a pediatric nephrology clinic in North Carolina, 29% of surveyed parents gave their children cranberry products, but only 23% of those who used cranberry products had discussed their use with the physician [22].

In addition to the outpatient setting, children and adolescents use dietary supplements in inpatient settings as well. Reports from an inpatient holistic pediatric consultation service noted that, in 70 consultations, 80% of patients had at least one question about using an herb or dietary supplement. Herbs of interest to families included essiac (an herbal combination), cat's claw, noni juice, astragalus, chamomile, echinacea, ginger, goldenseal, green tea, milk thistle, and various Chinese herbs and mushrooms [23]. Finally, several studies report concurrent use of prescription medications and dietary supplements in children. Drug and supplement interactions are a concern [6,24,25].

Several surveys have looked at the use of dietary supplements and homeopathy before surgery [26]. In a survey of 1021 pediatric patients, 29.5% indicated they had tried one or more CAM therapies in the year before surgery, and 12.8% of the pediatric patients had used herbal remedies before surgery. The most popular herbs included echinacea, aloe vera, cranberry, St. John's wort, and goldenseal [27]. In another multiregional preoperative survey of 894 pediatric patients, 42% had used some form of vitamins, nutritional supplements, herbs, or homeopathy. The most prevalent dietary supplement given to children presenting for elective surgery was echinacea [28].

Moving away from supplement use in the hospital setting, a discussion of supplement use by teenagers is important. Dietary supplements are increasingly marketed to teenagers to enhance athletic performance or personal appearance, maintain health, and treat specific conditions. These supplements are commonly available to teenagers in sport drinks, weight-loss products, and functional foods in pharmacies and stores and through the Internet.

The 1999–2000 National Health and Nutrition Examination Survey reported that approximately one in four adolescents aged 12 to 15 years used dietary supplements, and rates were higher for those between the ages of 16 and 19 years [1]. More recently, a 2002 online survey documented that 46% of teenagers reported using vitamins, and 29% reported using least one other dietary supplement within the last month. Commonly used supplements included ginseng, zinc, echinacea, ginkgo biloba, creatine, and weight-loss supplements [7].

Patient use of dietary supplements and homeopathy

In 1996, Vincent [29] identified reasons that patients seek complementary therapies, including dietary supplements and homeopathy. These reasons included a positive value associated with complementary treatment, the ineffectiveness of orthodox treatment for a patient's complaint, concern about the adverse effects of orthodox medicine, concerns about communication with doctors, and, finally, the availability of complementary medicine. Homeopathy patients were most strongly influenced by the ineffectiveness of orthodox medicine for their complaints. Jain and Astin [30], in 2001, found that people are less likely to use CAM if they believe that the therapies are in general ineffective or inferior to conventional methods or if they perceive that their doctor does not support the use of CAM.

Parents give their children dietary supplements or use homeopathic remedies for many reasons, including maintaining health, preventing disease, and treating a chronic or acute disease. Additionally, several clinical surveys have demonstrated a strong cultural influence in the use of folk medicine (herbs) in children [20,31–35]. Therefore, to make effective recommendations, it is important to be aware of the reasons families and patients use these treatments (ie, their culture, socioeconomic status, parental beliefs about healing and wellness, and previous treatments).

Parents get their information about dietary supplements from numerous places: friends, family, the popular press, the Internet, and, finally, health care professionals. In 2003, of 142 families surveyed in an emergency room, 45% of caregivers reported giving their child an herbal product. Of those who used these therapies, 80% reported either friends or relatives as their primary source of information. Only 45% of those who gave their children herbal products reported discussing this use with their child's primary health care provider [7].

The low rate of disclosure of dietary supplements has been reported many times in the pediatric literature [9,36]. For example, in a survey of 117 parents of children and adolescents who had ADHD or depression, 15% had used herbal medicine in the last year. Seventy-eight percent of these caregivers supervised the administration of herbal therapy in their children; 70% of the children's psychiatrists, 56% of their pediatricians, and 74% of pharmacists were not aware of this use [12].

Homeopathy—what is it?

Homeopathy is a popular form of CAM globally and is part of the official health care systems in a number of countries. It is 200 years old, and its core is based on the idea of "treating like with like" (*Similia similibus curentur*), aiming to stimulate self-healing processes. This principle also is applied in some areas of conventional medicine, such as allergy desensitization. The doses used in homeopathy range from those that are similar in concentration to conventional medicines to very high dilutions containing no material trace of the starting substance. There is no currently understood way that homeopathic medicines in "ultra-molecular" dilutions could have any physiologic effects. Homeopathic medicines are of botanical, chemical, mineral, zoologic, or human origin and are prepared by a process of successive dilution and agitation (succussion), known as "potentization." They are commonly available as single or complex remedies. Although there are challenges relating to underreporting and mistaken identity (herbal medicines identified as homeopathic), the level of direct risk resulting from the use of homeopathic medicinal products is low [37].

Homeopathic medications are manufactured by beginning with a "mother tincture" for soluble substances followed by a process known as "potentization"—serial dilution with shaking (succussion). Homeopathic potencies usually are labeled with a combination of a number and a letter. The number refers to the number of successive dilutions to which the starting material has been subjected to prepare that homeopathic medicine. The letter refers to the scale on which the dilution has been performed. The letter "X" or "D" denotes the decimal method (ie, one part of liquid is added to nine parts of diluent). The letter "C" indicates the centesimal method (ie, 1 part of liquid is added to 99 parts of diluent).

There are several distinct types of homeopathic practice. Two of the main types are "classical" and "clinical" homeopathy. In classical homeopathy a single homeopathic medicine is commonly selected, based on the total symptom picture of a patient, including mental, general, and constitutional features. In clinical homeopathy, one or more single or complex homeopathic medicines are administered for standard clinical situations or conventional diagnoses. Homeopathic medicines also are used in other therapeutic approaches such as anthroposophical medicine and homotoxicology.

Research background

Hierarchies for the evaluation of evidence of clinical research usually give the greatest weight to systematic reviews of controlled trials, followed by randomized, controlled trials. Other forms of evidence also are used to establish the effectiveness and safety of a therapy. The World Health Organization and many regulatory agencies use the hierarchy in Box 1 for evaluating evidence [38].

Research in homeopathy

Currently more than 130 randomized, controlled clinical trials of homeopathy have been published in the peer-reviewed medical literature. Of those, more than 15 have focused on the pediatric population.

Systematic reviews

The Lancet published a meta-analysis analyzing 89 placebo-controlled studies of homeopathy [39]. The overall mean odds ratio for these 89

Box 1. Hierarchy of evidence for research and evaluation of traditional medicine

Ia: Systematic review of randomized, controlled trials
Ib: At least one randomized, controlled trial
IIa: At least one well-designed quasi-experimental trial
IIb: At least one other type of well-designed quasi-experimental study
III: Well-designed nonexperimental descriptive studies: comparative studies, correlation studies and case control studies
IV: Expert committee reports or opinions and/or clinical experience of authorities

clinical trials was 2.45 (95% confidence interval, 2.05–2.93) in favor of homeopathy. This finding indicated that the chance of homeopathy being useful was two to three times greater than that of placebo. Even after correction for several potential confounders, the results remained statistically significant. The authors concluded that the results "were not compatible with the hypothesis that the effects of homoeopathy are completely due to placebo." Several systematic reviews in the pediatric population have reported positive results for homeopathy. These reviews include studies of the homeopathic treatment of childhood diarrhea, influenza, postoperative ileus, seasonal allergic rhinitis, vertigo, and rheumatic diseases [40–45].

Clinical trials in homeopathy (pediatric examples)

In a crossover study of children who had ADHD, patients received homeopathy or placebo for 6 weeks and then crossed over to the other arm of the study for an additional 6 weeks [46]. A standard rating scale was used, and the results showed a statistically significant improvement in the homeopathic group. A placebo-controlled trial of homeopathy for otitis media in children demonstrated a significant effect in the homeopathic treatment group at 24 and 64 hours [47]. Some corroboration these results may be found in another small, randomized study of homeopathy versus standard care in children who had chronic serous otitis media in which a significantly higher proportion of children receiving homeopathy had normal tympanograms at 12 months [48]. A comparison of homoeopathic and conventional medicine in acute otitis media was reported in 103 children received homeopathic medicines [49]. Median duration of pain was 2 days in the homeopathy group and 3 days in the conventional group. Seventy percent of the children in the homeopathy group and 56% of the children treated conventionally were free of recurrence in the following year.

Homeopathy in the treatment of influenza has been investigated in two large randomized, controlled clinical trials of *Anas barbariae hepatis et cordis extractum* [50,51]. Symptoms of the participants at 48 hours in the verum group were reduced to a greater extent, and the difference between the groups was statistically significant.

Oberbaum and colleagues [52] have demonstrated a statistically significant reduction in chemotherapy-induced stomatitis in children using Traumeel S liquid during stem cell transplantation, and this therapy currently is under investigation in a second clinical trial conducted under the auspices of the National Cancer Institute. Zell and colleagues [53] evaluated the same homeopathic remedy, Traumeel, applied topically for ankle sprains, and found that on the tenth day the injured ankle joint was back to normal in 17 (51.5%) of the 33 patients in the verum group versus 9 (25.0%) of the 36 patients in the placebo group ($P = .03$).

Dietary supplement research

This section gives examples of commonly used pediatric dietary supplements. Vitamins and minerals that can be obtained from food or supplements include vitamin A, B, C, D, E, calcium, and iron. Survey data clearly indicate that multivitamins are the most commonly used supplements. The question arises: should all children take a vitamins and minerals, and, if so, at what age do they begin? There are numerous different opinions and recommendations about vitamins and minerals, but there is no clear answer. To date systematic reviews show mixed results. The results of efficacy and safety mirror the nutritional status in the population, geography, and socioeconomic status of the country [54–65].

Calcium plays is a critical factor in maintaining a healthy skeleton, and the questions of dietary calcium intake, supplementing diets with calcium, who should be supplemented, and when are being hotly debated. For example, Winzenberg and colleagues [66–68] looked at 19 trials that included 2859 participants, of whom 1367 were assigned randomly to supplementation and 1426 to placebo. They found no effect of calcium supplementation on femoral neck or lumbar spine bone mineral density (BMD) and only a small effect on total body bone mineral content and upper limb BMD. This effect is approximately equivalent to a 1.7% greater increase in supplemented groups, which at best would reduce the absolute fracture risk in children by 0.1% to 0.2% per annum. The authors concluded "while there is a small effect of calcium supplementation in the upper limb, the increase in BMD which results is unlikely to result in a clinically significant decrease in fracture risk. The results do not support the use of calcium supplementation in healthy children as a public health intervention. These results cannot be extrapolated to children with medical conditions affecting bone metabolism" [68].

Numerous systematic reviews and guidelines address the use of vitamin D in children, especially breastfeeding infants (Box 2) [69–73].

Omega fatty acids have some of the most promising research. Omega-3s, such as eicosapentaenoic acid and docosahexaenoic acid (DHA), are long-chain polyunsaturated fatty acids that are found in the tissues of oily fish. Epidemiologic studies in adults and children have reported beneficial associations between dietary omega-3 fatty acids and many diseases. The results of interventional supplementation studies in established disease have been mixed, however. For example, a meta-analysis identified 34 controlled trials including 5 trials of fish oil and concluded that essential fatty acid supplementation did not show a large effect on the severity of atopic dermatitis [74]. For children who have chronic disease, fish oil has only marginal benefits in the treatment of cystic fibrosis [75]. Additionally, no clear and concrete conclusions can be made regarding the use of fish oil for children who have asthma [76,77].

There is some suggestive evidence that children who have ADHD may have low omega-3 fatty acids [78]. A recent placebo-controlled, double-blind

---

Box 2. Sources for American Academy of Pediatricians guidelines on complementary and alternative medicine and dietary supplements

Vitamin D: http://www.aap.org/policy/s010116.html
Folic acid: http://www.aap.org/policy/re9834.html
Calcium: http://www.aap.org/policy/re9904.html

---

study in which 40 children who had ADHD received either 3.6 g DHA/week from these foods for 2 months or placebo foods without fish oil concluded, however, that DHA supplementation did not improve ADHD-related symptoms [79].

Finally, there is a long tradition of families using herbal medicine to treat children (eg, chamomile and peppermint for upset tummies, and garlic and onions for colds and flu.) The scientific evaluation of efficacy and safety continues to lag behind popular and historical use, but there is a slow but growing body of evidence supporting the use of herbal medicine in children. For example, clinical trials and systematic reviews of the use of herbs in children can be found in mainstream medical journals [80–85]. Table 1 reviews commonly used herbs and their efficacy and safety.

Research challenges for dietary supplements and homeopathy

Patient preference

The use of dietary supplements and homeopathy, particularly in clinical research, often is associated with strong issues of patient preference. When subjects refuse to be randomized, it sometimes is possible to compensate for the challenges of recruitment by using of quasi-experimental designs, but then other methodologic challenges emerge. On the other side of the spectrum of patient preference is parental concern about the safety of non-pharmaceutical and pharmaceutical medicinal products for which the mechanism of action is not well established.

Specific and nonspecific effects

Specific effects are classified as the effects resulting from a treatment (eg, the pharmacologic effects of a drug). Nonspecific effects are all the other effects of treatment and range from reassurance to placebo effects. It is commonly assumed in conventional medical research that specific and nonspecific effects are simply additive and do not interact. This assumption has never been proven for conventional medicine, much less for dietary supplement and homeopathic medicinal therapies.

Table 1
Commonly used pediatric herbs

Dietary supplements	Scientific studies	Potential side effects and contraindications
Echinacea	Randomized, controlled trial of 524 children who had upper respiratory tract infection found no significant difference in duration or symptoms of those receiving Echinacea purpurea [86]	Side effects: allergic reactions
German chamomile (*Matricaria recutita*)	In controlled trials, chamomile and its constituents have positive effects as a mild sedative. Chamomile/pectin combinations have positive effects on diarrhea [87,88] Chamomile in combination with other herbs is effective for treating colic [89,90]	Individuals allergic to other members of the Compositae family (ragweed, asters, and chrysanthemums) may be allergic to chamomile [91]. Chamomile can cause atopic and contact dermatitis. There have been rare cases of anaphylaxis to chamomile [83]
Ginger	Clinical trials had mixed results for ginger as a treatment for motion sickness, postsurgical nausea, and vomiting. Ginger has proven helpful in treating hyperemesis gravidarum [92,93]	Side effects: heartburn Contraindications: patients who have gallstones because of ginger's cholagogue effect
Lemon balm (*Melissa officinalis*)	Animal data suggest sedative hypnotic effects. Randomized, controlled trials have examined lemon balm/valerian combinations; most show enhanced sleep quality [94–96]	Side effects: allergic reactions are possible
Valerian (*Valeriana officinalis*)	Clinical trials in children and adults show decreased sleep latency and improved sleep quality [96]	Side effects: headaches, insomnia

Chronic illness

Many children who seek treatment, particularly with herbal medicines or homeopathy, suffer from chronic illnesses and hope for long-term benefit rather than short-term symptom control. In chronic illness any change is likely to be relatively slow, so long-term follow-up is needed for results to be meaningful. Such follow-up is expensive and is not often done in a randomized, controlled trial. With the low (some might say homeopathic) economic returns from dietary supplements, herbs, and homeopathy, long-term studies in chronic disease or epidemiologic studies are unlikely.

Individualization

Therapeutic interventions using dietary supplements and homeopathic medicines are often individualized. Classical homeopathy, in particular, is often highly individualized: the same homeopathic remedies are not prescribed for all children who have the same clinical diagnosis. This individualization creates difficulties in research methodology, because treatment homogeneity cannot be assumed.

Funding issues and skepticism

In common with many other forms of CAM and traditional medicine, homeopathy and dietary supplements lack research funding and infrastructure. This lack of funding arises in part because most dietary supplements and homeopathic medicines are generic, and no intellectual property rights or patents are available. The lack of research funding and skepticism in the academic community continues to limit research and inhibit collaboration. The National Center for Complementary and Alternative Medicine and other institutes within the National Institutes of Health are funding more studies in integrative medicine, however.

Other issues confounding research

A final confounder, particularly prevalent in the dietary supplement arena, is that positive clinical trial evidence, when available, is commonly based on research conducted on a single ingredient, one hopes with a specific plant characterization and manufactured in a specific fashion. In the marketplace that single ingredient with positive research results may just be one of many ingredients in the range of products available to consumers, and it may have a different plant characterization (if it has one at all) or a different extraction process. Comparing trial results is often problematic, making it difficult in clinical practice to recommend specific products to families and patients.

Summary

Many pediatric patients and their families, especially those who have chronic or recurrent conditions, use dietary supplements and homeopathy. Families do not always disclose this information to their health care professionals. It is critical that health care practitioners have an open a dialogue with their patients about the use of dietary supplements and homeopathic medicinal products. As part of that dialogue, clinicians must consider what level of evidence or efficacy is acceptable to support the use of a medicinal plant or homeopathy by pediatric patients. This appraisal must take into consideration the relative efficacy and safety of the product, the medical condition being treated, and the personal beliefs and preferences of patients and their families.

References

[1] Briefel RR, Johnson CL. Secular trends in dietary intake in the United States. Annu Rev Nutr 2004;24:401–31.

[2] Eichenberger Gilmore JM, Hong L, Broffitt B, et al. Longitudinal patterns of vitamin and mineral supplement use in young white children. J Am Diet Assoc 2005;105:763–72.

[3] Ervin RB, Wright JD, Kennedy-Stephenson J. Use of dietary supplements in the United States, 1988–94. Vital Health Stat 1999;(244):1–14.

[4] Ervin RB, Wright JD, Reed-Gillette D. Prevalence of leading types of dietary supplements used in the Third National Health and Nutrition Examination Survey, 1988–94. Adv Data 2004;(349):1–7.

[5] Ervin RB, Wright JD, Wang CY, et al. Dietary intake of selected vitamins for the United States population: 1999–2000. Adv Data 2004;(339):1–4.

[6] Wilson KM, Klein JD, Sesselberg TS, et al. Use of complementary medicine and dietary supplements among U.S. adolescents. J Adolesc Health 2006;38:385–94.

[7] Lanski SL, Greenwald M, Perkins A, et al. Herbal therapy use in a pediatric emergency department population: expect the unexpected. Pediatrics 2003;111:981–5.

[8] Ottolini MC, Hamburger EK, Loprieato JO, et al. Complementary and alternative medicine use among children in the Washington, DC area. Ambul Pediatr 2001;1:122–5.

[9] Sawni-Sikand A, Schubiner H, Thomas RL. Use of complementary/alternative therapies among children in primary care pediatrics. Ambul Pediatr 2002;2:99–103.

[10] Angsten JM. Use of complementary and alternative medicine in the treatment of asthma. Adolesc Med 2000;11:535–46.

[11] Ball SD, Kertesz D, Moyer-Mileur LJ. Dietary supplement use is prevalent among children with a chronic illness. J Am Diet Assoc 2005;105:78–84.

[12] Cala S, Crismon ML, Baumgartner J. A survey of herbal use in children with attention-deficit-hyperactivity disorder or depression. Pharmacotherapy 2003;23(2):222–30.

[13] Chan E, Rappaport LA, Kemper KJ. Complementary and alternative therapies in childhood attention and hyperactivity problems. J Dev Behav Pediatr 2003;24:4–8.

[14] Gardiner P, Dvorkin L, Kemper KJ. Supplement use growing among children and adolescents. Pediatr Ann 2004;33:227–32.

[15] Gardiner P, Wornham W. Recent review of complementary and alternative medicine used by adolescents. Curr Opin Pediatr 2000;12:298–302.

[16] Heuschkel R, Afzal N, Wuerth A, et al. Complementary medicine use in children and young adults with inflammatory bowel disease. Am J Gastroenterol 2002;97:382–8.

[17] Johnston G. The use of complementary medicine in children with atopic dermatitis in secondary care in Leicester. Br J Dermatol 2003;149:566.

[18] Mazur LJ, De Ybarrondo L, Miller J, et al. Use of alternative and complementary therapies for pediatric asthma. Tex Med 2001;97:64–8.

[19] Orhan F, Sekerel BE, Kocabas CN, et al. Complementary and alternative medicine in children with asthma. Ann Allergy Asthma Immunol 2003;90:611–5.

[20] Sinha D, Efron D. Complementary and alternative medicine use in children with attention deficit hyperactivity disorder [see comment]. J Paediatr Child Health 2005;41(1–2):23–6.

[21] Slader CA, Reddel HK, Jenkins CR, et al. Complementary and alternative medicine use in asthma: who is using what? Respirology 2006;11:373–87.

[22] Super EA, Kemper KJ, Woods C, et al. Cranberry use among pediatric nephrology patients. Ambul Pediatr 2005;5:249–52.

[23] Kemper KJ, Wornham WL. Consultations for holistic pediatric services for inpatients and outpatient oncology patients at a children's hospital. Arch Pediatr Adolesc Med 2001;155:449–54.

[24] Braun JM, Schneider B, Beuth HJ. Therapeutic use, efficiency and safety of the proteolytic pineapple enzyme Bromelain-POS in children with acute sinusitis in Germany. In Vivo 2005; 19:417–21.

[25] Gardiner P, Graham RE, Legedza A, et al. Factors associated with dietary supplement use among prescription medication users. Arch Intern Med 2006;166:1968–74.

[26] Noonan K, Arensman RM, Hoover JD. Herbal medication use in the pediatric surgical patient. J Pediatr Surg 2004;39:500–3.

[27] Lin YC, Bioteau AB, Ferrari LR, et al. The use of herbs and complementary and alternative medicine in pediatric preoperative patients. J Clin Anesth 2004;16:4–6.

[28] Everett LL, Birmingham PK, Williams GD, et al. Herbal and homeopathic medication use in pediatric surgical patients. Paediatr Anaesth 2005;15:455–60.

[29] Vincent C, Furnham A. Why do patients turn to complementary medicine? An empirical study. Br J Clin Psychol 1996;35:37.

[30] Jain N, Astin J. Barriers to acceptance: an exploratory study of complementary/alternative medicine disuse. J Altern Complement Med 2001;7:689–96.

[31] Bearison DJ, Minian N, Granowetter L. Medical management of asthma and folk medicine in a Hispanic community. J Pediatr Psychol 2002;27(4):385–92.

[32] Flores G, Vega LR. Barriers to health care access for Latino children: a review [review] [35 refs]. Fam Med 1998;30(3):196–205.

[33] Geissler PW, Harris SA, Prince RJ, et al. Medicinal plants used by Luo mothers and children in Bondo district, Kenya. J Ethnopharmacol 2002;83(1–2):39–54.

[34] Pachter LM, Sumner T, Fontan A, et al. Home-based therapies for the common cold among European American and ethnic minority families: the interface between alternative/complementary and folk medicine. Arch Pediatr Adolesc Med 1998;152(11):1083–8.

[35] Wilson AH, Robledo L. Listening to Hispanic mothers: guidelines for teaching [Review] [10 refs]. J Soc Pediatr Nurs 1999;4(3):125–7.

[36] Martin KJ, Jordan TR, Vassar AD, et al. Herbal and nonherbal alternative medicine use in Northwest Ohio. Ann Pharmacother 2002;36:1862–9.

[37] Dantas F, Rampes H. Do homeopathic medicines provoke adverse effects? A systematic review. Br Homeopath J 2000;89(Suppl 1):S35.

[38] World Health Organization. General guidelines for methodologies on research and evaluation of traditional medicine. Geneva (Switzerland): World Health Organization; 2001.

[39] Linde K, et al. Are the clinical effects of homeopathy placebo effects? A meta-analysis of placebo-controlled trials. Lancet 1997;350:834–43.

[40] Barnes J, et al. Homeopathy for postoperative ileus? A meta-analysis. J Clin Gastroenterol 1997;25:628–33.

[41] Jacobs J, Jonas WB, Jimenez-Perez M, et al. Homeopathy for childhood diarrhea: combined results and metaanalysis from three randomized, controlled clinical trials. Pediatr Infect Dis J 2003;22:229–34.

[42] Jonas WB, Linde K, Ramirez G. Homeopathy and rheumatic disease. Rheum Dis Clin North Am 2000;26:117–23.

[43] Schneider B. Treatment of vertigo with a homeopathic complex remedy compared with usual treatments: a meta-analysis of clinical trials. Arzneimittelforschung 2005;55.

[44] Taylor MA, Reilly D, Llewellyn-Jones RH, et al. Randomised controlled trial of homoeopathy versus placebo in perennial allergic rhinitis with overview of four trial series. BMJ 2000;321:471–6.

[45] Vickers AJ, Smith C. Homoeopathic oscillococcinum for preventing and treating influenza and influenza-like syndromes. Cochrane Database Syst Rev 2006;3:CD001957.

[46] Frei H, Everts R, von Ammon K, et al. Homeopathic treatment of children with attention deficit hyperactivity disorder: a randomised, double blind, placebo controlled crossover trial. Eur J Pediatr 2005;164:758–67.

[47] Jacobs J, Springer DA, Crothers D. Homeopathic treatment of acute otitis media in children: a preliminary randomized placebo-controlled trial. Pediatr Infect Dis J 2001;20:177–83.

[48] Harrison H, Fixsen A, Vickers A. A randomized comparison of homoeopathic and standard care for the treatment of glue ear in children. Complement Ther Med 1999;7:132–5.

[49] Friese K. The homoeopathic treatment of otitis media in children—comparisons with conventional therapy. Int J Clin Pharmacol Ther 1997;35:296–301.

[50] Ferley J, et al. [Evaluation in ambulatory medicine of the effect of a homeopathic complex remedy in the prevention of flu and flu-like syndromes]. Immunologie Médical 1987;20:22–8.

[51] Papp R. Oscillococcinum® in patients with influenza-like syndromes: a placebo controlled double-blind evaluation. Br Homeopath J 1998;87:69–76.

[52] Oberbaum M, et al. A randomized, controlled clinical trial of the homeopathic medication Traumeel S in the treatment of chemotherapy-induced stomatitis in children undergoing stem cell transplantation. Cancer 2001;92:684.

[53] Zell J, Connert WD, Mau J, et al. [Treatment of acute sprains of the ankle joint. Double-blind study assessing the effectiveness of a homeopathic ointment preparation]. Fortschr Med 1988;106:96–100 [in German].

[54] Abrams SA, Griffin IJ, Hawthorne KM, et al. Relationships among vitamin D levels, parathyroid hormone, and calcium absorption in young adolescents. J Clin Endocrinol Metab 2005;90:5576–81.

[55] Gera T, Sachdev HPS. Effect of iron supplementation on incidence of infectious illness in children: systematic review [see comment]. BMJ 2002;325:1142.

[56] Hartman JJ. Vitamin D deficiency rickets in children: prevalence and need for community education. Orthop Nurs 2000;19:63–7.

[57] Idindili B, Masanja H, Urassa H, et al. Randomized controlled safety and efficacy trial of 2 vitamin A supplementation schedules in Tanzanian infants. Am J Clin Nutr 2007;85:1312–9.

[58] Mahawithanage STC, Kannangara KKNP, Wickremasinghe R, et al. Impact of vitamin A supplementation on health status and absenteeism of school children in Sri Lanka. Asia Pac J Clin Nutr 2007;16:94–102.

[59] Menon P, Ruel MT, Loechl CU, et al. Micronutrient Sprinkles reduce anemia among 9- to 24-mo-old children when delivered through an integrated health and nutrition program in rural Haiti. J Nutr 2007;137:1023–30.

[60] Ram FSF, Rowe BH, Kaur B. Vitamin C supplementation for asthma [Update of Cochrane Database Syst Rev 2001;(4):CD000993; PMID: 11687089]. Cochrane Database Syst Rev 2004;CD000993.

[61] Sachdev H, Gera T, Nestel P. Effect of iron supplementation on mental and motor development in children: systematic review of randomised controlled trials. Public Health Nutr 2005; 8:117–32.

[62] Salman M. Systematic review of the effect of therapeutic dietary supplements and drugs on cognitive function in subjects with Down syndrome. Eur J Paediatr Neurol 2002;6: 213–9.

[63] Sichert-Hellert W, Wenz G, Kersting M. Vitamin intakes from supplements and fortified food in German children and adolescents: results from the DONALD study. J Nutr 2006; 136:1329–33.

[64] Valery PC, Torzillo PJ, Boyce NC, et al. Zinc and vitamin A supplementation in Australian Indigenous children with acute diarrhoea: a randomised controlled trial. Med J Aust 2005; 182:530–5.

[65] Varma JL, Das S, Sankar R, et al. Community-level micronutrient fortification of a food supplement in India: a controlled trial in preschool children aged 36–66 mo. Am J Clin Nutr 2007;85:1127–33.

[66] Winzenberg T, Shaw K, Fryer J, et al. Effects of calcium supplementation on bone density in healthy children: meta-analysis of randomised controlled trials. BMJ 2006;333:775.

[67] Winzenberg TM, Shaw K, Fryer J, et al. Calcium supplementation for improving bone mineral density in children. Cochrane Database Syst Rev 2006;CD005119.

[68] Winzenberg TM, Shaw K, Fryer J, et al. Calcium supplementation for improving bone mineral density in children [systematic review]. Cochrane Database Syst Rev 2007;(2).

[69] Gartner LM, Greer FR. Section on Breastfeeding and Committee on Nutrition. American Academy of Pediatrics. Prevention of rickets and vitamin D deficiency: new guidelines for vitamin D intake [see comment]. Pediatrics 2003;111:908–10.

[70] Hochberg Ze, Bereket A, Davenport M, et al. Consensus development for the supplementation of vitamin D in childhood and adolescence. Horm Res 2002;58:39–51.

[71] Munns C, Zacharin MR, Rodda CP, et al. Prevention and treatment of infant and childhood vitamin D deficiency in Australia and New Zealand: a consensus statement. Med J Aust 2006;185:268–72.

[72] Raiten DJ, Picciano MF. Vitamin D and health in the 21st century: bone and beyond. Executive summary. Am J Clin Nutr 2004;80:1673S–7S.

[73] Thacher TD, Fischer PR, Strand MA, et al. Nutritional rickets around the world: causes and future directions. Ann Trop Paediatr 2006;26:1–16.

[74] van Gool CJ, Zeegers MP, Thijs C. Oral essential fatty acid supplementation in atopic dermatitis—a meta-analysis of placebo-controlled trials. Br J Dermatol 2004;150:728–40.

[75] Beckles Willson N, Elliott TM, Everard ML. Omega-3 fatty acids (from fish oils) for cystic fibrosis. Cochrane Database Syst Rev 2002;CD002201.

[76] Thien FCK, De Luca S, Woods R, et al. Dietary marine fatty acids (fish oil) for asthma in adults and children [systematic review]. Cochrane Database Syst Rev 2007.

[77] Woods RK, Thien FC, Abramson MJ. Dietary marine fatty acids (fish oil) for asthma in adults and children [update of Cochrane Database Syst Rev 2000;(4):CD001283; PMID: 11034708]. Cochrane Database Syst Rev 2002;CD001283.

[78] Antalis CJ, Stevens LJ, Campbell M, et al. Omega-3 fatty acid status in attention-deficit/hyperactivity disorder. Prostaglandins Leukot Essent Fatty Acids 2006;75:299.

[79] Hiriyama S, Hamazaki T, Terasawa K. Effect of docosahexaenoic acid-containing food administration on symptoms of attention deficit/hyperactivity disorder—a placebo-controlled double-blind study. Eur J Clin Nutr 2004;58(3):46–73.

[80] Charrois TL, Hrudey J, Gardiner P, et al. Peppermint oil. Pediatr Rev 2006;27:E49.

[81] Charrois TL, Hrudey J, Vohra S, et al. Echinacea. Pediatr Rev 2006;27:385.

[82] Charrois TL, Sadler C, Vohra S, et al. Complementary, holistic, and integrative medicine: St. John's wort. Pediatr Rev 2007;28:69.

[83] Gardiner P. Complementary, holistic, and integrative medicine: chamomile. Pediatr Rev 2007;28:E16.

[84] Hrastinger A, Dietz B, Bauer R, et al. Is there clinical evidence supporting the use of botanical dietary supplements in children? J Pediatr 2005;146:311.

[85] Shamseer L, Charrois TL, Vohra S, et al. Complementary, holistic, and integrative medicine: garlic. Pediatr Rev 2006;27:E77.

[86] Taylor JA, Weber W, Standish L, et al. Efficacy and safety of echinacea in treating upper respiratory tract infections in children: a randomized controlled trial. JAMA 2003;290:2824.

[87] Becker B, Kuhn U, Hardewig-Budny B. Double-blind, randomized evaluation of clinical efficacy and tolerability of an apple pectin-chamomile extract in children with unspecific diarrhea. Arzneimittelforschung 2006;56:387.

[88] de la Motte S, Bose-O'Reilly S, Heinisch M, et al. [Double-blind comparison of an apple pectin-chamomile extract preparation with placebo in children with diarrhea]. Arzneimittelforschung 1997;47:1247 [in German].

[89] Savino F, Cresi F, Castagno E, et al. A randomized double-blind placebo-controlled trial of a standardized extract of Matricariae recutita, Foeniculum vulgare and Melissa officinalis (ColiMil) in the treatment of breastfed colicky infants. Phytother Res 2005;19:335.

[90] Weizman Z, Alkrinawi S, Goldfarb D, et al. Efficacy of herbal tea preparation in infantile colic [see comments]. J Pediatr 1993;122:650.

[91] Paulsen E. Contact sensitization from Compositae-containing herbal remedies and cosmetics. Contact Dermatitis 2002;47:189.

[92] Borrelli F, Capasso R, Aviello G, et al. Effectiveness and safety of ginger in the treatment of pregnancy-induced nausea and vomiting. Obstet Gynecol 2005;105:849.

[93] Jewell D, Young G. Interventions for nausea and vomiting in early pregnancy. Cochrane Database Syst Rev 2007.

[94] Bent S, Padula A, Moore D, et al. Valerian for sleep: a systematic review and meta-analysis. Am J Med 2006;119:1005.

[95] Koetter U, Schrader E, Kaufeler R, et al. A randomized, double blind, placebo-controlled, prospective clinical study to demonstrate clinical efficacy of a fixed valerian hops extract combination (Ze 91019) in patients suffering from non-organic sleep disorder. Phytother Res 2007;21:847.

[96] Muller SF, Klement S. A combination of valerian and lemon balm is effective in the treatment of restlessness and dyssomnia in children. Phytomedicine 2006;13:383.

ELSEVIER
SAUNDERS

PEDIATRIC CLINICS
OF NORTH AMERICA

Pediatr Clin N Am 54 (2007) 875–884

Ethics of Complementary and Alternative Medicine Use in Children

Sunita Vohra, MD, MSc[a,b,*],
Michael H. Cohen, JD, MBA[c]

[a]Complementary and Alternative Research and Education (CARE) Program,
Stollery Children's Hospital, Edmonton, AB, Canada
[b]Department of Pediatrics, Faculty of Medicine, 8213 Aberhart Centre #1,
11402 University Avenue, University of Alberta, Edmonton, AB T6G 2J3, Canada
[c]Law Offices of Michael H. Cohen, 777 Massachusetts Avenue, PO Box 391108,
Cambridge, MA 02193, USA

Complementary and alternative medicine (CAM) has enjoyed tremendous public interest in North America in recent years. Usage data confirm that CAM is sought by a broad section of society, including children and adolescents [1–4]. Breuner and colleagues [5] found that 70% of homeless youth (n = 157) reported CAM use, helping to dispel the myth that CAM use is exclusive to those who have greater disposable income. CAM use extends beyond ethnic stereotypes, although its use may be higher in immigrant families. For example, Lohse and colleagues [6] sampled 2562 caregivers and found that although 48.4% of Latino children used herbs, so did 31.4% of non-Latino children. Many of the ethical considerations regarding CAM use in the pediatric population are the same as those for conventional medicine.

CAM is used most often by those who have serious, chronic, or recurrent illness, sometimes for symptom control and sometimes to combat the primary disease. Others use CAM to promote wellness or as a prophylaxis. For example, in Canada, Hagen and colleagues [7] found that 64% of pediatric rheumatology patients (n = 141) reported using at least one form of CAM. These results were similar to a United States study of 503 children who had chronic illness, of whom 61.6% reported dietary supplement use

---

* Corresponding author. CARE Program, Department of Pediatrics, 8213 Aberhart Centre #1, 11402 University Avenue, Edmonton, AB T6G 2J3, Canada.
E-mail address: care@med.ualberta.ca (S. Vohra).

[8]. Rates of CAM use have approximated 50% in several studies conducted in pediatric emergency departments [3,9], suggesting that pediatric CAM use is common in general, although it may be even more so in specific subpopulations of children. Usage rates seem to vary widely across studies, depending on how CAM is defined, whether usage describes current versus lifetime exposure, the nature of the population under study, and the method of inquiry (eg, mailed survey versus interview).

A phenomenon led by the public, CAM has caught the attention of conventional medicine, including academic hospitals. Complementary therapies are increasingly being offered in conventional medical settings, and dedicated funding for CAM research has been created within the National Institutes of Health (NIH), primarily at the National Center for Complementary and Alternative Medicine (NCCAM) but also at various other centers and institutes such as the Office of Cancer Complementary and Alternative Medicine at the National Cancer Institute. This article explores the major ethical principles involved in pediatric CAM use and how they affect clinical care and research.

Ethical principles

According to the 2005 Institute of Medicine (IOM) report on CAM in the United States [10], the relevant ethical commitments or values that must be considered are (1) social commitment to public welfare, or beneficence; (2) duty of nonmaleficence; (3) respect for patient autonomy/consumer choice; (4) recognition of medical pluralism; and (5) public accountability. The legal and policy implications of pediatric CAM use are being explored in the peer-reviewed literature, providing additional perspectives for consideration [11–14]. An overarching theme that has emerged is that the same standards for evaluation of safety and efficacy should apply whether a therapy is labeled "conventional" or "CAM," particularly because the label may change over time [10,15]. Furthermore, legal and ethical principles that apply to conventional medicine can, by and large, be applied across the board whether an emerging therapy is labeled "conventional," "innovative," or "CAM."

Although the IOM framework forms the basis for this article, it is worth noting that these IOM "value commitments" reflect familiar values injected in a new way. More often, ethicists refer to autonomy, nonmaleficence, beneficence, and justice. The IOM, however, leaves out justice, perhaps rephrasing it in terms of public accountability, and adds a fifth value—medical pluralism—a valuable contribution in and of itself because it inherently validates the judicious inclusion of therapies that historically have been outside conventional clinical care.

Social commitment to public welfare (beneficence)

Health care providers have a duty of beneficence to the individual patient and to the public, which can be interpreted to mean that health care providers are compelled to provide therapies based on best available evidence, regardless of whether the therapy is complementary, alternative, or conventional. According to the IOM, this commitment to public welfare translates into an obligation to generate and provide access to the best information available on the efficacy of CAM therapies to health care practitioners, policy makers, and the public [10].

To promote such access, a number of academic institutions have initiated "integrative" medicine programs, bringing complementary and conventional medicine together under one roof. A leading example is the Consortium of Academic Health Centers for Complementary and Integrative Medicine (CAHCIM) [16]. Launched in 1999, CAHCIM grew within 8 years to include 38 medical schools in the United States and Canada, with such notable institutions as Harvard, Yale, Duke, Stanford, and others. The primary mission for academic integrative medicine programs is to advance research, education, and clinical care in complementary and integrative therapies. Dedicated pediatric integrative medicine programs are also developing across the United States and Canada, as are pediatric CAM networks, to foster new research, education, and clinical initiatives [16–23]. These initiatives allow for academics and community providers (conventional and complementary) to come together to identify promising therapies, share knowledge, and exchange ideas due to their common social commitment to public welfare. A recent pediatrician survey acknowledges the relevance of these initiatives: 87% report being asked by patients or parents about CAM therapies, and 83% desired additional information or education about CAM [24]. CAM is of broad interest to families, making it important and relevant for conventional health care providers who wish to provide family-centered care. Consideration of the family's values, beliefs, and preferences are part of acting in a child's best interests and are therefore consistent with the ethical value of public accountability.

Nonmaleficence

Health care providers are duty-bound to protect their patients from harm. This obligation has multiple implications for clinical care and research as it relates to CAM: (1) there must be a commitment of resources and effort to identify harms; (2) such harms must be communicated to health care providers and the public in an efficient manner (effective knowledge translation becomes part of the ethical obligation of researchers); and (3) when harms are known, patients must be protected, suggesting that CAM can be abusive or neglectful when a known effective life-saving therapy is denied. Children who have life-threatening illness are also some of the highest users of CAM [25,26]. If choosing CAM denies the child access to a life-saving conventional therapy that has been proved effective, the courts may not take a lenient view of parental decision making that substitutes a CAM therapy with less evidence of efficacy. Although there are some cases of judicial leniency for religious choice, courts do not favor abandoning necessary medical care. The selection of therapies based on religious grounds does not necessarily apply to the choice of nonstandard, CAM therapies because these therapies may involve value choices and personal judgments outside the religious domain [11]. Recent work also suggests that CAM therapies should ideally be "sensibly incorporated into a conventional treatment plan" [11]. Rather than forcing parents to choose between CAM and conventional medicine, it may be most helpful to allow them to chart a course that incorporates the best of both and to provide clinical guidance that allows them to draw meaningful conclusions. This integration is most easily done when the relative risks and benefits have been well delineated.

Safety research can be politically charged. Some CAM providers may believe it is unfair to scrutinize their field, examining it for potential harms. The IOM report on patient safety in conventional medicine [10] is a cautionary tale, demonstrating that patient safety is not necessarily assured by good intentions alone. Patient safety would be furthered if the CAM practitioner community were similarly willing to take a self-critical view to identify potential harms associated with its therapies and mitigate them accordingly. Such initiatives are beginning and need to be supported and encouraged [27–29]. Such research is not necessarily popular among all practitioners, yet these data are vital to ensure that preventable harms are identified and avoided.

Lack of adequate safety data can be a major obstacle when considering approaches recommended to pediatricians with regard to their patients' CAM use. The pediatrician should "determine whether the CAM therapies selected are known to be unsafe and/or ineffective" [11]; however, one cannot make this determination when the primary data are lacking. Although it is not reasonable to assume that lack of harms reporting is equivalent to data confirming safety, it also is not reasonable to overestimate risk about therapies that have been used by millions of people over hundreds, even thousands, of years.

Because safety cannot be assumed, it seems that the best, most ethical course of action is to invest some energy into documenting safety. When this approach is taken, useful data are obtained, allowing health care providers to refer with greater ease and allowing patients to provide truly informed consent [28,29]. If the CAM therapy is safe, then patients, referring health care providers, policy makers, and other stakeholders can be reassured. If it is not safe, then it is better for all concerned to know this and to take appropriate steps to mitigate risk. Patient interests are not served when these issues are oversimplified: safety is relative, not absolute, and must be considered in combination with potential benefits; that is, how much risk is tolerable for how much potential benefit? There is no single "right" answer but one that each family and health care provider must come to terms with, given the individual circumstances of the specific child in question.

Patient autonomy

Respect for patient autonomy and consumer choice promotes the right of individuals to make free and informed decisions. Whether the therapy is conventional or CAM, such decisions need to be informed about risks and benefits [10].

Evidence about CAM therapies may be more challenging to accumulate, for a variety of reasons. Industry does not have the same financial incentive to invest in research due to difficulties in patenting natural remedies. If research is to be done, the burden often rests with public agencies such as the NIH NCCAM, the Canadian Institutes of Health Research, and publicly funded universities who ultimately serve the public, not their shareholders. Some may argue that this approach benefits the public good in a manner that industry research cannot. Others believe that this is a "waste" of taxpayer dollars, because they have already concluded that CAM is ineffective [30].

Even though CAM evidence may be more challenging to develop, health care providers need to be aware of current evidence with regard to CAM therapies and not to assume such evidence does not exist or is of inferior quality. Moher and colleagues [31] have identified more than 1400 pediatric CAM randomized controlled trials and more than 45 pediatric CAM systematic reviews. Although CAM research could benefit from improved methodological rigor, the quality of CAM randomized controlled trials and systematic reviews met or surpassed that of conventional medicine [32–34].

Respect for patient autonomy and consumer choices demands open discussion and shared decision making, whereby the patient can be presented with the best available evidence, regardless of whether the therapy is conventional or complementary. Liability might be premised on the theory of failed informed consent if clinicians fail to raise reasonable feasible alternatives or ignore evidence supporting the efficacy of integrating complementary therapies [12,35]. At present, only half of pediatricians agree that "pediatricians should consider use of all potential therapies, not just those of mainstream medicine, when treating patients" [24]. There is room for improvement in our evidence-based era when we strive to provide family-centered care, but how can we do that if pediatric health care providers are not yet prepared to take the family's preferences and values into consideration?

The few instances in which courts have been involved support this framework. United States courts are generally reluctant to overrule parental decisions about treatment, except in life-threatening situations [12]. A few courts have supported parental choices for CAM therapies when supported by some medical authority, as long as the child's life was not in danger [12].

Issues of autonomy are made even more complex when there is conflict between the child's wishes and those of the parents. The developing autonomy, values, and independence of children and adolescents implies that as children mature, they are owed not only confidentiality and privacy but also respect for treatment decisions [36].

Recognition of medical pluralism

The IOM report recognizes medical pluralism, as it honors social plural-ism, acknowledging that many forms of achieving health and healing exist in the world. This principle implies a moral commitment to openness and a commitment to innovative ways of finding evidence [10]. This approach is very much in keeping with current moves in medicine to ensure that health care providers demonstrate cultural competency [37–39]. There is a need to respect individual and cultural differences and to consider the effect of socio-cultural-religious beliefs on health care practices. The World Health Organi-zation estimates that 80% of the world's population uses CAM, not conventional medicine, as first-line therapy [40]. Given today's "global vil-lage," including the presence of large immigrant populations, health care pro-viders must recognize that their patients may use many approaches to achieve health. Asking about CAM use in an open, nonjudgmental fashion should be incorporated into routine history taking for all patients at every visit.

Public accountability

Because health care and health care research are publicly funded, it seems reasonable that CAM, in the context of clinical and research issues, should be held publicly accountable. This thinking raises many important yet complex issues: Who can own knowledge of indigenous traditions? Who should own such knowledge? Under what circumstances should this knowledge be trans-ferred, developed, commercialized, or maintained as private (or in some tradi-tions, held as sacred, and thereby beyond public dissemination?) [10]. Aboriginal peoples have rarely been consulted about the commercialization of their traditional knowledge, nor have they necessarily benefited from it. An example of this is the current marketing of traditional plant medicines [41]. Many aboriginal people consider this marketing an exploitation of tradi-tional knowledge at the hands of European settlers because it is sometimes used without any form of compensation [42]. As a result of the mistrust built from such research methods, Aboriginal peoples have struggled with ownership over their own knowledge, practices, and bodies. These barriers must be ac-knowledged and overcome. It is fortunate that this important work is starting to be done and that guidelines for ethical research involving Aboriginal people have been developed [41,43,44]. These approaches to promote public account-ability and respectful collaboration might be relevant in a broader context for the interaction between conventional Western medicine and CAM because the basis for many CAM therapies may be grounded in other cultures.

Public accountability may be most important in vulnerable populations, including children. An ethical approach must include values such as trust and respect for different social and cultural perspectives; therefore, health care systems must find ways to recognize and accommodate different views while providing responsible advice and treatment [36]. Because the health care system is accountable to the public that funds it, it must satisfy that it is meeting the best interests of its patients. As discussed earlier, this standard should be informed by the best available evidence, which may include conventional, complementary, or integrative approaches.

Impact on clinical care and research

Clinical care

Perhaps the greatest challenge with regard to ethical approaches to including CAM in conventional settings is the overall lack of policies within health care institutions [11]. Some model guidelines are provided by the Federation of State Medical Boards for physician use of CAM therapies in medical practice, including criteria for discipline, guidelines to evaluate patients and treatment plans, documentation of medical records, and sale of goods from physician offices [45]. These guidelines, however, do not necessarily address institutional concerns such as how to handle inpatient desire to continue the use of dietary supplements.

It is important to consider that most families use CAM in conjunction with conventional care, not instead of it [46]. It then becomes imperative for pediatric health care providers to (1) ask questions regarding CAM use (to promote open discussion, preferably in nonjudgmental fashion, else families will not disclose use); (2) become knowledgeable about CAM therapies; (3) refer to a pediatric integrative medicine specialist if they lack this expertise (such expertise is now increasingly available); and (4) develop a communications strategy with their patients' CAM providers. Communicating with CAM providers does not necessarily imply referral or approval of a given therapy; rather, in the patient's best interests, an "integrative" approach—whereby each provider knows the care plan of the other, coordinating their efforts and minimizing potential interactions—seems preferable to the "dis-integrative" approach whereby the patient is abandoned to chart his or her course alone while the health care providers knowingly and willfully choose not communicate. According to Adams and colleagues [14], a careful balance must be constructed, such that health care providers are encouraged to provide continuity of care through their legal and ethical obligation of nonabandonment while avoiding the false perception that remaining in the relationship provides reassurance to the patient about his or her health care decisions (ie, health care providers should not unduly overemphasize their ongoing role if their patient has made choices with full awareness of the possible consequences). Patient safety also demands open communication, suggesting that patients might benefit if conventional care practitioners were more willing to engage in dialog with CAM counterparts about different diagnostic and therapeutic methods.

Adams and colleagues [14] suggested seven factors that should be considered when assessing the ethics of whether to offer CAM therapies: (1) severity and acuteness of illness; (2) curability with conventional treatment; (3)

risks of conventional treatment (eg, invasiveness, adverse effects); (4) evidence with regard to the safety and efficacy of the proposed CAM therapy (including assessment of quality of the evidence); (5) degree of understanding regarding the risks/benefits of conventional and CAM therapies; (6) acceptance of those risks (by the patient); and (7) persistence of the patient's intention to use CAM therapy. A risk/benefit approach to guide therapeutic decision making is a useful construct for patients and health care providers [15].

Principles of social justice are challenged by the lack of access to CAM therapies demonstrated to be safe and effective. Lack of access and lack of coverage pose major barriers, creating a tiered health care system that serves the needs of some better than others.

Research

The relative lack of funding for CAM research in comparison to funding spent on pharmaceutic research has been a cause of debate. Some believe that publicly funded institutions have a moral responsibility to fund research according to the priorities of the public they serve. Others argue that investigating CAM is unethical because it wastes public resources on therapies of little value [30]. Certainly, CAM research is relevant to the public, and important questions of efficacy and safety remain that demand answers if patient needs are to be met. Such research must be conducted in a collaborative and respectful fashion.

Summary

The ethics of CAM use is founded in principles of beneficence, nonmaleficence, and autonomy to which the IOM has added medical pluralism and public accountability. There is an urgent and compelling case for research to evaluate the safety and efficacy of pediatric therapies and for clinical practice to adopt the best available evidence, whether the therapy under consideration is conventional, complementary, alternative, or integrative. Safety and efficacy are relative and must be interpreted in light of a child's health state and the family's beliefs, values, and preferences. An ethical approach to the pediatric use of CAM is a complex, multifaceted issue that demands open communication between families and all their health care providers to meet the best interests of the child.

Acknowledgments

The authors gratefully acknowledge the contributions and thoughtful advice provided by Sheena Sikora, Connie Winther, Lynne Lacombe, Cecelia Bukutu, Pierre Haddad, Liz Estey, and Daniel Roth.

References

[1] Barnes PM, Powell-Griner E, McFann K, et al. Complementary and alternative medicine use among adults: United States, 2002. Advance Data: From Vital and Health Statistics; 343.

[2] Braun CA, Bearinger LH, Halcon LL, et al. Adolescent use of complementary therapies. J Adolesc Health 2005;37(1):761–9.

[3] Lanski SL, Greenwald M, Perkins A, et al. Herbal therapy use in a pediatric emergency department population: expect the unexpected. Pediatrics 2003;111(5 Pt 1):981–5.

[4] Hughes SC, Wingard DL. Children's visits to providers of complementary and alternative medicine in San Diego. Ambul Pediatr 2006;6(5):293–6.

[5] Breuner CC, Barry PJ, Kemper KJ. Alternative medicine use by homeless youth. Arch Pediatr Adolesc Med 1998;152(11):1071–5.

[6] Lohse B, Stotts JL, Priebe JR. Survey of herbal use by Kansas and Wisconsin WIC participants reveals moderate, appropriate use and identifies herbal education needs. J Am Diet Assoc 2006;106(2):227–37.

[7] Hagen LE, Schneider R, Stephens D, et al. Use of complementary and alternative medicine by pediatric rheumatology patients. Arthritis Rheum 2003;49(1):3–6.

[8] Ball SD, Kertesz D, Moyer-Mileur LJ. Dietary supplement use is prevalent among children with a chronic illness. J Am Diet Assoc 2005;105(1):78–84.

[9] Goldman RD, Dickens R, Vohra S. Do family physicians and pediatricians know about complementary and alternative medicine use by children they care for? Paediatric Child Health 2007;12(Suppl A):44A.

[10] Report Brief. To err is human: building a safer health system. Available at: http://www.iom. edu/CMS/8089/5575/4117.aspx. Accessed August 13, 2007.

[11] Cohen MH, Kemper KJ, Stevens L, et al. Pediatric use of complementary therapies: ethical and policy choices. Pediatrics 2005;116(4):E568–75.

[12] Cohen MH, Kemper KJ. Complementary therapies in pediatrics: a legal perspective. Pediatrics 2005;115(3):774–80.

[13] Cohen MH. Legal issues in caring for patients with kidney disease by selectively integrating complementary therapies. Adv Chronic Kidney Dis 2005;12(3):300–11.

[14] Adams KE, Cohen MH, Eisenberg D, et al. Ethical considerations of complementary and alternative medical therapies in conventional medical settings [see comment]. Ann Intern Med 2002;137(8):660–4.

[15] Cohen MH, Eisenberg DM. Potential physician malpractice liability associated with complementary and integrative medical therapies. Ann Intern Med 2002;136(8):596–603.

[16] Consortium of Academic Health Centers for Integrative Medicine. Available at: http://www. imconsortium.org/cahcim/home.html. Accessed August 13, 2007.

[17] American Academy of Pediatrics (AAP) Provisional Section on Complementary, Holistic, and Integrative Medicine (SCHIM). Available at: www.aap.org/sections/chim/default. cfm. Accessed August 13, 2007.

[18] Canadian Pediatric Complementary and Alternative Medicine Network. Available at: www. pedcam.ca. Accessed August 13, 2007.

[19] Complementary and Alternative Research and Education Program (CARE). Available at: www.care.ualberta.ca. Accessed August 13, 2007.

[20] National Center for Complementary and Alternative Medicine (NCCAM). Available at: www.nccam.noh.gov. Accessed August 13, 2007.

[21] Canadian Interdisciplinary Network for Complementary and Alternative Medicine Research (IN-CAM). Available at: http://www.incamresearch.ca/. Accessed August 13, 2007.

[22] CAMline. Available at: www.camline.ca. Accessed August 13, 2007.

[23] National Library for Health (NHS). Complementary and Alternative Medicine Specialist Library. Available at: www.library.nhs.uk/cam. Accessed August 13, 2007.

[24] Kemper KJ, O'Connor KG. Pediatricians' recommendations for complementary and alternative medical (CAM) therapies. Ambul Pediatr 2004;4(6):482–7.

[25] Kelly KM, Jacobson JS, Kennedy DD, et al. Use of unconventional therapies by children with cancer at an urban medical center [see comment]. J Pediatr Hematol Oncol 2000; 22(5):412–6.

[26] McCurdy EA, Spangler JG, Wofford MM, et al. Religiosity is associated with the use of complementary medical therapies by pediatric oncology patients. J Pediatr Hematol Oncol 2003; 25(2):125–9.

[27] Vohra S, Johnston BC, Cramer K, et al. Adverse events associated with pediatric spinal manipulation: a systematic review [see comment erratum that appears in Pediatrics 2007;119(4):867]. Pediatrics 2007;119(1):e275–83.

[28] White A, Hayhoe S, Hart A, et al. Adverse events following acupuncture: prospective survey of 32,000 consultations with doctors and physiotherapists. BMJ 2001;323(7311):485–6.

[29] MacPherson H, Thomas K. Short term reactions to acupuncture—a cross-sectional survey of patient reports. Acupunct Med 2005;23(3):112–20.

[30] Colquhoun D. Should NICE evaluate complementary and alternative medicines? [see comment]. BMJ 2007;334(7592):507.

[31] Moher D, Sampson M, Campbell K, et al. Assessing the quality of reports of randomized controlled trials in pediatric complementary and alternative medicine. BMC Pediatr 2002; 2(2):1–8.

[32] Pham Ba, Klassen TP, Lawson ML, et al. Language of publication restrictions in systematic reviews gave different results depending on whether the intervention was conventional or complementary. J Clin Epidemiol 2005;58(8):769–76.

[33] Moher D, Soeken K, Sampson M, et al. Assessing the quality of reports of systematic reviews in pediatric complementary and alternative medicine. BMC Pediatr 2002;2:3.

[34] Lawson ML, Pham B, Klassen TP, et al. Systematic reviews involving complementary and alternative medicine interventions had higher quality of reporting than conventional medicine reviews. J Clin Epidemiol 2005;58(8):777–84.

[35] Ernst E, Cohen MH. Informed consent in complementary and alternative medicine. Arch Intern Med 2001;161(19):2287–92.

[36] Harrison C. Primum non nocere is only the beginning. J Paediatr Child Health 2007;12(5): 379–80.

[37] Beach MC, Cooper L, Robinson KA, et al. Strategies for improving minority healthcare quality: Evidence Report/Technology Assessment No. 90. AHRQ Evidence Report 2004;04-E008-02.

[38] Hixon AL. Beyond cultural competency. Acad Med 2003;78(6):634.

[39] Skelton JR, Kai J, Loudon RF. Cross-cultural communication in medicine: questions for educators. Med Educ 2001;35(3):257–61.

[40] World Health Organization. World Health Organization (WHO) traditional medicine strategy 2002–2005. Available at: http://whqlibdoc.who.int/hq/2002/WHO_EDM_TRM_2002. 1.pdf. Accessed August 13, 2007.

[41] Canadian Institutes of Health Research. CIHR Guidelines for Health Research Involving Aboriginal People. 2007. Available at: http://www.cihr-irsc.gc.ca/e/29134.html. August 13, 2007.

[42] Brigham T, Ralph J. Non-timber forest products—no easy answers: the commercialization of traditional medicinal plants. Available at: http://web2.uvcs.uvic.ca/courses/ntfp/commerce/sect4.htm. Accessed August 13, 2007.

[43] First Nations Centre @ NAHO. OCAP principles. Available at: www.naho.ca/firstnations/english/ocap_principles.php. Accessed August 13, 2007.

[44] World Intellectual Property Organization. Traditional knowledge. Available at: http://www.wipo.int/tk/en/tk/index.html. Accessed August 13, 2007.

[45] Federation of State Medical Boards. Available at: http://www.fsmb.org. Accessed August 13, 2007.

[46] Eisenberg DM, Davis RB, Ettner SL, et al. Trends in alternative medicine use in the United States, 1990–1997: results of a follow-up national survey [see comment]. JAMA 1998; 280(18):1569–75.

ELSEVIER
SAUNDERS

Pediatr Clin N Am 54 (2007) 885–899

PEDIATRIC CLINICS
OF NORTH AMERICA

Acupuncture for Pediatric Pain and Symptom Management

Anjana Kundu, MBBS, MD[a],*, Brian Berman, MD[b]

[a]Department of Anesthesiology and Pain Medicine, Complementary and Integrative Medicine Program, Children's Hospital and Regional Medical Center, University of Washington School of Medicine, 4800 Sand Point Way NE, M/S W9824, Seattle, WA 98105, USA
[b]Program in Complementary Medicine, Center for Integrative Medicine, University of Maryland School of Medicine, Kernan Hospital Mansion, 2200 Kernan Drive, Baltimore, MD 21207-6697, USA

Over 2 million people in the United States are estimated to use acupuncture annually [1,2], primarily for musculoskeletal complaints and pain management [3–5]. Most chronic pain clinics, including some pediatric pain clinics in the United States, offer acupuncture therapy [6,7]. Acupuncture is widely used throughout the world, including Asia, Europe, and the United States. It is increasingly becoming part of the health care system in the United States, where there are over 6000 physician acupuncturists, of whom most are actively performing acupuncture in their practices.

Acupuncture as defined by the National Center for Complementary and Alternative Medicine describes a family of procedures involving stimulation of specific anatomic locations on the skin by a variety of techniques. There are various approaches to diagnosis and treatment in American acupuncture that incorporate medical traditions from China, Japan, Korea, and other countries. The most-studied mechanism of stimulation of acupuncture points employs penetration of the skin by hair-thin, solid, metallic needles, which are manipulated manually or by electrical stimulation with the aim of restoring health by correcting an imbalance in qi (vital energy or force; pronounced *chee*). Stimulation of these areas by moxibustion, pressure, heat, and lasers is used in acupuncture practice, but because of the paucity of studies, these techniques are more difficult to evaluate.

The effectiveness of acupuncture for chronic pain relief remains in question despite (1) laboratory evidence documenting a biologic basis for acupuncture

* Corresponding author.
E-mail address: anjana.kundu@seattlechildrens.org (A. Kundu).

analgesia, (2) the increasing use of acupuncture by people in pain, and (3) the widespread availability of acupuncture at chronic pain clinics. Three systematic reviews [8–10] examining the efficacy of acupuncture for the relief of chronic pain demonstrate inconclusive results. The consistent emerging theme from these reviews is a call for well-designed, high-quality studies. However, more recent systematic reviews in acupuncture for specific pain conditions have produced evidence of effectiveness [11–19]. The use of complementary and alternative medicine and acupuncture is not limited to the adult population: the prevalence of use in children is 30% to 84% [5,20–22]; however, one factor that is clear from the reviews is the lack of data in the pediatric population.

This review aims to highlight the evidence for use of acupuncture in pain and symptom management.

History of acupuncture

It is commonly believed that the origins of acupuncture lie in ancient Chinese culture; however, the documentation of its origin is somewhat unclear and even controversial [23,24]. Most believe that the practice of acupuncture has been prevalent in China for over 3 millennia. Some instruments made from sharpened bones and stones were discovered around 6000 BC, but there was no written text to associate their use with acupuncture. These instruments may have been used for bloodletting or lancing abscesses. Conversely, it has been speculated that the tattoos on the body of "Ice Man," who is believed to have died about 3300 BC and was excavated when the Alpine glacier melted, represent the practice of acupuncture, independent of its believed origins in China [25]. The first written record of practice of acupuncture exists in the *Huang Di Nei Jing* (*Yellow Emperor's Classic of Internal Medicine*). It suggested that *Nei Jing* was passed verbally from generation to generation for centuries and finally recorded around 100 BC as written text. It is a narration of questions and answers between the Yellow Emperor and his minister, Chhi-Po. The text comprises two parts: *Su Wen* (plain questions) and *Lin Shu* (focus on acupuncture). Subsequently, various texts emerged, such as *Nan Jing* (*The Book of Difficult Questions*), which was thought to have been written around 100 BC, and *The Great Compendium of Acupuncture and Moxibustion,* which was published during the Ming Dynasty (1368–1644) and provided clear descriptions of the full set of 365 acupuncture points along the channels (meridians) where insertion of needles could modify the flow of qi. This concept of meridians, Qi, and acupuncture points form the basis of modern acupuncture practice.

The development of acupuncture continued through various dynasties and centuries and eventually became the main form of medical practice in China by the seventeenth century, along with practice of herbal medicine, massage, dietary practices, and moxibustion. In the eighteenth and nineteenth centuries, however, acupuncture lost popularity to the extent of being outlawed in 1929 along with other traditional Chinese medicine (TCM) modalities. During this period, there was increasing acceptance of Western medicine. With Chairman

Mao's support, acupuncture and TCM were reinstated where it would be offered within Western-style hospitals, and acupuncture research institutes received support [26].

Acceptance of acupuncture in the West occurred slowly, with France leading the way. Britain and the United States were slower to accept its application in health care. It was not until James Reston, a journalist for the *New York Times*, went to China before President Nixon's visit and received acupuncture in the postoperative period from appendectomy that acupuncture received much attention in the United States [27]. This experience opened the gateway for many physician scientists to investigate its role in surgical analgesia. In 1976, the Food and Drug Administration (FDA) labeled acupuncture needles as "investigational devices" (class III). Subsequently in 1994, a National Institutes of Health (NIH) and FDA workshop on the efficacy and safety of acupuncture led to the reclassification of acupuncture needles as "medical devices" (class II) in 1996.

In 1997, a consensus statement was released by the NIH about the efficacy of acupuncture for various medical conditions [28]. Consensus findings revealed clear and convincing evidence for the efficacy of acupuncture in adult postoperative pain, postoperative or chemotherapy-related nausea and vomiting, and postoperative dental pain. In addition, some promising evidence was found with the use of acupuncture as an acceptable alternative or included in the comprehensive management program when treating headache, menstrual cramps, tennis elbow, fibromyalgia, myofascial pain, osteoarthritis, carpal tunnel syndrome, low back pain, poststroke rehabilitation, tendonitis, and asthma. In 2003, the World Health Organization published a brief review of the published literature on acupuncture practice based on controlled clinical trials up to 1999. They reported that acupuncture was proven effective for 28 conditions [29].

Concepts in acupuncture

The term *acupuncture* is derived from the Latin words *acus* (meaning needle) and *pungere* (meaning pricking). The original terminology from China is *zhen jiu* (Chinese characters representing needle and moxibustion).

The practice of acupuncture in TCM is governed by the concept of balance and harmony of the perfectly opposing forces yin and yang. This balance determines an unobstructed flow of qi along the meridians. Qi is equated to energy or a vital force in our bodies. Obstruction in the flow of qi results in an illness; a state of health can be restored by stimulating specific points along the meridians called acupuncture points.

Mechanism of acupuncture analgesia

Several hypotheses and mechanisms for acupuncture analgesia have been postulated. One popular theory explaining how acupuncture modulates pain is the neurohumoral hypothesis of acupuncture analgesia. This hypothesis, based on information obtained from more than 100 scientific articles, states that analgesic properties of acupuncture are mediated, in part, by a cascade of peptides such as endorphins, encephalin, and monoamines that are activated by stimulating acupuncture points and creating a sensation of "de qi" (a sensation of fullness, heaviness, achiness) [30,31]. Stimulation of acupuncture points leads to the stimulation of A delta afferents that set the cascade in motion by way of the anterolateral tract of the spinal cord, midbrain periaquaductal gray, and raphe nucleus, which leads to the release of the inhibitory peptides norepinephrine and serotonin in the spinal cord. Systemic release of β-endorphins and corticotropin occurs by way of stimulation of the hypothalamic-pituitary axis. The role of endogenous opioids in acupuncture analgesia was further supported by demonstration of the reversal of acupuncture analgesia after administration of naloxone, an opioid antagonist [32].

Another mechanism for acupuncture analgesia indicates the role of polymodal receptors, which are responsive to acupuncture and moxibustion (thermal) stimuli [33].

Acupuncture influences regional brain activity and is demonstrated by way of functional MRI and positron emission tomography studies as deactivation or activation of corresponding areas of brain on stimulation of specific acupuncture points on the body [16,34–37].

Repeated or continuous acupuncture over a short period may lead to tolerance of analgesic effects from acupuncture. It has been speculated that acupuncture also provokes the release of antanalgesic substances like cholecystokinin octapeptide, and its antisense RNA increases the analgesic effects [17,38–40]. Although most evidence focuses on its analgesic effects, acupuncture leads to a wide range of systemic effects such as changes in central and peripheral blood flow regulation [13], changes in secretion of neurotransmitters and neurohormones, alterations in immune function [11], acceleration of nerve generation [41], and neuroplasticity [42].

Evidence base for use of acupuncture in clinical practice

Systematic reviews of randomized controlled trials (RCTs) are considered the gold standard for providing the best evidence with the least amount of bias in assessment of the efficacy of any therapy. It is unfortunate that in the past, research of acupuncture has largely consisted of uncontrolled trials. Despite demonstration of frequent positive results, the flawed design of many studies gives limited value to the results. With increased funding available, the quality of acupuncture studies has improved over the past 10 years.

Acupuncture in management of pediatric pain

Management of chronic pain in children requires a multidisciplinary approach. Many pediatric pain management services commonly provide various therapies including pharmacologic and nonpharmacologic interventions such as physical therapy, occupational therapy, counseling for behavioral medicine, guided imagery, biofeedback, relaxation therapy, massage therapy, music therapy, art therapy, yoga, and acupuncture. Reports indicate that more than 30% of pediatric pain centers offer acupuncture for pain management [7,43].

Efficacy, safety, and acceptance of acupuncture for pain management is well established in the adult population (Table 1); however, there is a paucity of evidence for acupuncture therapy in the management of pediatric conditions. This lack of pediatric data may be related to the perception of fear of needles in children, which can be a barrier to acceptance of acupuncture among the pediatric population. Three studies have indicated that in many cases, children are open to this intervention, especially for chronic illnesses [44–46], and that this fear may be overcome by careful explanation and demonstration before introducing acupuncture therapy.

One study of 243 children (167 girls, 76 boys; mean age, 14.3 years) treated with acupuncture for various pain complaints (lower back, hip, and lower-extremity complaints, 30%; abdomen pain, 25%; or headache, 23%). Patients received an average of 8.4 sessions of acupuncture therapy over a 6-week period [43].

A visual analog scale (VAS) of 0 to 10 was used to assess severity of pain at baseline and after each session. The VAS score decreased significantly from a mean of 8.3 at the initial visit to 3.3 at the completion of 6 weeks of therapy. In addition to reduced pain sores, the children experienced "overall improvement of well-being" while being treated. Patients also reported increased attendance at school, improved sleep patterns, and the ability to take part in more extracurricular activities. No side effects or complications related to treatment were reported. The limitation of this study was that it did not include randomization or control subjects.

Table 1
Systematic reviews on acupuncture and pain disorders

Disorder	Review	No. of trials	Results
Low back pain	Manheimer et al, 2005 [14]	33	Positive
	Furlan 2005 [91]	35	Positive
Osteoarthritis	Manheimer et al, 2007 [13]	13	Positive/inconclusive
	White et al, 2007 [11]	13	Positive
Dental pain	Ernst 1998 [92]	16	Positive
Headache	Melchart et al, 2001 [15]	26	Positive trend
Chronic pain	Patel et al, 1989 [9]	14	Inconclusive
	Ter Riet et al, 1990 [10]	51	Inconclusive
	Ezzo et al, 2000 [8]	51	Inconclusive
Fibromyalgia	Berman et al, 1999 [93]	7	Positive
Elbow pain	Gree et al, 2002 [94]	4	Inconclusive
	Trinh et al, 2004 [95]	6	Positive

Another study enrolled 33 children aged 6 to 18 years who had chronic pain (myofascial and migraine headaches, 46%; abdominal pain, 21%; fibromyalgia, 11%; and type I complex regional pain syndrome of an extremity, 11%) in whom effectiveness and acceptance of acupuncture and hypnotherapy was evaluated [46]. Over a 6-week period, 31 children accepted acupuncture along with a 20-minute hypnotherapy session; only 2 children refused. Reports of pain-associated disability (in physical activity and social interactions) from subjects and parents and the subjects' pain ratings were assessed before and after each of the six weekly sessions. The subjects experienced an average of a 46% reduction in pain and a 32% reduction in pain-related disability. The authors acknowledge that this study was limited, in that acupuncture and hypnotherapy were not evaluated individually and there was no control group.

When perceived efficacy and acceptance of acupuncture in 47 adolescent subjects (average age, 16 years; 79% girls) presenting with migraines, endometriosis, and reflex sympathetic dystrophy was reviewed, 70% of subjects reported that the treatments helped their symptoms and 67% rated the therapies as pleasant [45].

Headaches

Acupuncture for chronic headache can improve health-related quality of life at a small additional cost: this therapy is relatively cost effective compared with a number of other interventions [47].

A reasonable amount of literature exists to support the efficacy of acupuncture in the management of headaches [18]. Acupuncture was found to be more effective than no acupuncture (but not minimal acupuncture) in an RCT for tension-type headache [48] and recurrent headaches [49]. In a review of 26 trials for idiopathic headache, existing evidence was found to support the value of acupuncture for the treatment [15].

In trials comparing acupuncture with prophylactic medications, acupuncture was found as effective in migraine patients [50,51]. The comparison of semistandardized acupuncture with sham acupuncture in migraine prophylaxis, however, exhibited similar reductions in the percentage of patients who had reduction of migraine ($\geq 40\%$ and $\geq 50\%$, respectively) regarding frequency of migraine attacks, days with migraine, average duration of a migraine attack, rate of rescue medication used, severity rate of average headache, and other parameters compared with the baseline period in both groups [52].

Twenty-two patients aged 7 to 15 years who had migraine headaches received true acupuncture or placebo acupuncture (superficial needling) in 10 weekly treatments [53]. Along with clinical symptoms, plasma panopioid activity and levels of β-endorphin were monitored. The true acupuncture group had clear reductions in migraine frequency and severity along with a rise in plasma panopioid activity and β-endorphin levels, whereas the placebo group failed to show any of these changes. Despite a rigorous design, the sample sizes were relatively small and the long-term effects were unknown because no follow-up data were presented. Nevertheless, these findings support the efficacy of acupuncture in the treatment of pediatric migraine.

In a recent study, 50 pediatric patients aged 9 to 18 years (40 girls, 10 boys) underwent a mean of 6.0 ± 3.5 acupuncture treatments according to TCM principles [54]. Analysis of the VAS pain score at every visit revealed a marked downward trend in the pain score, with a mean VAS score of 7.4 ± 2.0 for all patients at the beginning of the consultation and a score of 4.1 ± 2.0 ($P < .01$) after 6 weeks. Thirty-one patients (62%) had at least a 50% reduction in the pain score on completion of treatment. In this study, pediatric patients who had tension-type headaches had a better response to acupuncture than those who had migraine-type headaches. The limitations of this study included a small sample size, no control group, no information about concurrent therapies, and no follow-up data.

Abdominal pain/pelvic pain

In a placebo-controlled clinical trial consisting of 43 female subjects who had primary dysmenorrhea, Helms [55] compared real acupuncture, placebo acupuncture at random points, no treatment, and physician visits administered weekly for 3 consecutive menstrual periods. The subjects were followed for over 1 year. The results showed pain relief in 90.9% (10/11) of the real acupuncture group, in 36.4% (4/11) of the placebo acupuncture group, in 18.2% (2/11) of the no treatment group, and in only 10% (1/10) in the physician visit group. Analgesic medication use was reduced by 41% in the real acupuncture group, with no change or increased use of medication in the other groups. A limitation of this study was its small sample size.

A small case series provided preliminary evidence that acupuncture may be an acceptable and safe adjunct treatment therapy for some adolescents who have endometriosis-related pelvic pain refractory to standard endometriosis therapies [56]. These patients experienced modest improvement in pain as measured by oral self-reports of pain on a scale from 1 to 10; however, no randomized control trials have been done to date.

Proctor and colleagues [57] showed that acupuncture was more effective than placebo acupuncture and two control groups in a study of acupuncture for primary dysmenorrhoea.

Evidence in favor of acupuncture for irritable bowel syndrome cannot be considered definite. One small study recorded improvements in bloating and general well-being [58]. An Austrian study in which acupuncture or sham acupuncture was used for irritable colon demonstrated benefit at 1 month (43.7% versus 26.7% relief; $P < .01$) [59]. Other studies, however, report no statistically significant benefit from true acupuncture over sham acupuncture [60,61]. Forbes and colleagues [60] demonstrated improvement in mean global symptom scores including pain and bloating with acupuncture and sham/placebo acupuncture for irritable bowel syndrome in a blinded placebo-controlled study of 67 participants aged 17 to 79 years. The difference in the two groups was not statistically significant, perhaps due to an inadequate sample size for demonstration of small difference. The review by Lim and colleagues [12] on the effectiveness of acupuncture in management of symptoms such as abdominal pain and bloating remains inconclusive due to the poor quality and low power of studies in this area.

Acupuncture for medication use, tolerance of endoscopy, and pain related to gastrointestinal endoscopy in adult patients was evaluated in a systematic review that included six RCTs. Acupuncture was shown to be as effective as medication use and superior to sham acupuncture; however, no studies have been conducted in the pediatric population thus far [62].

In a double-blinded, sham-controlled study in children undergoing unilateral hernia repair, it was concluded that application of capsicum plaster at Zusanli points (ST 36) reduces pain and postoperative opioid consumption after 6 hours [63].

Sickle cell pain

In one small crossover study, it was shown that acupuncture may be helpful in treating sickle crisis pain. Ten subjects who had sickle cell anemia received true acupuncture or sham acupuncture at nonacupuncture points during 16 painful crises involving extremities. During 15 of 16 treatments, subjects in the sham and real acupuncture groups reported equal pain relief. The conclusion was that needling of acupuncture or sham sites may be an effective tool for pain relief [64].

Cystic fibrosis

A pilot study evaluated the effects of acupuncture for pain management and associated illnesses in patients who had cystic fibrosis [65]. Acupuncture was found to be effective in decreasing pain on a VAS. No side effects or complications were reported in relation to the acupuncture treatment. The investigators recommended further RCTs to evaluate additional efficacy in pain management and the improvement of the quality of life of patients who have cystic fibrosis.

Cancer pain

With improved survival rate from cancer therapies, there is an increase in morbidity related to the disease or therapies used for treatment of cancer. Cancer pain, although managed well with analgesics, can be very difficult to manage in 10% to 20% of patients due to resistance to opioids, and these patients may require alternative treatments [66]. In addition, patients are deterred by the high side effect profile of opioids that are commonly used for pain management in cancer patients. These patients have often turned to the use of alternative therapies such as acupuncture. A systematic review of RCTs of various complementary and alternative medicine and acupuncture therapies indicated the merit of acupuncture for pain management in cancer pain [67]. Three RCTs were included in this review that compared acupuncture therapy to standard analgesic treatment [68], sham acupuncture, and control treatment [69,70]. These trials all showed improvement in pain control in the acupuncture groups compared with standard, sham, or control treatment groups. In an uncontrolled study in a palliative care setting, excellent to good pain control using acupuncture was documented in 62% of patients who had cancer-related pain. Acupuncture therapy was especially remarkable in pain related to myofascial etiologies [71]. A response rate up to 82% was reported in an uncontrolled study of 183 patients who had malignant pain undergoing acupuncture treatment. Muscle spasms and bladder spasms were also ameliorated in these patients [72]. There are no trials to date in the pediatric population that document the feasibility, safety, and efficacy of acupuncture in cancer-related pain in pediatric patients. This lack of evidence related to acupuncture in pediatric cancer pain may be partly related to the paucity of literature supporting the acceptability of acupuncture in these patients.

Myofascial/musculoskeletal pain

In the United States, back pain is the most common cause of activity limitation in patients younger than 45 years and is most common reason for visits to an acupuncturist [73]. Several systematic reviews have been done to evaluate whether acupuncture is effective in the alleviation of back pain, with variable results [74–76].

In a more recent meta-analysis consisting of 33 RCTs, the efficacy of acupuncture compared with sham or control treatment for management of back pain due to various etiologies was evaluated [14]. Acupuncture was deemed significantly better than sham treatment in this analysis.

Overall, the outcomes of 14 RCTs looking at the efficacy of acupuncture for neck pain were equally balanced between positive and negative. Acupuncture was superior to wait list and equal or superior to physiotherapy, but needle acupuncture was not found to be superior to sham/superficial needling [19]. No RCTs evaluating acupuncture for management of back or neck pain have been done in the pediatric population; however, evidence of the use, efficacy, and acceptability of acupuncture in pediatric chronic myofascial pain (including back pain) is documented in a few uncontrolled studies [43,46].

Osteoarthritis is the leading cause of disability among older adults. With significant concern about the long-term adverse effects and morbidity associated with various standard medical therapies for osteoarthritis (nonsteroidal anti-inflammatory drugs); a need for safer alternatives has led to the extensive exploration of safer alternative therapies including acupuncture. In a meta-analysis of 11 RCTs of more than 6 weeks' duration using acupuncture compared with sham, usual care, or wait list control, acupuncture was found superior for pain control and improved function to sham control and wait list control but only clinically relevant in wait list control [13]. This finding is perhaps due to the variability in the sham control methods and to placebo or expectation effects.

Rheumatoid arthritis is an autoimmune disorder affecting the joints, especially in the hands, and may affect young children in addition to adults. Compared with osteoarthritis, there are limited data that evaluate acupuncture therapy in rheumatoid arthritis. In two systematic reviews in 2002 and 2005 with a limited number of studies, the needle effects of acupuncture and electroacupuncture on pain scores, C-reactive protein, and erythrocyte sedimentation rate were evaluated [77,78]. Although not statistically significant, pain in the treatment group improved versus no improvement in the placebo group. In the electroacupuncture study, a significant decrease in knee pain was reported in the experimental group at 24 hours and 4 months post treatment compared with the placebo group, but no effect on erythrocyte sedimentation rate, C-reactive protein, pain, patient's global assessment, number of swollen joints, number of tender joints, general health, disease activity, or reduction of analgesics was found.

Acute pain

Acupuncture can potentially serve as an important adjuvant for postoperative analgesia and for relieving opioid-related adverse effects in the postoperative period. Controversial results, dissimilar study designs, and diverse acupuncture techniques, however, pose difficulty in obtaining consistency of outcomes. The NIH consensus statement shows clear efficacy of acupuncture in postoperative dental pain [28]. A randomized, double-blind, placebo-controlled trial demonstrated the efficacy of acupuncture for reducing pain and postoperative analgesic consumption after an oral surgery procedure [79]. In this study, acupuncture or a well-designed noninsertion placebo treatment was administered twice: immediately after the surgical procedure and after the patient reported moderate pain. The results showed that pain-free postoperative time was significantly longer in the acupuncture group (173 minutes) than in the placebo group (94 minutes). Average pain medication consumption was significantly less in the acupuncture group.

In a study comparing acupuncture anesthesia and analgesia in 20 patients undergoing recurrent hernia repair, acupuncture reduced the amount of local anesthetic required and was effective in pain relief and inhibiting gastrointestinal upset [80]. In children undergoing unilateral inguinal hernia repair, acupuncture reduced pain scores and postoperative opioid requirement in a double-blinded RCT involving 108 patients [63]. There is debate, however, about the effectiveness of acupuncture intraoperatively for anesthetic and analgesic requirements [81–85].

Safety of acupuncture

Despite the occasional case reports of serious adverse effects associated with acupuncture, such as pneumothorax, cardiac tamponade, or infections [86,87], acupuncture has been demonstrated to be a reasonably safe therapy in the hands of experienced and qualified individuals as evidenced by several large prospective studies [88,89]. Mild transient adverse effects such as bleeding at needling sites or mild needling discomfort may occur in 1% to 3%; the incidence of any nonserious events is 7% to 11% of cases. The largest study, including 190,924 chronic pain patients, revealed 2.4 serious adverse events per 10,000 acupuncture cases [90]. The investigators conclude that there may have been a reporting bias, but overall, acupuncture seems to be a safe modality.

With increasing evidence in the quality of trials demonstrating the efficacy and safety of acupuncture in medicine, it is evident that integration of acupuncture in the Western health care system is increasing. Not unlike other conventional therapies, pediatric acupuncture literature lacks the quantity and quality of the same body of evidence. As mentioned by several investigators, the acceptability of acupuncture in pediatric patients may be contributing to this paucity of evidence. There is an urgent need for high-quality RCTs on the use of acupuncture in the pediatric population.

References

[1] Burke A, Upchurch D, Dye C, et al. Acupuncture use in the United States: findings from the National Health Interview Survey. J Altern Complement Med 2006;12(7):639–48.

[2] Paramore L. Use of alternative therapies: estimates from the Robert Wood Johnson Foundation national access to care survey. J Pain Symptom Manage 1996;13:83–9.

[3] Bullock ML, Pheley AM, Kiresuk TJ, et al. Characteristics and complaints of patients seeking therapy at a hospital-based alternative medicine clinic. J Altern Complement Med 1997; 3(1):31–7.

[4] Bausell RB, Lee WL, Berman BM. Demographic and health-related correlates to visits to complementary and alternative medical providers. Med Care 2001;39(2):190–6.

[5] Ernst E. Prevalence of complementary/alternative medicine for children: a systematic review. Eur J Pediatr 1999;158(1):7–11.

[6] Woollam CH, Jackson AO. Acupuncture in the management of chronic pain. Anaesthesia 1998;53(6):593–5.

[7] Lin Y-C, LA, Kemper K, et al. Integrating complementary and alternative medicine in pediatric pain management. Anesthesiology 1999;91:939.

[8] Ezzo J, Berman B, Hadhazy VA, et al. Is acupuncture effective for the treatment of chronic pain? A systematic review. Pain 2000;86(3):217–25.

[9] Patel M, et al. A meta-analysis of acupuncture for chronic pain. Int J Epidemiol 1989;18(4): 900–6.

[10] ter Riet G, Kleijnen J, Knipschild P. Acupuncture and chronic pain: a criteria-based meta-analysis. J Clin Epidemiol 1990;43(11):1191–9.

[11] White A, Foster NE, Cummings M, et al. Acupuncture treatment for chronic knee pain: a systematic review. Rheumatology (Oxford) 2007;46(3):384–90.

[12] Lim B, Manheimer E, Lao L, et al. Acupuncture for treatment of irritable bowel syndrome. Cochrane Database Syst Rev 2006;4:CD005111.

[13] Manheimer E, Linde K, Lao L, et al. Meta-analysis: acupuncture for osteoarthritis of the knee. Ann Intern Med 2007;146(12):868–77.

[14] Manheimer E, White A, Berman B, et al. Meta-analysis: acupuncture for low back pain. Ann Intern Med 2005;142(8):651–63.

[15] Melchart D, Linde K, Fischer P, et al. Acupuncture for idiopathic headache. Cochrane Database Syst Rev 2001;(1): CD001218.

[16] Wu MT, Hsieh JC, Xiong J, et al. Central nervous pathway for acupuncture stimulation: localization of processing with functional MR imaging of the brain–preliminary experience. Radiology 1999;212(1):133–41.

[17] Han JS. Cholecystokinin octapeptide (CCK-8): a negative feedback control mechanism for opioid analgesia. Prog Brain Res 1995;105:263–71.

[18] Manias P, Tagaris G, Karageorgiou K. Acupuncture in headache: a critical review. Clin J Pain 2000;16(4):334–9.

[19] White AR, Ernst E. A systematic review of randomized controlled trials of acupuncture for neck pain. Rheumatology (Oxford) 1999;38(2):143–7.

[20] Grootenhuis MA, Last BF, de Graaf-Nijkerk JH, et al. Use of alternative treatment in pediatric oncology. Cancer Nurs 1998;21(4):282–8.

[21] Wang SM, Caldwell-Andrews AA, Kain ZN. The use of complementary and alternative medicines by surgical patients: a follow-up survey study. Anesth Analg 2003;97(4): 1010–5.

[22] Kelly KM, Jacobson JS, Kennedy DD, et al. Use of unconventional therapies by children with cancer at an urban medical center. J Pediatr Hematol Oncol 2000;22(5):412–6.

[23] White A, Ernst E. A brief history of acupuncture. Rheumatology (Oxford) 2004;43(5):662–3.

[24] Ernst E. Acupuncture–a critical analysis. J Intern Med 2006;259(2):125–37.

[25] Dorfer L, et al. A medical report from the stone age? Lancet 1999;354(9183):1023–5.

[26] Ceniceros S, Brown GR. Acupuncture: a review of its history, theories, and indications. South Med J 1998;91(12):1121–5.

[27] Reston J. Now about my operation in Peking? New York: The New York Times; July 26, 1971.

[28] National Center for Complementary and Alternative Medicine. Research report: acupuncture; 1997. Available at: http://nccam.nih.gov/health/acupuncture/.

[29] World Health Organization. Acupuncture: Review and Analysis of Reports on Controlled Clinical Trials 2003.

[30] Pomeranz B. Scientific research into acupuncture for the relief of pain. J Altern Complement Med 1996;2(1):53–60 [discussion 73–5].

[31] Sims J. The mechanism of acupuncture analgesia: a review. Complement Ther Med 1997;5: 102–11.

[32] Pomeranz B, Chiu D. Naloxone blockade of acupuncture analgesia: endorphin implicated. Life Sci 1976;19(11):1757–62.

[33] Kawakita K, Shinbara H, Imai K, et al. How do acupuncture and moxibustion act? Focusing on the progress in Japanese acupuncture research. J Pharmacol Sci 2006;100(5):443–59.

[34] Biella G, Sotgiu ML, Pellegata G, et al. Acupuncture produces central activations in pain regions. Neuroimage 2001;14(1 Pt 1):60–6.

[35] Cho ZH, Oleson TD, Alimi D, et al. Acupuncture: the search for biologic evidence with functional magnetic resonance imaging and positron emission tomography techniques. J Altern Complement Med 2002;8(4):399–401.

[36] Cho ZH, Son YD, Kang CK, et al. Pain dynamics observed by functional magnetic resonance imaging: differential regression analysis technique. J Magn Reson Imaging 2003; 18(3):273–83.

[37] Peyron R, Laurent B, Garcia-Larrea L. Functional imaging of brain responses to pain. A review and meta-analysis. Neurophysiol Clin 2000;30(5):263–88.

[38] Han JS, Li SJ, Tang J. Tolerance to electroacupuncture and its cross tolerance to morphine. Neuropharmacology 1981;20(6):593–6.

[39] Liu NJ, Xu T, Xu C, et al. Cholecystokinin octapeptide reverses mu-opioid-receptor-mediated inhibition of calcium current in rat dorsal root ganglion neurons. J Pharmacol Exp Ther 1995;275(3):1293–9.

[40] Tang NM, Dong HW, Wang XM, et al. Cholecystokinin antisense RNA increases the analgesic effect induced by electroacupuncture or low dose morphine: conversion of low responder rats into high responders. Pain 1997;71(1):71–80.

[41] Chen YS, Yao CH, Chen TH, et al. Effect of acupuncture stimulation on peripheral nerve regeneration using silicone rubber chambers. Am J Chin Med 2001;29(3–4):377–85.

[42] Napadow V, Kettner N, Ryan A, et al. Somatosensory cortical plasticity in carpal tunnel syndrome–a cross-sectional fMRI evaluation. Neuroimage 2006;31(2):520–30.

[43] Lin Y-C, Bioteau A, Lee AC. Acupuncture for the management of pediatric pain: a pilot study. Medical Acupuncture 2002;14(1):45–6.

[44] Lin Y-C, Ly H. Acupuncture And Needlephobia: The Pediatric Patient's Perspective. Medical Acupuncture 2003;14(3):15–6.

[45] Kemper KJ, Sarah R, Silver-Highfield E, et al. On pins and needles? Pediatric pain patients' experience with acupuncture. Pediatrics 2000;105(4 Pt 2):941–7.

[46] Zeltzer LK, Tsao JC, Stelling C, et al. A phase I study on the feasibility and acceptability of an acupuncture/hypnosis intervention for chronic pediatric pain. J Pain Symptom Manage 2002;24(4):437–46.

[47] Wonderling D, Vickers AJ, Grieve R, et al. Cost effectiveness analysis of a randomised trial of acupuncture for chronic headache in primary care. BMJ 2004;328(7442):747.

[48] Melchart D, Streng A, Hoppe A, et al. Acupuncture in patients with tension-type headache: randomised controlled trial. BMJ 2005;331(7513):376–82.

[49] Melchart D, Linde K, Fischer P, et al. Acupuncture for recurrent headaches: a systematic review of randomized controlled trials. Cephalalgia 1999;19(9):779–86 [discussion 765].

[50] Melchart D, Thormaehlen J, Hager S, et al. Acupuncture versus placebo versus sumatriptan for early treatment of migraine attacks: a randomized controlled trial. J Intern Med 2003; 253(2):181–8.

[51] Allais G, De Lorenzo C, Quirico PE, et al. Acupuncture in the prophylactic treatment of migraine without aura: a comparison with flunarizine. Headache 2002;42(9):855–61.

[52] Alecrim-Andrade J, Maciel-Junior JA, Cladellas XC, et al. Acupuncture in migraine prophylaxis: a randomized sham-controlled trial. Cephalalgia 2006;26(5):520–9.

[53] Pintov S, Lahat E, Alstein M, et al. Acupuncture and the opioid system: implications in management of migraine. Pediatr Neurol 1997;17(2):129–33.

[54] Lin YC. Acupuncture for the Management of Childhood Headache Disorders, a Pilot Study. ASA Annual Meeting Abstract. San Francisco (CA), October 13–17, 2007.

[55] Helms JM. Acupuncture for the management of primary dysmenorrhea. Obstet Gynecol 1987;69(1):51–6.

[56] Highfield ES, Laufer MR, Schnyer RN, et al. Adolescent endometriosis-related pelvic pain treated with acupuncture: two case reports. J Altern Complement Med 2006;12(3): 317–22.

[57] Proctor ML, Smith CA, Farquhar CM, et al. Transcutaneous electrical nerve stimulation and acupuncture for primary dysmenorrhoea. Cochrane Database Syst Rev 2002;1: CD002123.

[58] Chan J, Carr I, Mayberry JA. The role of acupuncture in the treatment of irritable bowel syndrome: a pilot study. Hepatogastroenterology 1997;44(17):1328–30.

[59] Kunze M, Seidel M, Stube G. Comparative studies of the effectiveness of brief psychotherapy, acupuncture and papaverin therapy in patients with irritable bowel syndrome. Z Gesamte Inn Med 1990;45(20):625–7.

[60] Forbes A, Jackson S, Walter C, et al. Acupuncture for irritable bowel syndrome: a blinded placebo-controlled trial. World J Gastroenterol 2005;11(26):4040–4.

[61] Fireman Z, Segal A, Kopelman Y, et al. Acupuncture treatment for irritable bowel syndrome. A double-blind controlled study. Digestion 2001;64(2):100–3.

[62] Lee H, Ernst E. Acupuncture for GI endoscopy: a systematic review. Gastrointest Endosc 2004;60(5):784–9.

[63] Kim KS, Kim DW, Yu YK. The effect of capsicum plaster in pain after inguinal hernia repair in children. Paediatr Anaesth 2006;16(10):1036–41.

[64] Co LL, Schmitz TH, Havdala H, et al. Acupuncture: an evaluation in the painful crises of sickle cell anaemia. Pain 1979;7(2):181–5.

[65] Lin YC, Ly H, Golianu B. Acupuncture pain management for patients with cystic fibrosis: a pilot study. Am J Chin Med 2005;33(1):151–6.

[66] Charlton JE. Cancer pain management. Cah Anesthesiol 1993;41(6):621–4.

[67] Bardia A, Barton DL, Prokop LJ, et al. Efficacy of complementary and alternative medicine therapies in relieving cancer pain: a systematic review. J Clin Oncol 2006;24(34):5457–64.

[68] Xia YQ, Zang D, Yang CX, et al. An approach to the effect on tumors of acupuncture in combination with radiotherapy or chemotherapy. J Tradit Chin Med 1986;6:23–6.

[69] Alimi D, Rubino C, Pichard-Leandri E, et al. Analgesic effect of auricular acupuncture for cancer pain: a randomized, blinded, controlled trial. J Clin Oncol 2003;21(22):4120–6.

[70] Dang W, Yang J. Clinical study on acupuncture treatment of stomach carcinoma pain. J Tradit Chin Med 1998;18(1):31–8.

[71] Leng G. A year of acupuncture in palliative care. Palliat Med 1999;13(2):163–4.

[72] Filshie J, Redman D. Acupuncture and malignant pain problems. Eur J Surg Oncol 1985; 11(4):389–94.

[73] Cherkin DC, Deyo RA, Sherman KJ, et al. Characteristics of visits to licensed acupuncturists, chiropractors, massage therapists, and naturopathic physicians. J Am Board Fam Pract 2002;15(6):463–72.

[74] Ernst E, White AR. Acupuncture for back pain: a meta-analysis of randomized controlled trials. Arch Intern Med 1998;158(20):2235–41.

[75] Smith LA, Oldman AD, McQuay HJ, et al. Teasing apart quality and validity in systematic reviews: an example from acupuncture trials in chronic neck and back pain. Pain 2000; 86(1–2):119–32.

[76] Tulder MV, Cherkin DC, Berman B, et al. Acupuncture for low back pain. Cochrane Database Syst Rev 2000;2:CD001351.

[77] Casimiro L, Barnsley L, Brosseau L, et al. Acupuncture and electroacupuncture for the treatment of rheumatoid arthritis. Cochrane Database Syst Rev 2005;4:CD003788.

[78] Casimiro L, Brosseau L, Milne S, et al. Acupuncture and electroacupuncture for the treatment of RA. Cochrane Database Syst Rev 2002;3:CD003788.

[79] Lao L, Bergman S, Hamilton GR, et al. Evaluation of acupuncture for pain control after oral surgery: a placebo-controlled trial. Arch Otolaryngol Head Neck Surg 1999;125(5):567–72.

[80] Chu DW, Lee DT, Chan TT, et al. Acupuncture anaesthesia in inguinal hernia repair. ANZ J Surg 2003;73(3):125–7.

[81] Greif R, Laciny S, Mokhtarani M, et al. Transcutaneous electrical stimulation of an auricular acupuncture point decreases anesthetic requirement. Anesthesiology 2002;96(2):306–12.

[82] Gupta S, Francis JD, Tillu AB, et al. The effect of pre-emptive acupuncture treatment on analgesic requirements after day-case knee arthroscopy. Anaesthesia 1999;54(12):1204–7.

[83] Morioka N, Akca O, Doufas AG, et al. Electro-acupuncture at the Zusanli, Yanglingquan, and Kunlun points does not reduce anesthetic requirement. Anesth Analg 2002;95(1): 98–102, table of contents.

[84] Sim CK, Xu PC, Pua HL, et al. Effects of electroacupuncture on intraoperative and postoperative analgesic requirement. Acupunct Med 2002;20(2–3):56–65.

[85] Taguchi A, Sharma N, Ali SZ, et al. The effect of auricular acupuncture on anaesthesia with desflurane. Anaesthesia 2002;57(12):1159–63.

[86] Ernst E, Sherman KJ. Is acupuncture a risk factor for hepatitis? Systematic review of epidemiological studies. J Gastroenterol Hepatol 2003;18(11):1231–6.

[87] Ernst E, White A. Life-threatening adverse reactions after acupuncture? A systematic review. Pain 1997;71(2):123–6.

[88] Melchart D, Weidenhammer W, Streng A, et al. Prospective investigation of adverse effects of acupuncture in 97,733 patients. Arch Intern Med 2004;164(1):104–5.

[89] White A, Hayhoe S, Hart A, et al. Adverse events following acupuncture: prospective survey of 32,000 consultations with doctors and physiotherapists. BMJ 2001;323(7311):485–6.

[90] Endres HG, Molsberger A, Lungenhausen M, et al. An internal standard for verifying the accuracy of serious adverse event reporting: the example of an acupuncture study of 190,924 patients. Eur J Med Res 2004;9(12):545–51.

[91] Furlan AD, van Tulder M, Cherkin D, et al. Acupuncture and dry-needling for low back pain: an updated systematic review within the framework of the cochrane collaboration. Spine 2005;30(8):944–63.

[92] Ernst E, Pittler MH. The effectiveness of acupuncture in treating acute dental pain: a systematic review. Br Dent J 1998;84(9):443–7.

[93] Berman BM, Ezzo J, Hadhazy V, et al. Is acupuncture effective in the treatment of fibromyalgia? J Fam Pract 1999;48(3):213–8.

[94] Green S, Buchbinder R, Barnsley L, et al. Acupuncture for lateral elbow pain. Cochrane Database Syst Rev 2002;1:CD003527.

[95] Trinh KV, Phillips SD, Ho E, et al. Acupuncture for the alleviation of lateral epicondyle pain: a systematic review. Rheumatology (Oxford) 2004;3(9):1085–90.

ELSEVIER
SAUNDERS

Pediatr Clin N Am 54 (2007) 901–926

Complementary and Alternative Medicine Therapies to Promote Healthy Moods

Kathi J. Kemper, MD, MPH[a],*, Scott Shannon, MD[b]

[a]Pediatrics and Public Health Sciences, Wake Forest University School of Medicine,
Medical Center Boulevard, Winston-Salem, NC 27157, USA
[b]Northern Colorado Center for Holistic Medicine, 7603 Colland Drive,
Fort Collins, CO 80525, USA

Pediatric mood disorders (unipolar depression and bipolar disorder) are serious, common, persistent, and recurrent medical conditions. The US National Institute of Mental Health and the World Health Organization estimate that depression is the leading cause of disability in the United States, and worldwide, it is the second-leading contributor to the global burden of disease for persons 15 to 44 years old [1].

Mood disorders have several nonmodifiable risk factors, including family history, gender, and race. Major depression and suicide are associated with fewer serotonin transporter sites in the prefrontal cortex of the brain. Lower norepinephrine levels are associated with dysphoria and apathy. Central nervous system dopamine levels are also reduced in depression. Before puberty, the prevalence of depression is higher in boys than in girls; after puberty, the rates in girls are about twice those in boys. Native Americans have higher rates of depression, whereas Asians report fewer depressive symptoms than Caucasians.

Mood disorders have a high rate of comorbidity with mental health and medical problems. For example, many children and adolescents suffering from attention-deficit/hyperactivity disorder, anxiety, or substance abuse also suffer from depression, and vice versa. Depressive disorders are also common among patients who have chronic medical conditions, including

Dr. Kemper is supported in part by the Kohlberg Foundation, by NIH NCCAM K24 AT002207 and NIH NCAM R21 AT001901, and by the Caryl Guth Fund for Holistic and Integrative Medicine. The views expressed in this article are those of the authors and do not necessarily represent the views of the Kohlberg Foundation, the NIH, or Dr. Guth.

* Corresponding author.

E-mail address: kkemper@wfubmc.edu (K.J. Kemper).

doi:10.1016/j.pcl.2007.09.002

pediatric.theclinics.com

any condition causing chronic pain, obesity, endocrine disorders, inflammatory disorders, cancer, anemia, viral infections, and brain injury. Depression can also be caused by medications, including antihypertensive medications and oral contraceptives. Depression recurs in 70% of those affected. Therefore, even patients who have improved should actively pursue activities to promote positive moods and prevent recurrences.

Mainstream therapies, such as medications, cognitive behavioral therapies, electroconvulsive therapy, and vagal nerve stimulators have been discussed extensively in other reviews [2–5]. Furthermore, given the side effects and stigmatization of standard antidepressant medications, many families turn to complementary therapies. In fact, depression is one of the most common reasons for adolescents and adults to seek complementary therapies [6].

Therefore, the focus of this article is the fundamental lifestyle approaches and complementary therapies that enhance mental health, particularly those that help achieve and maintain healthy moods. The emerging term to describe the use of lifestyle and complementary therapies in combination with traditional, scientific medicine is "integrative medicine." Integrative medicine is informed by science and is based on four core concepts:

- Patient-centered care (individualized, consistent with patient values and goals)
- Sustainable, healing environment
- Comprehensive approach to therapies
- Health promotion and wellness; promotion of the innate healing potential

Health: physical and mental

Mental health is closely tied to physical health. A successful athlete exhibits strength, flexibility, endurance, coordination, focus, resilience, teamwork, and sport-specific skills. Similarly, a mentally healthy person exhibits confidence, courage, cheerfulness, coping abilities, hardiness, and focused attention. It's not that the fit athlete never stumbles or that he/she always hits a home run, but that, barring a catastrophe, he/she can get up and try again. Similarly, a mentally healthy person occasionally experiences sadness, worry, misery, exhilaration, ecstasy, and the full range of human emotions, recognizing that "into each life, some rain must fall," but views the rain as a challenge rather than an insurmountable obstacle. Holistic physicians also consider spiritual health as a critical element of overall health. Table 1 shows some of the characteristics of physical, mental, and spiritual health.

Because the mind–body connection is real, promotion of mental health, including healthy moods, relies on very similar strategies to those promoting physical health.

Table 1
Physical, mental, and spiritual health characteristics

Physical fitness	Mental health	Spiritual health
Strength	Confidence and courage	Faith
Flexibility	Adaptability	Forgiveness
Endurance	Cheerfulness	Hope
Focus	Focus and attention	Love
Coordination	Harmony	Kindness
Resilience	Hardiness	Charity and generosity
Teamwork	Social network, communication skills, and connection to community	Connection with a higher power

Therapeutic options for achieving healthy moods fall into four major categories:

- Lifestyle
- Biochemical
- Biomechanical
- Bioenergetic

Lifestyle essentials: the fundamentals for healthy moods

Successful athletic coaches emphasize the fundamental skills of their sport. When it comes to mental and physical health, the fundamentals are excellent nutrition (including avoiding toxic ingestions and inhalations while optimizing the intake of essential nutrients); exercise balanced with restful sleep; a healthy environment (such as plenty of sunshine; mood-boosting music; minimal environmental and psychosocial toxins; and supportive family, friends, and community); and mind–body therapies and techniques (such as meditation and relaxation) [7]. In a German study, intensive lifestyle therapy was as effective as counseling and medication in improving depressive symptoms [8].

Nutrition

Healthy nutrition means taking in optimal amounts of essential nutrients while avoiding or minimizing the intake of toxic substances. Individual genetic variability, previous dietary patterns, medical illnesses, medications, allergies, and environmental exposures may increase the need for specific nutrients in the form of supplements.

Evidence-based guidance includes the following suggestions:

- Promote stable blood sugar by encouraging foods with a low glycemic index, such as proteins and complex carbohydrates [9].
- Encourage patients to eat breakfast, including some protein, to promote stable blood sugar throughout the day [10–12].
- Minimize the use of processed foods.

- Emphasize drinking plenty of pure water and eating fresh fruits and vegetables, legumes, whole grains, fish, and, if dairy and meat are eaten, organic, locally raised products whenever possible.
- Avoid sweetened beverages, processed foods, fatty foods, fried foods, and junk food.

Approximately 6% to 10% of children have allergies or sensitivities to foods, including 1% who cannot tolerate gluten [13]. The most common food sensitivities are to wheat, corn, soy, dairy, eggs, tree nuts, shell fish, and peanuts. Food sensitivities can cause mood problems in addition to rashes, asthma, and rhinorrhea [14,15]. Detection of food sensitivities begins with keeping a careful food diary. In some cases, blood testing, skin testing, endoscopic biopsy (for gluten sensitivity), and elimination diets may be useful in diagnosing food sensitivities. Eliminating the triggering food or foods from the diet can improve mood [14,15] and other symptoms such as chronic headaches, rashes, and gastrointestinal upset. Children with multiple food sensitivities may benefit from nutritional counseling to ensure adequate intakes of essential nutrients [16].

One should avoid toxic ingestions. Some people try to manage their moods by smoking, drinking alcohol, or taking other drugs. Although these may improve mood in the short term, over the longer term, they contribute to many miseries. Rarely, people are sensitive to petrochemicals, artificial flavors, artificial colors, and artificial sweeteners; these food additives are not essential nutrients and can easily be avoided by most people. Choosing organic food is a good way to ensure freedom from chemical residues. Pediatricians can advocate for farm, nutrition, and environmental policies that are health promoting.

One should ensure an adequate intake of the nutrients essential to healthy mood. Nutrients are essential for optimal production of neurotransmitters affecting mood, such as serotonin (made from tryptophan, with B vitamins and zinc as cofactors). The easiest way for most bodies to absorb nutrients is through unprocessed, locally grown, organic foods. Table 2 provides a listing of food sources for nutrients essential for mental health.

Exercise and rest

For many people, vigorous physical exercise is as effective as, or more effective than, antidepressant medications in promoting positive moods. Children who are sedentary report higher levels of depression [12,17,18]. Depressed mood and fatigue are common in individuals deprived of the usual exercise activities (whether from an injury or acute illness), and may be partially mediated by reduced fitness levels [19]. Getting kids away from the television, computer, and electronic games in favor of vigorous activity can improve mood. In a meta-analysis of yoga therapy, five randomized controlled trials (RCTs) in adults suffering from depression all reported positive effects of exercise [20]. No adverse effects were reported, with the

Table 2
Nutrients essential for mental health and their food sources

Nutrient	Food sources
Essential fatty acids (omega-3 fatty acids such as linolenic acid)	Fish (tuna, salmon, and mackerel) fish oil, flax seeds, flax oil, canola oil, walnut oil, dark green leafy vegetables
Vitamin B_6	Beans, nuts, legumes Eggs, meats, fish Whole grains and fortified breads and cereals
Vitamin C	(All fruits and vegetables contain some amount of vitamin C.) Green and red peppers, citrus fruits and juices, strawberries, tomatoes, broccoli, turnip greens and other leafy greens, sweet and white potatoes, cantaloupe, papaya, mango, watermelon, Brussels sprouts, cauliflower, cabbage, winter squash, raspberries, blueberries, cranberries, and pineapples
Folate	Beans and legumes Citrus fruits and juices Wheat bran and other whole grains Dark green leafy vegetables Poultry, pork, shellfish Liver
Calcium	Milk, yogurt, buttermilk, cheese Calcium-fortified orange juice Green leafy vegetables (broccoli, collards, kale, mustard greens, turnip greens, and bok choy or Chinese cabbage) Canned salmon and sardines canned with their soft bones Shellfish Almonds, Brazil nuts Dried beans
Vitamin D	Fish, fish oils, oysters Fortified foods such as cow milk, soy milk, and rice milk, and some cereals
Tryptophan	Turkey, chicken, fish Milk, cheese Eggs Soy, tofu Sesame seeds Pumpkin seeds Tree nuts, peanuts, peanut butter
Zinc	Beef, pork, lamb, oysters, dark meat of poultry Peanuts, peanut butter, nuts, and legumes (beans) Fortified cereals

exception of fatigue and breathlessness in participants in one study. The side effects of exercise include over-use injuries, decreased obesity, lower risk of heart disease, improved sleep, less chronic fatigue, improved academic performance, and decreased pain. Clinicians should advise patients suffering from depression to maintain a healthy lifestyle by exercising regularly.

Sleep deprivation can lead to poor mood, and insomnia is a common symptom of depression [21]. Many teenagers do not get sufficient sleep. Improving sleep hygiene (using the bed only for sleep, removing the television from the bedroom, ensuring that the bedroom is dark and cool, taking a hot bath before bed, listening to relaxing music, reading positive or inspiring books, receiving a brief massage from a trusted family member, and writing in a journal before bed) can help improve mood and set the tone for a restful sleep.

Environment

A healthy environment is of critical importance in promoting, maintaining, and restoring healthy mood. An environment that includes poverty, abuse, neglect, or absence of opportunities for work or school can have severe adverse effects on mood that cannot be corrected through medications alone. The key elements that affect mood in the physical environment (eg, light, nature), the psychologic environment (eg, television), the social and cultural environment (racism, sexism, poverty, and social isolation) are touched on here.

Songs, poems, stories, and folk wisdom support the association between sunshine and happiness, and lack of sunshine and sadness (the blues). Bright light suppresses daytime melatonin production and shifts circadian rhythms. Desynchronization of internal rhythms plays an important role in the pathophysiology of depressive disorders. Serotonin levels are lowest during the winter months. Seasonal affective disorder has been well described. Given the modern lifestyles of living indoors and traveling in enclosed vehicles, modern children and adolescents receive far less sunshine than our ancestors. Psychiatrists have noted that depressed patients hospitalized in sunny rooms have shorter lengths of stay than patients in less sunny rooms [22].

Sunlight is an essential component of our natural environment. Daylighting, the practice of enhancing direct daylight exposure for children in classrooms, enhances school performance, reduces illness, and improves attendance [23]. Bright light therapy plays an effective role in the treatment of mood disorders. In an RCT published in 2006, bright light was as effective as fluoxetine in improving symptoms of seasonal affective disorder (67% response rate for both) [24]. Phototherapy has also been as effective as antidepressant medication in treating depression during pregnancy [25]. A 2005 meta-analysis of RCTs of light therapy concluded that bright light treatment for nonseasonal depression is efficacious, with effect sizes equivalent to those in most antidepressant pharmacotherapy trials [26]. Light therapy can also enhance the effectiveness of other treatments [27].

Bright light early in the morning seems to be the most effective. In most trials of light therapy, the patient sits in front of a light box, exposed to 10,000 lux for 30 to 120 minutes daily. Trials comparing the effects of light boxes with outdoor activity (eg, 15–60 minutes of sunlight daily) and tanning booths are needed.

Nature

Recently, a new field of inquiry has emerged that explores the therapeutic effects of nature and the natural environment. Investigators have called this field biophilia, which emphasizes the connection to our natural environment [28]. This field of study includes both natural settings alone and those combined with contact with animals. One recent study from the *British Medical Journal* [29] explored the value of swimming with dolphins, a variation of animal-assisted therapy, controlled for the beneficial effect of the natural setting. A significant positive effect with this approach was found for 30 adult patients who had mild to moderate depression after 2 weeks of treatment in this single-blind RCT.

Minimizing environmental toxins

Heavy metals (eg, lead and mercury) [30] and carbon monoxide poisoning are also associated with depressive symptoms [31,32]. Checking for toxins and eliminating them may help improve mood. The benefit is well documented with lead and carbon monoxide, but the value for other heavy metals remains a frontier of knowledge at this point.

One of the easiest ways to become depressed is to compare oneself with someone who is more attractive and intelligent, or in possession of more friends, toys, desirable food, or clothing, or has better transportation or housing. Exposure to television and other sources of marketing increases the likelihood that children and adolescents will make these comparisons. Furthermore, the "If it bleeds, it leads" philosophy in the media has resulted in a preponderance of negative, disheartening news on television. Removing televisions from children's rooms and sharply reducing the time the television is on may contribute to improved mood. The elimination of marketing to children (already in place in several European countries), as a result of advocacy, could also contribute to enhanced mental health. At home, children and families can practice "appreciation audits," listing the elements in their lives for which they are grateful or keeping a daily journal of appreciation and kindness items (ie, ways the writer has been kind to others). (For more information on the appreciation audit, see Dan Baker's book, listed in Appendix 1).

Poverty and lack of opportunity adversely affect mood [33,34]. Racism, sexism, homophobia, and other social injustices also contribute to suffering and decreased access to care [35–39]. Problems within the family and local community, such as child abuse and neglect and child sexual abuse have significant long-term adverse effects on mood [40–42]. Physician advocacy for social justice, equal access to care, and family support services can have a profound impact on children's moods.

Mind–body therapies

Meditation

Meditation practice, particularly mindfulness meditation (moment-to-moment nonjudgmental awareness of breathing, physical sensations, emotions, and thoughts), can contribute to enhanced mood, and can change brain activation patterns in ways likely to support ongoing benefits.

Specifically, meditation training leads to significant increases in left-sided anterior activation, a pattern associated with positive affect [43]. Long-term meditators, compared with age-matched controls, exhibit increased cortical thickness in brain regions associated with attention and sensory processing, including the prefrontal cortex [44]. Side effects of meditation may include improved ability to cope with stress, reduced pain, reduced anxiety, and enhanced immune function.

Dialectic behavior therapy

Dialectic behavior therapy is a psychosocial therapy based in cognitive behavioral therapy and mindfulness. Originally designed for chronically suicidal patients with borderline personality disorder, dialectic behavior therapy helps people build awareness about their emotional states and about how to gain control over behavior. This technique works well for emotionally labile teens with mood issues and for chronically suicidal teens [45,46]. Recently, one preliminary study [47] found benefits in children with oppositional defiant disorder (who commonly have comorbid mood disorders). A 1-year open trial with bipolar youth also found promising beneficial effects [48].

Eye movement desensitization and reprocessing

Eye movement desensitization and reprocessing (EMDR) significantly improved depression in adult patients of childhood sexual abuse in an RCT of 880 patients [49]. In this study, EMDR was most effective for more recent trauma and significantly outperformed fluoxetine on various measures. Many clinicians who treat children are finding EMDR a safe, effective, and often faster treatment approach for angry, violent, or depressed youth who have suffered abuse.

Other

Various evidenced-based approaches that calm the mind may play a role in the care of children with mood disorders. Tai chi and mindfulness techniques have been applied successfully in a Boston public middle school [50] and resulted in the improvement of various measures, including general well-being. Gordon and colleagues [51] applied various mind–body techniques to improve symptoms in a group of war-weary Kosovo students. Music therapy improved mood and depressive scales in a group of grieving children [52]. In an RCT of 69 adult patients hospitalized for stem cell transplantation, music therapy significantly improved mood and anxiety [53]. In a study of 22 children with recurrent abdominal pain (commonly comorbid with depression), guided imagery was a more effective treatment than breathing exercises alone [54]. Reynolds and Coats [55] demonstrated in an RCT that relaxation therapy was as effective as cognitive behavior therapy (a well-researched, evidence-based treatment) for a group of 30 depressed adolescents. Relaxation therapy was also found to be more effective than antidepressant therapy for major depression in one adult trial [56].

Social support and spirituality

Children who attend church regularly have about a 20% lower risk of developing depression than nonattendees. Church may be protective because of inherent spiritual factors and because it provides a sense of social support and cohesiveness and opportunities for connecting with a trusted adult in whom to confide. Numerous studies document benefit from various spiritual paths. The positive factors seem to be faith and community, rather than a specific belief system. Primary care clinicians can also provide important psychosocial support that improves outcomes in depressed adolescents [57].

Biochemical therapies

Because of our individual uniqueness (genomic variability), diet, and environment, some individuals require additional nutrients or benefit from specific biochemical therapies to achieve healthy moods. For example, simple nucleotide polymorphisms represent a significant factor in biochemical individuality. The enzyme delta-5-desaturase converts omega-3 fatty acids such as alpha linolenic acid into eicosapentaenoic acid (EPA) and docosahexaenoic acid (DHA). If a simple nucleotide polymorphism impairs delta-5-desaturase, a child may require significantly higher levels of alpha linolenic acid, EPA, or DHA in his/her diet to maintain normal cell membrane function and healthy mood.

For this article, the authors focus on vitamins and minerals, herbs, and other dietary supplements. Given the fact that fewer than 1% of American children meet their recommended daily allowance of essential nutrients through diet alone [58], it is likely that many children would benefit from supplementation, in addition to striving to improve their overall diet. Supplementation is especially important for children who eat a restricted diet because of suspected food allergies or sensitivities. Also, any child who restricts calories, whether because he/she performs in such sports as wrestling, gymnastics, and so forth, or because he/she has self-image problems (ie, anorexia), will have enhanced needs. (Stress and conflict also significantly escalate nutrient demands).

Essential nutrients (vitamins, minerals, fatty acids, amino acids)

Here, the authors do not cover all essential nutrients, but focus on a few that are vitally important and often lacking in Americans, some of whom might benefit from nutrient supplementation.

Multivitamin–mineral preparations

Several investigators have concluded that multivitamin–mineral combinations can help improve mood and behavior. In a large British trial in 231 young offenders, violent acts and rule infractions were significantly reduced among those given micronutrient supplementation [59]. Several case studies and case series support the effectiveness of a proprietary multivitamin–mineral (EMPower) on young people with mood disorders (including depression and bipolar disorders) [60–62]. This product has numerous testimonials, but requires up to 15 capsules daily for a loading dose; it contains significant amounts of calcium, magnesium, and B vitamins. It has not been compared with supplementation with generic versions of these nutrients.

Individual vitamins

B vitamins, including folate

Vitamin B_6 is essential in metabolizing tryptophan to serotonin. Folate and vitamin B_{12} are major determinants of one-carbon metabolism, in which S-adenosylmethionine (SAMe, pronounced Sam-ee) is formed. SAMe donates methyl groups that are crucial for neurologic function. See later discussion on SAMe.

Low levels of pyridoxal phosphate are significantly associated with depressive symptoms [63]. A systematic review suggested that 100 to 200 mg daily supplementation with vitamin B_6 significantly benefits premenstrual depression [64]. The side effects of excessive doses of vitamin B_6 include nausea, vomiting, abdominal pain, anorexia, headache, somnolence, lower B12 levels, and sensory neuropathy. The last typically occurs with doses of more than 1000 mg daily, but can occur lower with lower doses.

Folate is a water-soluble vitamin that donates a methyl group in the one-carbon cycle needed for the production of SAMe and the remethylation of homocysteine. Folate deficiency is common and contributes to various psychiatric symptoms, including depression, psychosis, irritability, dementia, and impaired memory.

Considerable research evidence supports the value of folate in maintaining a healthy mood. Folate and B12 levels are lower in depressed than in nondepressed persons, and replacing deficient folate can lead to remarkable improvements in mood [65–67]. Low folate levels predict treatment resistance to fluoxetine [68]. In one study, folate supplementation was as effective as 150 mg of amitriptyline in treating depressed outpatients [69]. Adding 500 μg of folate to 20 mg of fluoxetine significantly improved the response rate in patients who had major depression [70]. One review concluded that folate supplementation is beneficial in treating depression, whether used as monotherapy or as an augmentation of conventional medications [71]. Primary care clinicians should ensure that children prone to mood disorders have an adequate intake of folate and should consider recommending a multivitamin or a B-vitamin complex containing folate. Given the safety of water-soluble vitamins, a dose of 1 mg per day in symptomatic children is reasonable. It should be given with B_{12} to avoid masking a B_{12} deficiency.

Vitamin D

A growing body of research suggests that American youth are vitamin D–deficient, even in older pediatric and adolescent populations that do not appear to have classic rickets [72–74]. This deficiency may be a particular problem in children taking anticonvulsant medications [75]; those with inflammatory bowel disease [76,77] or arthritis [78,79]; those with chronic renal disease [80]; those living in the inner city [81]; African-Americans [82]; or those who are veiled. Many adolescents have relatively low levels of vitamin D because of an indoor lifestyle and inadequate intake of vitamin D–fortified foods [83]. A recent study found that obese children have significantly depressed vitamin D levels [84], perhaps from inadequate outdoor time. Skin cancer concerns, inactivity, obesity, excessive screen time (eg, too much time watching television, playing electronic games, or working on a computer), and other issues may contribute to sun avoidance and vitamin D deficiency.

Low levels of vitamin D are associated with depressive symptoms, and treatment with vitamin D supplements is associated with improved mood. For example, 25-hydroxyvitamin D_3 and 1,25-dihydroxvitamin D_3 levels are significantly lower in psychiatric patients than in normal controls [85]. Vitamin D deficiency is associated with anxiety and depression in patients who have fibromyalgia [86]. In an RCT of vitamin D given to 44 Australian patients (none versus 400 IU versus 800 IU vitamin D), vitamin D_3 significantly enhanced mood in a dose-dependent fashion [87].

The recommended daily allowance for vitamin D was set to prevent rickets in young children and may be insufficient to prevent certain health problems in older adults. It may be worthwhile for adolescents to take vitamin D supplements, particularly during winter months, to ensure adequate vitamin D levels and prevent subclinical hypoparathyroidism; supplementation is also worthwhile for patients who have renal disease, inflammatory bowel disease, or juvenile arthritis, and those patients on anticonvulsant drugs that lower vitamin D levels.

Minerals

This section includes brief discussions on the role of calcium, magnesium, chromium, zinc, and iron in promoting and maintaining a healthy mood.

Calcium

Lower levels of calcium and higher levels of parathyroid hormone have been observed in depressed persons. Likewise, depression is commonly noted among patients suffering from hyperparathyroidism [88]. Quality of life and depressive symptoms improve when these patients receive appropriate treatment [89]. Estrogen regulates calcium and parathyroid hormone metabolism [90]; sometimes dysregulation occurs, which is particularly notable in women suffering from premenstrual symptoms. Epidemiologically, normal to high intakes of calcium and vitamin D are associated with a lower risk of depressive mood in patients who have premenstrual syndrome; conversely, lower intakes of calcium and vitamin D are associated with an increased risk of premenstrual syndrome [91]. Small studies suggest that calcium supplementation may benefit women with premenstrual syndrome-related depression [92,93].

Most adolescent girls do not meet their minimum daily requirement for calcium through diet alone. According to the Continuing Survey of Food Intakes of Individuals (1994-96), the following percentages of Americans do not meet their recommended intake for calcium:

- 44% of boys and 58% of girls aged 6 to 11
- 64% of boys and 87% of girls aged 12 to 19

It is important for clinicians counseling adolescents about mood to address adequate calcium intake (optimally 1200–1500 mg daily) to ensure bone health and promote a healthy mood.

Magnesium

Magnesium is second only to potassium in intracellular concentration. It facilitates the conversion of 5-hydroxytryptophan (5-HTP) into serotonin. Signs of magnesium deficiency include irritability, fatigue, loss of appetite, mental confusion, insomnia, and a predisposition to stress. Historically, magnesium has been used, like lithium, as a treatment for mania or severe agitation [94]. It is not used widely or recommended as a treatment for depression.

Magnesium, like lithium, suppresses hippocampal kindling, regulates N-methyl-D-aspartate receptors, and alters glutamate activity [95,96]. It has been a successful treatment for premenstrual mood changes [97]. Magnesium and verapamil were much more effective than verapamil alone in treating acute mania [98].

Magnesium deficiency is extremely common [99]. Research is currently underway on the value of magnesium supplementation in pediatric bipolar disorder. Ensuring an adequate intake of magnesium is important in maintaining a balanced mood.

Chromium

Chromium, a dietary trace mineral, has a crucial role in glucose and fat metabolism and neurotransmitter synthesis. Chromium improves insulin sensitivity and increases free brain levels of serotonin, norepinephrine, and melatonin. In an RCT of bipolar II patients and patients who had atypical depression, chromium had a significant benefit [100]. Five patients responded to chromium supplementation after failing conventional depression treatment [101]. An RCT of chromium picolinate (600 µg daily) in patients whose depression was characterized by carbohydrate craving showed significant improvement in craving and depressive symptoms [102].

Chromium is well tolerated but can have a stimulating effect. The recommended daily allowance for chromium is 120 µg. The daily dietary intake of chromium for a typical American adult is only 25 to 50 µg per day. The dose range in studies of its effects on mood is typically 200 to 600 µg per day.

Dietary sources rich in chromium include breads, cereals, spices, fresh vegetables, meats, fish, and brewer's yeast.

Zinc

Zinc is an essential mineral that is found in almost every cell. It stimulates the activity of approximately 100 enzymes. Low serum zinc levels have been linked to major depression. Zinc, an antagonist of the glutamate/N-methyl-D-aspartate receptor, exhibits antidepressant-like activity in rodent models of depression. Like antidepressants, zinc induces brain-derived neurotrophic factor gene expression and increases the level of the synaptic pool of zinc in the hippocampus [103]. Furthermore, zinc treatment has been shown to have an antidepressant effect [104].

The American recommended dietary allowance for zinc ranges from 5 mg daily for younger children to 11 mg daily for teenagers. Vegetarians may need as much as 50% more zinc than nonvegetarians because of the lower absorption of zinc from plant foods, so it is important for vegetarians to include good sources of zinc in their diet. Breastfeeding depletes zinc, and some experts suggest that because breast milk contains relatively low levels of zinc, breastfed infants should receive zinc supplementation after 7 months of age.

Low zinc status has been observed in 30% to 50% of alcoholics. Alcohol decreases the absorption of zinc and increases the loss of zinc in urine. In addition, many alcoholics do not eat an acceptable variety or amount of food, so their dietary intake of zinc may be inadequate. If an adolescent has a drinking problem in addition to a mood problem, it is especially important to ensure adequate mineral supplementation.

Zinc toxicity occurs with intakes of 150 to 450 mg of zinc per day and appears as low copper status, altered iron function, reduced immune function, and reduced levels of high-density lipoproteins.

Iron

Iron deficiency anemia is often accompanied by depression. Long-term iron deficiency in infancy and early childhood is associated with mood and learning problems, even years after the deficiency is corrected [105]. It is important to ensure that adolescents be checked for iron sufficiency, particularly female adolescents who may not be meeting their needs for iron to replace menstrual losses [106]. Primary care clinicians should ensure that their patients consume adequate amounts of iron through either diet or supplementation.

Fatty acids

Linolenic, eicosapentaenoic, and docosahexaenoic acids

The human brain is 60% fat, and the essential fatty acids contribute a substantial portion of that weight. Essential fatty acids are crucial to normal fetal and neonatal maturation of the brain. Three common essential fatty acids (EPA, DHA, and arachidonic acid), are crucial building blocks of neuronal membranes. Fatty acids also form the precursors of prostaglandins and leukotrienes. Fatty fish such as salmon, mackerel, and herring are excellent sources of EPA and DHA.

Fish consumption and levels of omega-3 fatty acids have a strong epidemiologic correlation with protection from depression and suicide [107–111]. Furthermore, clinical trials suggest that supplemental essential fatty acids (EPA and DHA) can improve mood and decrease hostility and violence, even in patients hospitalized for severe depression or suicidality [112–115]. The doses in these studies range from 1 g per day to 10 g per day.

The benefit of omega-3 supplementation for bipolar disorder is less clear [116]. Stoll and colleagues' [117] double-blind study augmenting treated bipolar patients with fish oil (9.6 g per day) or placebo found significant reductions in relapse and all other outcome measures with fish oil. However, another trial with 120 bipolar patients found no significant treatment effect [118]. A 2007 study of pediatric bipolar disorder [119] found a modest, but statistically significant, improvement in an open-label trial of 20 children, 6 to 17 years of age. The intervention was 1290 to 4300 mg of an EPA–DHA combination.

In children, the developmental requirements and absence of serious toxicity suggest that daily supplementation with 1 to 3 g of fish oil (EPA–DHA) can support healthy mood. Product testing has revealed no significant contamination with mercury, dioxins, or other contaminants in molecularly distilled fish oil products. More potent and palatable forms of molecularly distilled fish oils make these dietary recommendations easier to swallow. Small children can take one of the liquid forms often easily hidden in food. Recently, a prescription brand of fish oil entered the scene, further increasing treatment options.

Amino acids

L-tryptophan

5-HTP is the immediate precursor of serotonin in its metabolism from dietary L-tryptophan (L-trp). Unlike tryptophan, which faces competitive inhibition in its absorption, 5-HTP does not, and it appears to be a better choice for increasing central nervous system levels of serotonin.

Tryptophan depletion leads to depressive symptoms in rats and humans. Various smaller (open and controlled) studies [120–125] have found 5-HTP useful in depression. A Cochrane meta-analysis of trials involving 64 patients suggested 5-HTP and L-trp are better than placebo in treating depression [126]. The doses given in most trials start at 50 mg three times a day. The typical dosing is 50 mg, slowly increasing to 150 mg, two or three times daily on an empty stomach, based on size. A large single dose of 200 to 400 mg can be used by slowly increasing the dose. The maximum recommended dose is 1200 mg daily.

Side effects of 5-HTP and L-trp include nausea and drowsiness (which may make it useful at bedtime); they may cause serotonergic syndrome if used in combination with selective serotonin reuptake inhibitor (SSRI) medications; they may also be associated with decreased carbohydrate intake and weight loss [127]. Eosinophilia-myalgia syndrome was reported in numerous people taking L-trp, which led to its removal from the American market; however, investigations revealed that the problem was related to a contaminated lot from one manufacturer, and L-trp is again available. During the time it was off the market, many people turned to 5-HTP supplements instead to ensure safety. Experts now recommend using products that are tested and free of a "Peak X" contaminant.

S-Adenosylmethionine

SAMe is a methyl donor in more than 35 reactions in the brain and body. It plays a crucial role in the production of monoamine neurotransmitters, nucleotides, and neuronal membrane phospholipids. SAMe has been found to be the most potent chemical trigger for the induction of mania in bipolar patients, a reflection of its antidepressant potency.

More than 25 controlled trials have evaluated the effectiveness of SAMe for patients with mood disorders. A 2002 review by the Agency for Health care Quality and Research (AHRQ) concluded that, compared with placebo, 3 weeks of treatment with SAMe was associated with a significant improvement in depression [128]. Several studies published since the AHRQ 2002 report confirm its effectiveness in improving mood, and suggest it has a potency similar to tricyclic antidepressants [129–132]. It may also be helpful in patients for whom antidepressant medications have been ineffective [133]. Furthermore, it can also be a useful adjunctive treatment, along with conventional antidepressant medications [133].

Typical doses are 800 to 1600 mg of SAMe daily. Benefits typically appear within 2 weeks of starting the medication. Although product variability is a major problem in many dietary supplements, a review of SAMe products by ConsumerLabs revealed that only 1 out of 11 tested products failed their rigorous standards.

SAMe has fewer side effects than conventional antidepressant medications and works more quickly. Side effects include triggering mania and increasing the risk of serotonergic syndrome in patients taking SSRI medications. It should not be used by patients who have bipolar disorder. Furthermore, it is expensive (50 cents to $1 per 200 mg tablet) and is not usually covered by insurance.

Herbs for mood

St. John's wort

The herb most commonly used as a complementary or alternative remedy for depression is St. John's wort. Studies on its effectiveness have had mixed results, with most of the positive studies coming from European trials using standard extracts [134]. See Table 3 for a listing of the compounds used in the studies with positive results and the American imports containing these

Table 3
St. John's wort products used in studies reporting positive effects

Products with positive results in clinical studies	Brand name (manufacturer)
LI 160 and LI 160S	Quanterra Emotional Balance (Warner-Lambert); Kira (Lichtwer Pharma US/Germany)
WS 5570 and WS 5572	Neuroplant (Schwabe Pharmaceuticals) Perika (Schwabe Pharmaceuticals, imported by Nature's Way Products, Inc)
Ze 117	Remotiv (Bayer Vital GmbH and Zeller AG)

Courtesy of Paula Gardiner, MD, Boston, MA.

compounds. For example, in a German RCT, St. John's wort was as effective as sertraline in improving depressive symptoms [135]. A similar German study showed its comparability to citalopram [136]. Two open-label trials in adolescents showed improvement within 2 weeks in 25 out of 33, and 9 out of 11 patients in separate studies [137,138]; patients who improved in these studies generally showed improvement within 2 weeks of starting therapy. It is reasonable to stop treatment or change to a higher dose or a different product if no benefit has been noted within 3 weeks.

St. John's wort is generally safer than most antidepressant medications. A meta-analysis of 16 post-marketing surveillance studies including 34,804 patients recorded an incidence of adverse events between 0% and 6%; of the four large-scale surveillance studies with a total of 14,245 patients, the rate of adverse events ranged from 0.1% to 2.4% and a drop-out rate due to adverse events of 0.1% to 0.9% [139]. This finding is at least ten-fold lower than that recorded with synthetic antidepressants. The adverse events associated with St. John's wort were mild and transient in nearly all cases.

St. John's wort can, however, have direct adverse effects and serious interactions with commonly used medications. The most common direct effects are phototoxicity and stomach upset. The most serious adverse effects are drug interactions in which St. John's wort reduces the serum levels of other medications including contraceptives, digoxin, immunosuppressants, theophylline, clarithromycin, erythromycin, cyclosporine, tacrolimus, protease inhibitors, and certain chemotherapeutic agents. It should not be used in conjunction with SSRIs because such use may increase the risk of serotonergic syndrome.

St. John's wort preparations have substantial variability in quality. Patients who wish to use it may use a product tested in a large RCT or refer to product testing conducted by ConsumerLabs (see Appendix 1).

Other dietary supplements

Inositol

Inositol, an isomer of glucose, works as an intracellular messenger that relays the neurotransmitter message to the cell nucleus. One review found that inositol was useful in panic disorder, obsessive-compulsive disorder, and depression [140]. In a large comparative study of treatments for bipolar depression, the recovery rate was 23.8% for lamotrigine, 4.6% for risperdone, and 17.4% for inositol [141]. It has been suggested that inositol can trigger mania episodes in patients who have bipolar disorder [142]. Inositol can be mildly sedating and has also been used as a sleep aid. Inositol had far fewer side effects in all comparison studies. As a sweet-tasting powder that can be mixed into any liquid, inositol offers a well-tolerated intervention for children with mood disorders. The typical starting dose is 1 to 2 g two or three times daily, increasing up to 12 to 18 g per day in divided doses.

Biomechanical therapies: massage

Massage is used widely to improve mood. In fact, therapeutic massage struggles to overcome an historical connection with the "entertainment" industry. Despite its marketing problems, massage has many medical uses. Therapeutic massage contributes to increased blood flow and lymphatic drainage; muscle relaxation; stress reduction; and social support. Physiologically, massage balances right and left prefrontal cortex activity in those with right dominance [143]. The left prefrontal cortex has been associated with positive mood, whereas dominance of the right prefrontal cortex is associated with depressed mood [144]. Furthermore, massage decreases cortisol levels and increases levels of serotonin and dopamine in patients who have depression [145]. In depressed women, massage, compared with progressive relaxation, led to higher dopamine and serotonin levels and lower levels of cortisol and norepinephrine [146]. Massage significantly reduced aggression in 17 adolescent psychiatric inpatients [147]. A simple 30-minute back rub daily reduced anxiety and improved cooperation in 52 pediatric psychiatric inpatients [148].

Considerable research has been published on the pervasive and persistent negative effects of maternal depression on childhood mental health [149]. The infants of depressed mothers who received massage scored higher on various measures in the Brazelton scale than mothers who only received light touch [150], thus reducing the ensuing emotional risk to the unborn child.

In the studies showing positive effects, massage has generally been provided 5 days a week. To achieve this frequency cost effectively, parents are generally trained to provide massage for children and adolescents. Massage is generally safe if care is taken to avoid wounds, burns, intravenous lines, pumps or other subcutaneous devices, and vigorous strokes in patients who have low platelet counts. Careful discussion and respect for individual patients is important for patients who have a history of physical or sexual abuse.

Bioenergetic therapies: acupuncture

Acupuncture involves the stimulation (using pressure, heat, needles, and magnets) of specific points on the body, with the intention of promoting healing. RCTs suggest that acupuncture has significant benefits for depressed adults and may be comparable in effectiveness to prescription antidepressant medications [151]. For example, in an RCT of true acupuncture, sham acupuncture, and massage provided to 61 pregnant women with major depressive disorder, response rates were statistically significantly higher for acupuncture (69%) than for massage (32%), with an intermediate sham acupuncture response rate (47%) [152]. In a meta-analysis published in 2005, the investigators concluded that "the effect of electroacupuncture may not be significantly different from antidepressant medication," with a weighted mean difference in comparison trials of -0.43 (95% CI -5.61 to 4.76) [153].

Acupuncture rarely causes bleeding, bruising, or infection; it causes sleepiness in about 5% of patients. In general, it has fewer side effects than medications. Serious side effects are rare. Pediatric patients will accept it, but it's not usually their first choice of therapies. Those who receive it generally report that it is helpful and, unlike their expectations, pleasant [154].

Resources

Research in this area is growing constantly. It is helpful to have a list of resources to address common questions and concerns and to keep abreast of emerging knowledge about the safety and effectiveness of therapies and approaches to promote healthy moods. See Appendix 1.

Summary

Depression is the second-leading cause of illness and disability among young people worldwide. A healthy lifestyle and healthy environment are the cornerstones for promoting positive moods. In addition, several complementary therapies, including nutritional supplements, herbs, mind–body therapies, massage, and acupuncture can be helpful. Various resources are available to clinicians to help patients and families promote mental health.

Appendix 1. Resources on integrative approaches to pediatric mood disorders

Internet resources

American Academy of Pediatrics Provisional Section for Complementary, Holistic and Integrative Medicine (http://www.aap.org/sections/chim/)

American Academy of Pediatrics, Committee on Environmental Health (http://www.aap.org/visit/cmte16.htm)

National Institutes of Health, Institute on Mental Health (information on depression in children and adolescents) (http://www.nimh.nih.gov/healthinformation/depchildmenu.cfm)

National Library of Medicine, Medline Plus (information on many medications, nutrients, and dietary supplements) (http://www.nlm.nih.gov/medlineplus/)

Natural Medicines Comprehensive Database (http://www.naturaldatabase.com/)

Natural Standard (http://www.naturalstandard.com/)

World Health Organization (information on depression) (http://www.who.int/mental_health/management/depression/definition/en/)

ConsumerLabs (comparison of dietary supplement brands) (www.consumerlabs.com)

Books

Baker D. What happy people know: how the new science of happiness can change your life for the better. New York: St. Martin's Press; 2003.

Baumel S. Dealing with depression naturally. Los Angeles (CA): Keats Publishing; 2000.

Emmons H. The chemistry of joy. New York: A Fireside Book (Simon and Schuster); 2006.

Hallowell EM. The childhood roots of adult happiness: five steps to help kids create and sustain lifelong joy. New York: Ballantine Books; 2002.

Lake J. Textbook of integrative mental health. New York: Thieme Medical Publishers; 2007.

Lake JH; Spiegel D. Complementary and alternative treatments in mental health care. Washington, DC: American Psychiatric Publishing; 2007.

Larson JM. Depression-free naturally. New York: Ballantine Books (Random House); 1999.

Shannon S, ed. Handbook of complementary and alternative therapies in mental health. San Diego (CA): Academic Press (Elsevier); 2001.

Shannon S. Please don't label my child. New York: Rodale Press; 2007.

Werbach MR. Nutritional influences on mental illness: a sourcebook of clinical research. Tarzana (CA): Third Line Press, Inc; 1999.

Williams M, Teasdale J, Segal Z, et al. The mindful way through depression: freeing yourself from chronic unhappiness. New York: Guilford Press; 2007.

References

[1] Murray L, Hipwell A, Hooper R, et al. The cognitive development of 5-year-old children of postnatally depressed mothers. J Child Psychol Psychiatry 1996;37(8):927–35.

[2] Birmaher B, Arbelaez C, Brent D. Course and outcome of child and adolescent major depressive disorder. Child Adolesc Psychiatr Clin N Am 2002;11(3):619–37, x.

[3] Zalsman G, Brent DA, Weersing VR. Depressive disorders in childhood and adolescence: an overview: epidemiology, clinical manifestation and risk factors. Child Adolesc Psychiatr Clin N Am 2006;15(4):827–41, vii.

[4] Kowatch RA, Fristad M, Birmaher B, et al. Treatment guidelines for children and adolescents with bipolar disorder. J Am Acad Child Adolesc Psychiatry 2005;44(3):213–35.

[5] Pavuluri MN, Birmaher B, Naylor MW. Pediatric bipolar disorder: a review of the past 10 years. J Am Acad Child Adolesc Psychiatry 2005;44(9):846–71.

[6] Grzywacz JG, Suerken CK, Quandt SA, et al. Older adults' use of complementary and alternative medicine for mental health: findings from the 2002 National Health Interview Survey. J Altern Complement Med 2006;12(5):467–73.

[7] Afifi M. Positive health practices and depressive symptoms among high school adolescents in Oman. Singapore Med J 2006;47(11):960–6.

[8] Hamre HJ, Witt CM, Glockmann A, et al. Anthroposophic therapy for chronic depression: a four-year prospective cohort study. BMC Psychiatry 2006;6:57.

[9] Ludwig DS. Clinical update: the low-glycaemic-index diet. Lancet 2007;369(9565):890–2.

[10] Kleinman RE, Hall S, Green H, et al. Diet, breakfast, and academic performance in children. Ann Nutr Metab 2002;46(Suppl 1):24–30.

[11] Fulkerson JA, Sherwood NE, Perry CL, et al. Depressive symptoms and adolescent eating and health behaviors: a multifaceted view in a population-based sample. Prev Med 2004; 38(6):865–75.

[12] Allgower A, Wardle J, Steptoe A. Depressive symptoms, social support, and personal health behaviors in young men and women. Health Psychol 2001;20(3):223–7.

[13] Bangash SA, Bahna SL. Pediatric food allergy update. Curr Allergy Asthma Rep 2005;5(6): 437–44.

[14] Bischoff SC. Role of mast cells in allergic and non-allergic immune responses: comparison of human and murine data. Nat Rev Immunol 2007;7(2):93–104.

[15] Teufel M, Biedermann T, Rapps N, et al. Psychological burden of food allergy. World J Gastroenterol 2007;13(25):3456–65.

[16] Christie L, Hine RJ, Parker JG, et al. Food allergies in children affect nutrient intake and growth. J Am Diet Assoc 2002;102(11):1648–51.

[17] Brown RS. Exercise and mental health in the pediatric population. Clin Sports Med 1982; 1(3):515–27.

[18] Anton SD, Newton RL Jr, Sothern M, et al. Association of depression with body mass index, sedentary behavior, and maladaptive eating attitudes and behaviors in 11 to 13-year old children. Eat Weight Disord 2006;11(3):e102–8.

[19] Hulens M, Vansant G, Claessens AL, et al. Health-related quality of life in physically active and sedentary obese women. Am J Hum Biol 2002;14(6):777–85.

[20] Pilkington K, Kirkwood G, Rampes H, et al. Yoga for depression: the research evidence. J Affect Disord 2005;89(1–3):13–24.

[21] Tsuno N, Besset A, Ritchie K. Sleep and depression. J Clin Psychiatry 2005;66(10):1254–69.

[22] Beauchemin KM, Hays P. Sunny hospital rooms expedite recovery from severe and refractory depressions. J Affect Disord 1996;40(1–2):49–51.

[23] Manuel JS. Solar flair. Environ Health Perspect 2003;111(2):A104–7.

[24] Lam RW, Levitt AJ, Levitan RD, et al. The Can-SAD study: a randomized controlled trial of the effectiveness of light therapy and fluoxetine in patients with winter seasonal affective disorder. Am J Psychiatry 2006;163(5):805–12.

[25] Epperson CN, Terman M, Terman JS, et al. Randomized clinical trial of bright light therapy for antepartum depression: preliminary findings. J Clin Psychiatry 2004;65(3): 421–5.

[26] Golden RN, Gaynes BN, Ekstrom RD, et al. The efficacy of light therapy in the treatment of mood disorders: a review and meta-analysis of the evidence. Am J Psychiatry 2005; 162(4):656–62.

[27] Martiny K. Adjunctive bright light in non-seasonal major depression. Acta Psychiatr Scand Suppl 2004;(425):7–28.

[28] Frumkin H. Beyond toxicity: human health and the natural environment. Am J Prev Med 2001;20(3):234–40.

[29] Antonioli C, Reveley MA. Randomised controlled trial of animal facilitated therapy with dolphins in the treatment of depression. BMJ 2005;331(7527):1231.

[30] Ross WD, Sholiton MC. Specificity of psychiatric manifestations in relation to neurotoxic chemicals. Acta Psychiatr Scand Suppl 1983;303:100–4.

[31] Schottenfeld RS, Cullen MR. Organic affective illness associated with lead intoxication. Am J Psychiatry 1984;141(11):1423–6.

[32] Johansson C, Castoldi AF, Onishchenko N, et al. Neurobehavioural and molecular changes induced by methylmercury exposure during development. Neurotox Res 2007; 11(3–4):241–60.

[33] Mikolajczyk RT, Bredehorst M, Khelaifat N, et al. Correlates of depressive symptoms among Latino and non-Latino white adolescents: findings from the 2003 California Health Interview Survey. BMC Public Health 2007;7:21.

[34] Galea S, Ahern J, Nandi A, et al. Urban neighborhood poverty and the incidence of depression in a population-based cohort study. Ann Epidemiol 2007;17(3):171–9.

[35] Siefert K, Finlayson TL, Williams DR, et al. Modifiable risk and protective factors for depressive symptoms in low-income African American mothers. Am J Orthopsychiatry 2007; 77(1):113–23.

[36] Igartua KJ, Gill K, Montoro R. Internalized homophobia: a factor in depression, anxiety, and suicide in the gay and lesbian population. Can J Commun Ment Health 2003;22(2): 15–30.

[37] Borrell LN, Kiefe CI, Williams DR, et al. Self-reported health, perceived racial discrimination, and skin color in African Americans in the CARDIA study. Soc Sci Med 2006;63(6): 1415–27.

[38] Whitbeck LB, McMorris BJ, Hoyt DR, et al. Perceived discrimination, traditional practices, and depressive symptoms among American Indians in the upper Midwest. J Health Soc Behav 2002;43(4):400–18.

[39] Szalacha LA, Erkut S, Garcia Coll C, et al. Discrimination and Puerto Rican children's and adolescents' mental health. Cultur Divers Ethnic Minor Psychol 2003;9(2):141–55.

[40] Salzinger S, Rosario M, Feldman RS, et al. Adolescent suicidal behavior: associations with preadolescent physical abuse and selected risk and protective factors. J Am Acad Child Adolesc Psychiatry 2007;46(7):859–66.

[41] Handwerker WP. Childhood origins of depression: evidence from native and nonnative women in Alaska and the Russian Far East. J Womens Health 1999;8(1):87–94.

[42] Widom CS, DuMont K, Czaja SJ. A prospective investigation of major depressive disorder and comorbidity in abused and neglected children grown up. Arch Gen Psychiatry 2007; 64(1):49–56.

[43] Davidson RJ, Kabat-Zinn J, Schumacher J, et al. Alterations in brain and immune function produced by mindfulness meditation. Psychosom Med 2003;65(4):564–70.

[44] Lazar SW, Kerr CE, Wasserman RH, et al. Meditation experience is associated with increased cortical thickness. Neuroreport 2005;16(17):1893–7.

[45] Rathus JH, Miller AL. Dialectical behavior therapy adapted for suicidal adolescents. Suicide Life Threat Behav 2002;32(2):146–57.

[46] Katz LY, Cox BJ, Gunasekara S, et al. Feasibility of dialectical behavior therapy for suicidal adolescent inpatients. J Am Acad Child Adolesc Psychiatry 2004;43(3): 276–82.

[47] Nelson-Gray RO, Keane SP, Hurst RM, et al. A modified DBT skills training program for oppositional defiant adolescents: promising preliminary findings. Behav Res Ther 2006; 44(12):1811–20.

[48] Goldstein TR, Axelson DA, Birmaher B, et al. Dialectical behavior therapy for adolescents with bipolar disorder: a 1-year open trial. J Am Acad Child Adolesc Psychiatry 2007;46(7): 820–30.

[49] van der Kolk BA, Spinazzola J, Blaustein ME, et al. A randomized clinical trial of eye movement desensitization and reprocessing (EMDR), fluoxetine, and pill placebo in the

treatment of posttraumatic stress disorder: treatment effects and long-term maintenance. J Clin Psychiatry 2007;68(1):37–46.

[50] Wall RB. Tai Chi and mindfulness-based stress reduction in a Boston public middle school. J Pediatr Health Care 2005;19(4):230–7.

[51] Gordon JS, Staples JK, Blyta A, et al. Treatment of posttraumatic stress disorder in post-war Kosovo high school students using mind-body skills groups: a pilot study. J Trauma Stress 2004;17(2):143–7.

[52] Hilliard RE. The effects of music therapy-based bereavement groups on mood and behavior of grieving children: a pilot study. J Music Ther 2001;38(4):291–306.

[53] Cassileth BR, Vickers AJ, Magill LA. Music therapy for mood disturbance during hospitalization for autologous stem cell transplantation: a randomized controlled trial. Cancer 2003;98(12):2723–9.

[54] Weydert JA, Shapiro DE, Acra SA, et al. Evaluation of guided imagery as treatment for recurrent abdominal pain in children: a randomized controlled trial. BMC Pediatr 2006; 6:29.

[55] Reynolds WM, Coats KI. A comparison of cognitive-behavioral therapy and relaxation training for the treatment of depression in adolescents. J Consult Clin Psychol 1986; 54(5):653–60.

[56] Murphy WJ, Talmadge CL, Tubis A, et al. Relaxation dynamics of spontaneous otoacoustic emissions perturbed by external tones. I. Response to pulsed single-tone suppressors. J Acoust Soc Am 1995;97(6):3702–10.

[57] Stein RE, Zitner LE, Jensen PS. Interventions for adolescent depression in primary care. Pediatrics 2006;118(2):669–82.

[58] Munoz KA, Krebs-Smith SM, Ballard-Barbash R, et al. Food intakes of US children and adolescents compared with recommendations. Pediatrics 1997;100(3 Pt 1):323–9.

[59] Gesch CB, Hammond SM, Hampson SE, et al. Influence of supplementary vitamins, minerals and essential fatty acids on the antisocial behaviour of young adult prisoners. Randomised, placebo-controlled trial. Br J Psychiatry 2002;181:22–8.

[60] Kaplan BJ, Simpson JS, Ferre RC, et al. Effective mood stabilization with a chelated mineral supplement: an open-label trial in bipolar disorder. J Clin Psychiatry 2001;62(12): 936–44.

[61] Popper CW. Do vitamins or minerals (apart from lithium) have mood-stabilizing effects? J Clin Psychiatry 2001;62(12):933–5.

[62] Simmons M. Nutritional approach to bipolar disorder. J Clin Psychiatry 2003;64(3):338 [author reply 338–9].

[63] Hvas AM, Juul S, Bech P, et al. Vitamin B6 level is associated with symptoms of depression. Psychother Psychosom 2004;73(6):340–3.

[64] Wyatt KM, Dimmock PW, Jones PW, et al. Efficacy of vitamin B-6 in the treatment of premenstrual syndrome: systematic review. BMJ 1999;318(7195):1375–81.

[65] Dimopoulos N, Piperi C, Salonicioti A, et al. Correlation of folate, vitamin B12 and homocysteine plasma levels with depression in an elderly Greek population. Clin Biochem 2007; 40(9–10):604–8.

[66] Tolmunen T, Voutilainen S, Hintikka J, et al. Dietary folate and depressive symptoms are associated in middle-aged Finnish men. J Nutr 2003;133(10):3233–6.

[67] Godfrey PS, Toone BK, Carney MW, et al. Enhancement of recovery from psychiatric illness by methylfolate. Lancet 1990;336(8712):392–5.

[68] Papakostas GI, Petersen T, Denninger JW, et al. Psychosocial functioning during the treatment of major depressive disorder with fluoxetine. J Clin Psychopharmacol 2004;24(5): 507–11.

[69] Bottiglieri T, Hyland K, Laundy M, et al. Folate deficiency, biopterin and monoamine metabolism in depression. Psychol Med 1992;22(4):871–6.

[70] Coppen A, Bailey J. Enhancement of the antidepressant action of fluoxetine by folic acid: a randomised, placebo controlled trial. J Affect Disord 2000;60(2):121–30.

[71] Crellin R, Bottiglieri T, Reynolds EH. Folates and psychiatric disorders. Clinical potential. Drugs 1993;45(5):623–36.

[72] Cashman KD. Vitamin D in childhood and adolescence. Postgrad Med J 2007;83(978): 230–5.

[73] Olmez D, Bober E, Buyukgebiz A, et al. The frequency of vitamin D insufficiency in healthy female adolescents. Acta Paediatr 2006;95(10):1266–9.

[74] Schnadower D, Agarwal C, Oberfield SE, et al. Hypocalcemic seizures and secondary bilateral femoral fractures in an adolescent with primary vitamin D deficiency. Pediatrics 2006; 118(5):2226–30.

[75] Bergqvist AG, Schall JI, Stallings VA. Vitamin D status in children with intractable epilepsy, and impact of the ketogenic diet. Epilepsia 2007;48(1):66–71.

[76] Pappa HM, Gordon CM, Saslowsky TM, et al. Vitamin D status in children and young adults with inflammatory bowel disease. Pediatrics 2006;118(5):1950–61.

[77] Sinnott BP, Licata AA. Assessment of bone and mineral metabolism in inflammatory bowel disease: case series and review. Endocr Pract 2006;12(6):622–9.

[78] Pepmueller PH, Cassidy JT, Allen SH, et al. Bone mineralization and bone mineral metabolism in children with juvenile rheumatoid arthritis. Arthritis Rheum 1996;39(5):746–57.

[79] Patel S, Farragher T, Berry J, et al. Association between serum vitamin D metabolite levels and disease activity in patients with early inflammatory polyarthritis. Arthritis Rheum 2007;56(7):2143–9.

[80] Khan S. Vitamin D deficiency and secondary hyperparathyroidism among patients with chronic kidney disease. Am J Med Sci 2007;333(4):201–7.

[81] Ford L, Graham V, Wall A, et al. Vitamin D concentrations in a UK inner-city multicultural outpatient population. Ann Clin Biochem 2006;43(Pt 6):468–73.

[82] Weng FL, Shults J, Leonard MB, et al. Risk factors for low serum 25-hydroxyvitamin D concentrations in otherwise healthy children and adolescents. Am J Clin Nutr 2007; 86(1):150–8.

[83] Calvo MS, Whiting SJ, Barton CN. Vitamin D fortification in the United States and Canada: current status and data needs. Am J Clin Nutr 2004;80(6 Suppl):1710S–6S.

[84] Reinehr T, de Sousa G, Alexy U, et al. Vitamin D status and parathyroid hormone in obese children before and after weight loss. Eur J Endocrinol 2007;157(2):225–32.

[85] Schneider B, Weber B, Frensch A, et al. Vitamin D in schizophrenia, major depression and alcoholism. J Neural Transm 2000;107(7):839–42.

[86] Armstrong DJ, Meenagh GK, Bickle I, et al. Vitamin D deficiency is associated with anxiety and depression in fibromyalgia. Clin Rheumatol 2007;26(4):551–4.

[87] Lansdowne AT, Provost SC. Vitamin D3 enhances mood in healthy subjects during winter. Psychopharmacology (Berl) 1998;135(4):319–23.

[88] Bohrer T, Krannich JH. Depression as a manifestation of latent chronic hypoparathyroidism. World J Biol Psychiatry 2007;8(1):56–9.

[89] Roman S, Sosa JA. Psychiatric and cognitive aspects of primary hyperparathyroidism. Curr Opin Oncol 2007;19(1):1–5.

[90] Thys-Jacobs S. Micronutrients and the premenstrual syndrome: the case for calcium. J Am Coll Nutr 2000;19(2):220–7.

[91] Bertone-Johnson ER, Hankinson SE, Bendich A, et al. Calcium and vitamin D intake and risk of incident premenstrual syndrome. Arch Intern Med 2005;165(11):1246–52.

[92] Dickerson LM, Mazyck PJ, Hunter MH. Premenstrual syndrome. Am Fam Physician 2003;67(8):1743–52.

[93] Thys-Jacobs S, Ceccarelli S, Bierman A, et al. Calcium supplementation in premenstrual syndrome: a randomized crossover trial. J Gen Intern Med 1989;4(3):183–9.

[94] Heiden A, Frey R, Presslich O, et al. Treatment of severe mania with intravenous magnesium sulphate as a supplementary therapy. Psychiatry Res 1999;89(3):239–46.

[95] Siwek M, Wrobel A, Dudek D, et al. [The role of copper and magnesium in the pathogenesis and treatment of affective disorders]. Psychiatr Pol 2005;39(5):911–20 [in Polish].

[96] Murck H. Magnesium and affective disorders. Nutr Neurosci 2002;5(6):375–89.

[97] Facchinetti F, Sances G, Borella P, et al. Magnesium prophylaxis of menstrual migraine: effects on intracellular magnesium. Headache 1991;31(5):298–301.

[98] Giannini AJ, Nakoneczie AM, Melemis SM, et al. Magnesium oxide augmentation of verapamil maintenance therapy in mania. Psychiatry Res 2000;93(1):83–7.

[99] Schimatschek HF, Rempis R. Prevalence of hypomagnesemia in an unselected German population of 16,000 individuals. Magnes Res 2001;14(4):283–90.

[100] Davidson JR, Abraham K, Connor KM, et al. Effectiveness of chromium in atypical depression: a placebo-controlled trial. Biol Psychiatry 2003;53(3):261–4.

[101] McLeod MN, Gaynes BN, Golden RN. Chromium potentiation of antidepressant pharmacotherapy for dysthymic disorder in 5 patients. J Clin Psychiatry 1999;60(4):237–40.

[102] Docherty JP, Sack DA, Roffman M, et al. A double-blind, placebo-controlled, exploratory trial of chromium picolinate in atypical depression: effect on carbohydrate craving. J Psychiatr Pract 2005;11(5):302–14.

[103] Nowak G, Szewczyk B, Pilc A. Zinc and depression. An update. Pharmacol Rep 2005;57(6): 713–8.

[104] Levenson CW. Zinc: the new antidepressant? Nutr Rev 2006;64(1):39–42.

[105] Lozoff B, Jimenez E, Hagen J, et al. Poorer behavioral and developmental outcome more than 10 years after treatment for iron deficiency in infancy. Pediatrics 2000;105(4):E51.

[106] Rangan AM, Blight GD, Binns CW. Iron status and non-specific symptoms of female students. J Am Coll Nutr 1998;17(4):351–5.

[107] Conklin SM, Harris JI, Manuck SB, et al. Serum omega-3 fatty acids are associated with variation in mood, personality and behavior in hypercholesterolemic community volunteers. Psychiatry Res 2007;152(1):1–10.

[108] Garland MR, Hallahan B, McNamara M, et al. Lipids and essential fatty acids in patients presenting with self-harm. Br J Psychiatry 2007;190:112–7.

[109] Hibbeln JR. Fish consumption and major depression. Lancet 1998;351(9110):1213.

[110] Hibbeln JR. Seafood consumption, the DHA content of mothers' milk and prevalence rates of postpartum depression: a cross-national, ecological analysis. J Affect Disord 2002; 69(1–3):15–29.

[111] Silvers KM, Scott KM. Fish consumption and self-reported physical and mental health status. Public Health Nutr 2002;5(3):427–31.

[112] Hallahan B, Hibbeln JR, Davis JM, et al. Omega-3 fatty acid supplementation in patients with recurrent self-harm. Single-centre double-blind randomised controlled trial. Br J Psychiatry 2007;190:118–22.

[113] Nemets B, Stahl Z, Belmaker RH. Addition of omega-3 fatty acid to maintenance medication treatment for recurrent unipolar depressive disorder. Am J Psychiatry 2002;159(3): 477–9.

[114] Peet M, Horrobin DF. A dose-ranging study of the effects of ethyl-eicosapentaenoate in patients with ongoing depression despite apparently adequate treatment with standard drugs. Arch Gen Psychiatry 2002;59(10):913–9.

[115] Su KP, Shen WW, Huang SY. Omega-3 fatty acids as a psychotherapeutic agent for a pregnant schizophrenic patient. Eur Neuropsychopharmacol 2001;11(4):295–9.

[116] Stoll AL, Locke CA, Marangell LB, et al. Omega-3 fatty acids and bipolar disorder: a review. Prostaglandins Leukot Essent Fatty Acids 1999;60(5–6):329–37.

[117] Stoll AL, Severus WE, Freeman MP, et al. Omega 3 fatty acids in bipolar disorder: a preliminary double-blind, placebo-controlled trial. Arch Gen Psychiatry 1999;56(5): 407–12.

[118] Keck PE Jr, McElroy SL. Carbamazepine and valproate in the maintenance treatment of bipolar disorder. J Clin Psychiatry 2002;63(Suppl 10):13–7.

[119] Wozniak J, Biederman J, Mick E, et al. Omega-3 fatty acid monotherapy for pediatric bipolar disorder: a prospective open-label trial. Eur Neuropsychopharmacol 2007;17(6–7): 440–7.

[120] Alino JJ, Gutierrez JL, Iglesias ML. 5-Hydroxytryptophan (5-HTP) and a MAOI (nial-amide) in the treatment of depressions. A double-blind controlled study. Int Pharmacopsy-chiatry 1976;11(1):8–15.

[121] Angst J, Woggon B, Schoepf J. The treatment of depression with L-5-hydroxytryptophan versus imipramine. Results of two open and one double-blind study. Arch Psychiatr Ner-venkr 1977;224(2):175–86.

[122] Byerley WF, Judd LL, Reimherr FW, et al. 5-Hydroxytryptophan: a review of its antide-pressant efficacy and adverse effects. J Clin Psychopharmacol 1987;7(3):127–37.

[123] Nolen WA, van de Putte JJ, Dijken WA, et al. L-5HTP in depression resistant to re-uptake inhibitors. An open comparative study with tranylcypromine. Br J Psychiatry 1985;147:16–22.

[124] Turner EH, Loftis JM, Blackwell AD. Serotonin a la carte: supplementation with the sero-tonin precursor 5-hydroxytryptophan. Pharmacol Ther 2006;109(3):325–38.

[125] van Hiele LJ. l-5-Hydroxytryptophan in depression: the first substitution therapy in psychi-atry? The treatment of 99 out-patients with 'therapy-resistant' depressions. Neuropsy-chobiology 1980;6(4):230–40.

[126] Shaw K, Turner J, Del Mar C. Tryptophan and 5-hydroxytryptophan for depression. Co-chrane Database Syst Rev 2002;1:CD003198.

[127] Das YT, Bagchi M, Bagchi D, et al. Safety of 5-hydroxy-L-tryptophan. Toxicol Lett 2004;150(1):111–22.

[128] AHRQ. S-Adenosyl-L-methionine for treatment of depression, osteoarthritis, and liver dis-ease. In: AHRQ, editor. 2002. Available at: www.ahrq.gov/clinic/epcsums/melatsun.htm.

[129] Pancheri P, Scapicchio P, Chiaie RD. A double-blind, randomized parallel-group, efficacy and safety study of intramuscular S-adenosyl-L-methionine 1,4-butanedisulphonate (SAMe) versus imipramine in patients with major depressive disorder. Int J Neuropsycho-pharmacol 2002;5(4):287–94.

[130] Hardy ML, Coulter I, Morton SC, et al. S-adenosyl-L-methionine for treatment of depres-sion, osteoarthritis, and liver disease. Evid Rep Technol Assess (Summ) 2003;64:1–3.

[131] Shippy RA, Mendez D, Jones K, et al. S-adenosylmethionine (SAM-e) for the treatment of depression in people living with HIV/AIDS. BMC Psychiatry 2004;4:38.

[132] Williams AL, Girard C, Jui D, et al. S-adenosylmethionine (SAMe) as treatment for depres-sion: a systematic review. Clin Invest Med 2005;28(3):132–9.

[133] Alpert JE, Papakostas G, Mischoulon D, et al. S-adenosyl-L-methionine (SAMe) as an ad-junct for resistant major depressive disorder: an open trial following partial or nonresponse to selective serotonin reuptake inhibitors or venlafaxine. J Clin Psychopharmacol 2004;24(6):661–4.

[134] Linde K, Mulrow CD, Berner M, et al. St John's wort for depression. Cochrane Database Syst Rev 2005;2:CD000448.

[135] Gastpar M, Singer A, Zeller K. Efficacy and tolerability of hypericum extract STW3 in long-term treatment with a once-daily dosage in comparison with sertraline. Pharmacopsy-chiatry 2005;38(2):78–86.

[136] Gastpar M, Singer A, Zeller K. Comparative efficacy and safety of a once-daily dosage of hypericum extract STW3-VI and citalopram in patients with moderate depression: a dou-ble-blind, randomised, multicentre, placebo-controlled study. Pharmacopsychiatry 2006;39(2):66–75.

[137] Findling RL, McNamara NK, O'Riordan MA, et al. An open-label pilot study of St. John's wort in juvenile depression. J Am Acad Child Adolesc Psychiatry 2003;42(8):908–14.

[138] Simeon J, Nixon MK, Milin R, et al. Open-label pilot study of St. John's wort in adolescent depression. J Child Adolesc Psychopharmacol 2005;15(2):293–301.

[139] Schulz V. Safety of St. John's wort extract compared to synthetic antidepressants. Phyto-medicine 2006;13(3):199–204.

[140] Levine J. Controlled trials of inositol in psychiatry. Eur Neuropsychopharmacol 1997;7(2):147–55.

[141] Nierenberg AA, Ostacher MJ, Calabrese JR, et al. Treatment-resistant bipolar depression: a STEP-BD equipoise randomized effectiveness trial of antidepressant augmentation with lamotrigine, inositol, or risperidone. Am J Psychiatry 2006;163(2):210–6.

[142] Levine J, Witztum E, Greenberg BD, et al. Inositol-induced mania? Am J Psychiatry 1996; 153(6):839.

[143] Jones NA, Field T. Massage and music therapies attenuate frontal EEG asymmetry in depressed adolescents. Adolescence 1999;34(135):529–34.

[144] Accortt EE, Allen JJ. Frontal EEG asymmetry and premenstrual dysphoric symptomatology. J Abnorm Psychol 2006;115(1):179–84.

[145] Field T, Hernandez-Reif M, Diego M, et al. Cortisol decreases and serotonin and dopamine increase following massage therapy. Int J Neurosci 2005;115(10):1397–413.

[146] Field T, Diego MA, Hernandez-Reif M, et al. Massage therapy effects on depressed pregnant women. J Psychosom Obstet Gynaecol 2004;25(2):115–22.

[147] Diego MA, Field T, Hernandez-Reif M, et al. Aggressive adolescents benefit from massage therapy. Adolescence 2002;37(147):597–607.

[148] Field T, Morrow C, Valdeon C, et al. Massage reduces anxiety in child and adolescent psychiatric patients. J Am Acad Child Adolesc Psychiatry 1992;31(1):125–31.

[149] Weissman MM, Wickramaratne P, Nomura Y, et al. Offspring of depressed parents: 20 years later. Am J Psychiatry 2006;163(6):1001–8.

[150] Field T, Hernandez-Reif M, Diego M. Newborns of depressed mothers who received moderate versus light pressure massage during pregnancy. Infant Behav Dev 2006;29(1):54–8.

[151] Leo RJ, Ligot JS Jr. A systematic review of randomized controlled trials of acupuncture in the treatment of depression. J Affect Disord 2007;97(1–3):13–22.

[152] Manber R, Schnyer RN, Allen JJ, et al. Acupuncture: a promising treatment for depression during pregnancy. J Affect Disord 2004;83(1):89–95.

[153] Mukaino Y, Park J, White A, et al. The effectiveness of acupuncture for depression–a systematic review of randomised controlled trials. Acupunct Med 2005;23(2):70–6.

[154] Kemper KJ, Sarah R, Silver-Highfield E, et al. On pins and needles? Pediatric pain patients' experience with acupuncture. Pediatrics 2000;105(4 Pt 2):941–7.

ELSEVIER
SAUNDERS

PEDIATRIC CLINICS
OF NORTH AMERICA

Pediatr Clin N Am 54 (2007) 927–947

Integrative Approaches to Childhood Constipation and Encopresis

Timothy P. Culbert, MD[a],*, Gerard A. Banez, PhD[b]

[a]*Integrative Medicine Program, Children's Hospitals and Clinics of Minnesota, 2525 Chicago Avenue South, Minneapolis, MN 55404, USA*
[b]*Behavioral Pediatrics Treatment Service, Cleveland Clinic Children's Hospital, 9500 Euclid Avenue, Cleveland, OH 44195, USA*

Epidemiology

Constipation and encopresis (fecal soiling) are common childhood disorders that may lead to significant functional impairment. These problems account for 3% of general pediatric referrals and up to 30% of referrals to pediatric gastroenterologists [1,2]. The worldwide prevalence of constipation ranges in reports from 0.3% to 28% [3,4]. At least 1% to 3% of children experience encopresis (fecal soiling) [5–7]. The quality of life of children who have constipation and encopresis has been found to be lower than that of children who have more serious gastrointestinal (GI) disorders such as inflammatory bowel disease and gastroesophageal reflux. Youssef and colleagues [8] found that 80 children who had chronic constipation reported a lower quality of life than a healthy control group (n = 46), children who had inflammatory bowel disease (n = 42), and children who had gastroesophageal reflux (n = 56). Children who had constipation also rated themselves as less physically active. Although constipation and encopresis are no longer seen as indicative of serious psychologic disturbance, children who soil have been identified as experiencing more emotional/behavior problems than children who do not soil [9].

Constipation and encopresis typically are categorized as functional GI disorders. As discussed in detail later, increasing evidence suggests that dietary, lifestyle, cognitive, emotional/behavioral, and broader psychosocial factors may all play a role in the etiology, maintenance, and clinically effective treatment of functional GI disorders. Because of the multifactorial nature of constipation, a holistic approach to its assessment and treatment is

---

* Corresponding author.
E-mail address: timothy.culbert@childrensmn.org (T.P. Culbert).

0031-3955/07/$ - see front matter © 2007 Elsevier Inc. All rights reserved.
doi:10.1016/j.pcl.2007.09.001
pediatric.theclinics.com

critical. The application of holistic or integrative approaches that may include complementary/alternative medicine (CAM) to these problems can be clinically effective, often provides less-invasive options than traditional biomedical interventions, and can be blended/balanced safely with other necessary treatments.

The use of CAM therapies is becoming increasingly common among children and is gaining acceptance with pediatricians [10–12]. Use of CAM is particularly high in populations of children and adolescents who have chronic illness, including children who have inflammatory bowel disease [13,14]. In an Australian study, CAM use among 92 children ages 6 months to 16 years attending a pediatric gastroenterology clinic was evaluated by a parental survey [15]. Of the parents who responded, 35.9% reported using CAM therapies for their children, and 23.8% specifically reported using probiotics. Almost all parents (98.6%) stated they would be open to administering CAM to their child if recommended. These findings are consistent with adult studies, which also support the use of "integrative" approaches to GI problems, particularly for constipation [16–18].

Definitions

In children, bowel frequency ranges from four stools per day during the first week of life to 1.2 stools per day at 4 years of age [19]. Most authors agree that fewer than three stools per week is diagnostic of constipation in any age group [20–22].

Constipation is defined not only by abnormally reduced stool frequency but also by painful bowel movements, even when stool frequency is normal [23]. Encopresis refers to the passage of feces in inappropriate places, such as in clothing. In the majority of children, the inappropriate fecal passage is an overflow incontinence that results from constipation. For others, constipation is not present. Fecal soiling may be involuntary or intentional.

Existing systems for classifying constipation have focused on subtypes of functional constipation. The *Diagnostic and Statistical Manual of Mental Disorders, fourth edition* (DSM-IV) diagnostic criteria for encopresis include [24]

1. Repeated passage of feces into inappropriate places (eg, clothing or floor) whether involuntary or intentional
2. At least one such event a month for at least 3 months
3. Chronologic age (or equivalent developmental level) of at least 4 years
4. Behavior is not exclusively the direct physiologic effect of a substance (eg, laxative) or a general medical condition except through a mechanism involving constipation

The DSM-IV requires that constipation and overflow incontinence be coded as present or absent.

The multinational pediatric gastroenterology Rome Working Team has described two diagnostic categories: functional constipation and nonretentive fecal incontinence and has established symptom-based diagnostic criteria for these subtypes [25].

Functional constipation must include two or more of the following in a child with a developmental age of at least 4 years with insufficient criteria for diagnosis of irritable bowel syndrome:

1. Two or fewer defecations in the toilet per week
2. At least one episode of fecal incontinence per week
3. History of retentive posturing or excessive volitional stool retention
4. History of painful or hard bowel movements
5. Presence of a large fecal mass in the rectum
6. History of large-diameter stools that may obstruct the toilet

These criteria must be fulfilled at least once per week for at least 2 months before diagnosis.

Nonretentive fecal incontinence must include all of the following in a child with a developmental age at least 4 years:

Defecation into places inappropriate to the social context at least once per month

No evidence of an inflammatory, anatomic, metabolic, or neoplastic process that explains the subject's symptoms

No evidence of fecal retention

These criteria must also be fulfilled for at least 2 months before diagnosis.

Distinguishing between retentive and nonretentive encopresis, as in the Rome classification, can be particularly useful in treatment planning [26]. Distinguishing between these subtypes helps identify the specific behavioral and medical factors that need to be addressed in an integrative manner. This article focuses on constipation and overflow incontinence, or retentive encopresis, as it is more commonly seen.

Biopsychosocial model and pathophysiology

Like many pediatric GI disorders, the etiology and course of constipation and encopresis are increasingly conceptualized from a broad biopsychosocial perspective [27]. This model assumes that a child's condition is a function of multiple interacting determinants, including early life factors (eg, genetic predisposition, environmental factors), psychosocial factors (eg, life stress, psychologic state, coping, social support), and interactions between physiologic and psychologic factors via the central nervous system–enteric nervous system, or "brain–gut," axis. According to this model, a child who has constipation and encopresis and has no psychosocial problems and parental/familial support will have a better outcome than the child who has these problems as well as coexisting emotional difficulties, high life stress, and limited support. The child's clinical outcome (eg, daily function, quality of life) will, in turn, affect the severity of the defecation difficulties.

The etiology of constipation is multifactorial, including genetic predisposition, diet, withholding of stool, and psychologic/behavioral factors. No specific organic etiology is found in 90% to 95% of children [6,28]. Stool withholding, fear, and anxiety often play a significant role in the development of functional constipation. Constipation associated with stool withholding typically begins with painful defecation. In the effort to delay or prevent defecation, the child begins withholding at urge. Colon walls stretch, and the urge to have a bowel movement passes. Over time, repeated withholding leads to an accumulation of feces, and soft or liquid stool may seep down around the fecal mass into the clothing. Chronic withholding of stool stretches the rectum, resulting in habituation to the sensation of fullness or alteration of thresholds of detection [29], creating a vicious cycle that perpetuates the child's bowel problems.

Conventional treatment

Conventional, evidence-based treatment of constipation and encopresis typically consists of four components: education, disimpaction, maintenance therapy (preventing the reaccumulation of stool), and behavioral treatment [26,30]. A truly holistic approach to constipation and encopresis must engage the child and establish his or her personal interest in and motivation for resolving this condition. Effective education is an important first step in treatment and usually includes

- Developmentally appropriate discussion of the anatomy and physiology of defecation and its associated disorders, and education about the mind–body (brain–gut) connection
- Demystification and validation of the prevalence of constipation and encopresis and discussion of related shame, embarrassment, and social issues
- Exploration of readiness and motivation for change on the part of the patient and the role of parental frustration and concern in seeking treatment
- Reframing the child's perception of the potential for success
- Promoting internal as opposed to external perception of control over toileting difficulties and support for active versus passive coping and treatment strategies
- Parent/caregiver training on appropriate coaching and supportive roles

In the disimpaction or cleanout stage of treatment, enemas, suppositories, or cathartic oral agents are used to evacuate the large intestine. Youssef and DiLorenzo [28] suggest discussing the various options with patients and families. When impaction is severe, a hospital admission for cleanout may be needed. Without a thorough cleanout, the success of later treatment may be limited.

Following disimpaction, maintenance therapy with stool softeners and laxatives is necessary to prevent the reaccumulation of stool. The most commonly used agents are polyethylene glycol 3350 powder [31] and lactulose. These agents draw fluid into the large intestine, preventing stool from drying and facilitating more rapid transit. An increase in dietary fiber (discussed in more detail later) and improved water consumption are recommended also. Although dietary changes alone may not be sufficient to treat constipation and encopresis, they are an important part of a holistic treatment.

Behavioral strategies are an essential component of treatment for many children who have constipation and encopresis. These typically include a sitting schedule, reinforcement program, and a stooling chart or symptom diary to monitor progress. When establishing a behavioral program, it is important to start where the child is at the beginning of treatment. For example, compliance with recommendations and good effort, as opposed to actual stool toileting, may be appropriate initial target behaviors. If stool withholding and/or defecation anxiety contribute to the child's difficulties, positive sits and successive approximations are helpful [26].

Regularly scheduled follow-up visits, initially more frequent, are recommended. These visits address the needs for ongoing dietary modification, behavioral and lifestyle changes, monitoring of bowel activity, and the eventual tapering and discontinuation of medications. Scheduled follow-up allows problem solving and ensures that the treatment plan is being maintained.

Integrative approaches

The approaches described in the remainder of this article may be used concurrently with conventional treatment strategies. The authors' clinical experience suggests that some children and adolescents who have chronic constipation and encopresis may experience only partial success with conventional treatment. Children who have slow bowel motility and those whose toileting is complicated by other neurologic, biologic, psychologic, and social factors may struggle particularly [32]. Medications and traditional behavioral treatment may be insufficient for these children, and an expanded, integrative approach can be quite helpful. The authors' philosophy of care is that of integration: the blending of the best available conventional and CAM strategies in an approach that best fits each individual child and family. Safety of treatment is of paramount importance, and therapy choices are informed by existing empiric evidence, clinical experience, and patient preference. The authors implement treatment strategies in an integrative fashion and subsequently monitor and evaluate outcomes in discrete trial periods, typically 4 to 8 weeks at a time. In some cases, they have been able to use integrative approaches to avoid more invasive options such as anterograde continence enema surgery, multiple enemas, or anal sphincter injections of botulinum toxin.

The authors present integrative approaches to constipation and encopresis together because of their frequent co-occurrence. Treatment strategies are discussed according to the four-category organizational framework proposed by the National Center for Complementary and Alternative Medicine [33] with additional discussions of whole medical systems and lifestyle factors. In many cases, the approach described has a primary impact on constipation. As constipation improves, related fecal soiling decreases.

Mind–body medicine

Biofeedback

Biofeedback is defined as the use of electronic or electromechanical equipment to measure and provide information about specific physiologic functions that can then be controlled in therapeutic directions. Biofeedback often is recommended for children who have constipation and encopresis associated with specific physical, anatomic, or postsurgical complications. It also is recommended for children who exhibit pelvic floor dyssynergia or paradoxical contraction.

Biofeedback treatment of constipation and encopresis typically involves some combination of the following: training in discriminating the sensation of rectal distention, strengthening or controlled relaxation of the external anal sphincter through electromyography (EMG) training, training in the synchronization of internal and external anal sphincter responses, and, for those who have pelvic floor dyssynergia or paradoxical contraction, training in the coordination of abdominal and pelvic floor musculature for elimination. The type of biofeedback used is a function of the physiologic mechanisms hypothesized to underlie the child's soiling. For example, if a child's soiling is thought to be associated with poor sensation of the urge to stool, training aimed at improving rectal sensation is indicated. When soiling is associated with poor control caused by a weak external anal sphincter, sphincter strengthening through EMG biofeedback may be appropriate.

Most existing research seems to focus on biofeedback treatment of constipation and encopresis associated with pelvic floor dyssynergia. Pelvic floor dyssynergia is the abnormal closure of the anal canal during straining for defecation. Children who have dyssynergia squeeze the buttocks and hips during attempts to defecate and are unable to relax the external anal sphincter. These abnormal defecation dynamics are thought to develop in response to past painful bowel movements. To control the amount of stool being passed and to protect against pain, the child squeezes the anal canal during defecation. More than 60% of children who have encopresis may contract the external anal sphincter during defecation, impairing their ability to empty the rectum completely and compounding ongoing impaction [34]. Assessment of pelvic floor dyssynergia uses surface EMG electrodes to monitor abdominal muscles and an anal sensor (manometric sensor within anal canal or surface EMG electrodes just outside the anal opening) to evaluate the child's ability to maintain external anal sphincter relaxation while contracting abdominal muscle. If there is dyssynergia between the two muscle regions, biofeedback training is used to teach appropriate responses.

Numerous uncontrolled studies suggest that this type of biofeedback is an effective adjunctive treatment for encopresis [34,35]. The findings from controlled studies, however, have not been as positive. Although some controlled investigations have found that biofeedback is beneficial [36,37], other studies have reported that the addition of biofeedback to standard medical management does not increase effectiveness of treatment [38–41], even for children who positively evidence pelvic floor dyssynergia. In one study that suggested the benefits of biofeedback treatment [36], no statistically significant differences from the control group were found at long-term follow-up [7]. The results of controlled studies have been described as disappointing by some investigators, such as Loening-Baucke [34]. Others, such as McGrath, Mellon, and Murphy [29], point out methodologic problems (eg, subject selection, varying types/methods of training) that complicate the process of evaluating the efficacy of this treatment. At present, existing data do not support the use of biofeedback as the sole treatment for encopresis. In clinical practice, the authors encourage consideration of brief biofeedback training, typically no more than two to four sessions, for children who have pelvic floor dyssynergia and are not showing a positive response to standard medical management. To be most helpful, such training needs to be provided within the context of a comprehensive biobehavioral treatment of encopresis, including cleanout, medications, sitting schedule, and dietary restrictions/recommendations.

Relaxation strategies

For some children who have constipation, the fear of painful bowel movements leads to a conditioned aversion or more generalized condition referred to as "defecation anxiety." As a result of their anxiety, these children refuse to use the toilet for stooling and become habitual stool withholders. Consequently, they develop problems releasing the pelvic floor muscles and external anal sphincter and are unable to stool normally and completely. Clinically, the authors have found consistently that relaxation techniques, such as progressive muscle relaxation and diaphragmatic breathing, can help release the pelvic floor muscles, promote a general relaxation, and facilitate more comfortable and complete defecation.

Mental imagery/hypnosis

Mental imagery (or self-hypnosis) also is useful for reducing the feelings of anticipatory anxiety associated with defecation [42]. Imagery can be used to assist children in "visualizing" themselves with healthy, relaxed stooling in the bathroom and helps them feel confident about their ability to control their muscles "just the right way." For example, children can be coached to use "favorite place" imagery when sitting on the toilet as a means of relaxing and focusing on positive feelings. Another useful technique is to encourage pediatric patients to visualize themselves having "easy, comfortable" bowel movements in the toilet each day and noticing how "proud they feel" as they engage in this healthy activity.

Stress management

Clinical/anecdotal experience and perspectives from the field of neurophysiology suggest that chronic stress, which affects autonomic nervous system balance in the direction of sympathetic predominance, may lead to a disturbance of intestinal motility and contribute to constipation. One adult study found that adult women exhibited constipation as a psychophysiologic response to life stress [43]. In addition, psychologic distress scores have been found to be higher in patients who have slow-transit constipation than in controls and those who have normal-transit constipation [44]. Although it is difficult to establish that stress leads to constipation in children, at a minimum, emotional distress (eg, depression, anxiety, adjustment reaction) clearly can interfere with children's ability to engage optimally in a treatment plan for constipation.

Lifestyle factors

Diet

Management of dietary factors is a major component of effective management, in both the short and long term, for children who have constipation and encopresis. Dietary management includes attention to dietary fiber, dairy intake, hydration status, and food allergy/sensitivity/intolerance. A recent World Health Organization report on "diet, nutrition and the prevention of chronic diseases" points out that scientific evidence is "increasingly supporting the view that alterations in diets have strong effects, both positive and negative, on health throughout life" [45]. Studies examining the dietary intake of children who have chronic constipation indicate that these children have significantly lower fiber intake than healthy controls [46,47]. Fiber softens and enlarges the stool by pulling in water, resulting in decreased transit time and more frequent bowel movements [48]. Fiber also alters stooling patterns by significantly increasing microbial mass because it acts as a substrate for intestinal bacteria. Gas production from dietary fiber metabolism adds to stool bulk, assisting with smooth muscle contraction [49].

Two recent studies of specific fiber supplements (glucomannan and cocoa husk) underscore their potential benefits. Loening-Baucke and her colleagues [50] evaluated whether fiber supplementation with glucomannan (a fiber gel polysaccharide extract of the Japanese konjac root) was more beneficial than placebo in the treatment of children who had functional constipation with or without encopresis. In a double-blind, crossover study, fiber and placebo were given daily as 100 mg/kg body weight daily (maximal 5 g/d) with 50 mL fluid/500 mg for 4 weeks each. Parents were asked to have children sit on the toilet four times daily after meals and to maintain a stool diary. Age, frequency of bowel movements into the toilet and into the undergarment, presence of abdominal pain, dietary fiber intake, medications, and the presence of an abdominal and/or a rectal fecal mass were recorded at the time of recruitment and 4 weeks and 8 weeks later. Children were rated by the physician as successfully treated when they had three or more bowel movements per and one or fewer episodes of soiling per 3 weeks with no abdominal pain in the last 3 weeks of each 4-week treatment period. Parents provided a global assessment on whether they believed that the child was better during the first or second treatment period. Forty-six chronically constipated children were recruited, and 31 children completed the study. These 31 children (16 boys and 15 girls) were 4.5 to 11.7 years of age (mean age, 7 ± 2 years). All children had functional constipation, and 18 had encopresis when recruited for the study. The results found that children who had constipation alone were more likely to be treated successfully (69%) than those who had constipation and encopresis (28%). Overall, glucomannan was beneficial in the treatment of constipation with and without encopresis. Children who had encopresis and who were already being treated with laxatives also benefited from the additional fiber.

Another study using a parallel, randomized, double-blind, controlled design evaluated the use of fiber in the form of cocoa husk in a group of children who had constipation. After screening, patients were assigned randomly to receive either a cocoa husk supplement or placebo for a period of 4 weeks, along with standardized toilet training procedures. Before and at the conclusion of treatment, the investigators (1) performed anthropometry, a physical examination, and routine laboratory measurements; (2) determined total and segmental colonic transit time; (3) evaluated bowel movement habits and stool consistency with a diary; and (4) received a subjective evaluation from the parents regarding the efficacy of the treatment. Fifty-six chronically constipated children were assigned randomly into the study, but only 48 children completed the study. Study completers were between 3 and 10 years of age, and all had a diagnosis of chronic idiopathic constipation. Total transit time decreased by 45.4 ± 38.4 hours in the cocoa husk group and by 8.7 ± 28.9 hours in the placebo group. The average increase in bowel movement frequency was greater in children who received cocoa husk supplements than in children who received placebo. Patients receiving the cocoa husk treatment also reported a reduction in hard stools. No significant adverse effects were reported during the study. The authors concluded that their data supported the beneficial effect of a cocoa husk supplement rich in dietary fiber [51].

The dairy connection with constipation is complicated and may include allergic or intolerance phenomena that adversely affect the large intestine [52]. For example, Ianoco and colleagues [53] found that cow's milk intolerance can cause perianal lesions leading to painful defecation and subsequent constipation. In their study, lesions improved significantly with soymilk replacement. These researchers also reported that in some children who have constipation, cow's milk intolerance is associated with histologic and manometric changes that lead to constipation [54]. Olness and Tobin [55] described the successful management of 60 children who had constipation, ages 2 to 12 years, with a 6-week dietary program that eliminated dairy intake and included ingestion of a raw bran product.

Low fluid intake, which may lead to a chronic state of dehydration, is cited frequently in the medical and nursing literature as an antecedent of constipation [56]. Elderly patients who have altered fluid intake and decreased bowel motility are prone to experience constipation related to chronic dehydration [57]. To date, no child studies have demonstrated the benefits of increasing fluid intake in states other than severe dehydration.

Other dietary factors as a direct or primary cause of constipation are less clearly defined, but for children who have chronic, refractory constipation, a food allergy evaluation and/or elimination diet with rechallenge can be considered [58,59]. A clean diet with organic foods may also be desirable to avoid GI irritation or insult.

For patients who have constipation and/or retentive encopresis, the authors generally recommend a dairy-elimination diet for the first 4 to 6 weeks of treatment combined with high fiber intake (20–30 g/d) and good hydration to ensure soft stools that are easy to pass. One safe and effective dietary fiber recommendation for many children is the "age + 5" grams guideline [60]. According to this guideline, the amount of dietary fiber recommended daily is the sum of the child's year in age plus five.

Exercise and physical therapy

Although it is commonly taught that physical inactivity may lead to constipation and that exercise promotes bowel activity, there are few studies that actually link physical activity/exercise to increased frequency of bowel movements in children. Although some have suggested that decreased mobility contributes to the development of constipation [61,62], Stewart and colleagues [63] did not demonstrate an association between lack of exercise and constipation in their study of adults. A lack of exercise in children has not been shown to contribute to constipation unless the constipation is severe and protracted, as in persons who have neuromuscular defects [64]. Children who have constipation and encopresis, however, do report being less physically active than normal controls [8].

Toileting posture is one specific physical factor that has received some attention. Sikirov [65] suggested that the use of traditional toilet seats may create an alteration in the recto-anal angle that contributes to the development of constipation. Although this possibility has not been established, constipation that develops during early childhood may be influenced by a variety of precipitants [66], and proper positioning is one potential additional factor.

A study emphasizing the use of physical therapy techniques in children who have complex elimination disorders supports some role for physical therapy [67]. In this case series, 20 children who had voiding dysfunction, including 8 who had encopresis, benefited from a program that included training for proper toileting posture, a voiding calendar, instruction in relaxation of pelvic floor muscles, and strategies for home practice. The study suggested that these noninvasive approaches can be beneficial in a majority of children who have complex elimination disorders, including those who have encopresis.

The authors recommend regular physical activity as part of an overall treatment plan for constipation, along with attention to toileting posture, support of the feet during toilet sitting, and simple pelvic floor exercises [68]. Cox and his colleagues [39] have described a toilet-sitting routine and abdominal straining exercises that the authors have found particularly helpful.

Biologically based practices

Herbals/botanicals

Herbals and botanicals have been used in many cultures over hundreds of years for GI complaints in children, including colic, stomachaches, and nausea. Much of the information about herbals and botanicals has been handed down within specific cultural traditions. Although these agents may well have beneficial effects, good scientific evidence of their effectiveness with childhood constipation is sparse. Herbs and supplements with reported benefits in the treatment of constipation have included psyllium, magnesium, cascara, buckthorn, glycerol, olive oil, senna, aloe, castor oil, guar gum, wheat bran and xantham gum [69]. Other herbs, such as chamomile, lavender, and peppermint may have GI antispasmodic effects and can be used safely in children as essential oils or as herbal tea preparations. In a randomized, double-blind, controlled study, 42 children who had abdominal pain with irritable bowel syndrome were given pH-dependent, enteric-coated peppermint oil capsules or placebo [70]. After 2 weeks, 75% of those receiving peppermint oil had reduced severity of pain, supporting the use of peppermint oil as an antispasmodic.

A recent observational study investigated the use of a Japanese herbal medicine, Dai-Kenchu-To (DKT), in 15 children who had severe constipation over a 3- to 12-month period [71]. Outcomes were assessed with anorectal manometry as well as a clinical scoring system for constipation and fecal incontinence. Investigators concluded that DKT had a favorable effect on constipation as evidenced by improved rectal reservoir functions and sensation threshold as well as significantly improved constipation and incontinence ratings. It was postulated that this effect probably was mediated by DKT-simulated peristalsis of the intestine, resulting in a more regular bowel habit.

Historically, the botanical agents *Rhamni purshiana* and senna (*Sannae folum*) have been used as stimulant laxatives and are approved by the Food and Drug Administration for the treatment of constipation in children over 2 years of age [72]. Dried latex from the inner lining of aloe leaves traditionally has been used as an oral laxative, but additional studies are needed to establish safe and effective dosages. With its high fiber content, ground flaxseed also can work well as a natural laxative and is high in omega-3 fatty acid content. Psyllium (*Plantago Ovata*) is another good fiber source and can be stirred into juices or foods easily.

Probiotics

Probiotics, or "beneficial bacteria" can be defined as "non-pathogenic microbes ... that are used to improve or normalize the balance of gut microflora" [73]. Another description of probiotics is that they are "living microorganisms that affect the host in a beneficial manner by modulating mucosal and systemic immunity as well as improving nutritional and microbial balance in the intestinal tract" [74]. Probiotics are theorized to have a positive effect on intestinal motility and stool consistency, and they are being used increasingly in clinical settings. The most extensive studies to date have involved *Lactobacillus GG*, bifidobacteria, and saccharomyces in the treatment of GI problems such as irritable bowel syndrome, acute infectious gastroenteritis, and antibiotic-associated diarrhea [73,74].

Szajewska and colleagues [75] provided an excellent overview of the use of probiotics in the treatment of a broad range of pediatric GI disorders. Although randomized, controlled trials in adults have identified potential benefits to probiotic use in constipation [76,77], studies examining probiotics and childhood constipation are limited. One report suggested an imbalance of beneficial to harmful bacteria, termed "dysbiosis," in the intestinal flora of children who had chronic constipation [78]. Another study suggested that probiotics may improve intestinal motility in children [79]. A randomized, controlled trial of *Lactobacillus GG* with children was not as encouraging [80]. Participants in this research were 84 children, ages 2 to 16 years, who had constipation. *Lactobacillus GG* was combined with lactulose and compared with a placebo treatment over 12 weeks. Results suggested that the use of *Lactobacillus GG* did not result in clinically significant improvements in bowel movement frequency or fecal soiling when compared with the placebo.

Prebiotics are substances that facilitate the growth of desirable bacteria. A double-blinded, placebo-controlled study in healthy infants evaluated the use of the prebiotic, fructose oligosaccharide cereal. Fructose oligosaccharide is a soluble dietary fiber that increases the water-holding capacity of the stool and stimulates the growth of probiotic bifidobacteria. The use of fructose oligosaccharide resulted in significant increases in the mean number of stools per infant and softer stools [81].

Functional medicine

The field of functional medicine offers an intriguing and potentially useful holistic, biologic approach to GI disorders, including constipation. Functional medicine is defined as "a systems biology approach to health care: a comprehensive analysis of the manner in which all components of the human biological system interact functionally with the environment over time" [82]. In the *Textbook of Functional Medicine*, Lukaczer [83] proposed a general approach (the "four Rs") to GI disorders:

- Remove—What might need to be removed to support healthy GI function? This may include pathogenic bacteria, yeast or protozoa, as well as foods or dietary additives that result in allergic or intolerant responses.
- Replace—What factors may need to be replaced to support healthy GI function? This could include digestive enzymes or stomach acid.
- Re-inoculate—What is needed to restore a healthy balance of intestinal microflora? Probiotics and prebiotics may be needed for restoration purposes.
- Repair—What may be needed to support regeneration/repair of a healthy mucosal layer? This could involve providing specific nutrients such as zinc, glutamine, and essential fatty acids.

Manipulative and body-based practices

Massage

Massage is one of the oldest health care practices and has been used since ancient times in India, China, Arabia, Egypt, and Greece. The term "massage" is used to refer to a variety of techniques, some of which require significant training, including structural integration (Rolfing), movement integration (Feldenkreis, Alexander technique), and pressure point techniques (shiatsu, acupressure). Massage techniques manipulate, compress, and stretch the skin, muscles, and joints. Thee techniques activate a variety of health-promoting mechanisms, including

- Mechanical effects—enhancing blood flow to the muscles and soft tissues and promoting lymphatic flow
- Immunologic effects—enhancing specific immune cell functions such as natural killer cell activity
- Neurologic effects—triggering the relaxation response and lowering sympathetic nervous system arousal, reducing serum cortisol, enhancing endogenous serotonin and dopamine levels, and modulating pain perception

Ernst [84] reviewed four controlled trials of abdominal massage for chronic constipation and concluded that it is a very promising but not proven approach to treatment. He pointed out that massage was perceived as agreeable by most patients. Additional studies describe the successful use of abdominal massage for constipated adult patients in palliative care settings [85] and for patients who had spinal cord injury [86].

In the authors' experience, abdominal massage for constipation in children is clinically useful for promoting bowel activity and relaxing the abdomen and pelvic floor. Parents can be trained to use this technique in as little as one training session. The usual technique is imagining the abdomen with a clock face superimposed on it, with the navel as the center of the clock. Gentle, clockwise massage of the abdomen with a 2- to 3-inch span from the navel is administered with mild-to-moderate pressure, 30 seconds to 1 minute at each location [87].

Chiropractic and osteopathic manipulation

Although chiropractic and osteopathic manipulation techniques are quite popular, few studies support their use in treating chronic constipation and encopresis. Quist and Duray [88] described successful chiropractic manipulation for an 8-year-old who had chronic constipation. In this case study, the patient was determined to suffer from "sacral subluxation complex." Manipulation of the sacral area and external abdominal massage were performed over a 4-week period at a frequency of two visits per week, with benefits noted immediately following the initial session. Osteopathic manipulation also may be an option, but there are no published studies of its effectiveness. From the osteopathic standpoint, tissue stresses and dysfunction in the sacral and pelvic areas are common findings in childhood constipation and may be responsive to osteopathic manipulative techniques [89].

Energy medicine

Electrical nerve stimulation

Although some may not consider transcutaneous electrical nerve stimulation (TENS) to be a CAM modality, it can be classified as an energy therapy in that it involves the application of energy in the form of an electrical current to the body. In a pilot study, eight children who had treatment-refractory chronic constipation and soiling were provided TENS treatment three times per week for 3 to 4 weeks [90]. Four surface electrodes were used, with two placed on the paraspinal area of T9/T10 to L2 and one to either side of the anterior abdominal wall beneath the costal margin. The TENS treatment, using interferential current application, resulted in cessation of soiling in seven of the eight subjects and increased the frequency of spontaneous defecation in five of the eight subjects.

Sacral neuromodulation involves modifying the neural control of the lower bowel and pelvic floor through sacral nerve stimulation. In a recent case series, sacral neuromodulation with a surgically implanted device was used and evaluated. Participants were 23 children, ages 6 to 15 years, who had dysfunctional elimination syndromes including both bowel and bladder problems. After a mean follow-up period of 13.3 months after stimulation, the majority of patients who had constipation/soiling demonstrated significant improvements [91].

Reflexology

Reflexology can be defined as a therapy that uses manual pressure applied to specific areas or zones of the feet that are believed to correspond to different areas of the body, thereby effecting therapeutic change. Bishop and colleagues [92] described the use of reflexology in the successful treatment of 50 children, ages 3 to 14 years, who had chronic constipation and/or encopresis. In this study, children received six 30-minute sessions of reflexology treatment. Results supported a general increase in bowel movement frequency and decrease in soiling accidents.

The authors' clinical experience suggests that children who have chronic constipation can benefit from energy therapies such as Reiki and healing touch, but no published studies were identified.

Whole medical systems

Many systems of medicine and healing around the world have their own healing approaches in the assessment and treatment of disease including GI dysfunction [93]. The review of these alternative systems is limited to approaches for which the authors could access published studies.

Acupuncture/traditional Chinese medicine

Traditional Chinese medicine recognizes different types of constipation, specific etiologies for each condition (eg, spleen qi deficiency, liver qi stagnation, yin deficiency), and related treatments including dietary changes, massage, herbal therapies, and acupuncture. Yong [94] explains that within

Chinese culture, the term "hot qi" is used to describe various physical symptoms in children. In a cross-sectional survey at a private clinic and public hospital in Hong Kong, constipation was among the top five symptoms described as a component of "hot qi" [94]. Remedies included increased consumption of water, fruit, soup, and the use of herbal beverages.

Acupuncture, a component of traditional Chinese medicine, has become increasingly popular in the treatment of adult GI disorders [95,96]. Historical evidence and the experience of expert traditional Chinese medicine practitioners suggest its broad applicability to pediatric GI disorders as well [97].

Acupuncture may have multiple effects on GI function, including alteration of acid secretion, changes in GI motility, and effects on visceral pain [96]. Specific effects of certain acupoints, such as the stimulatory effects of ST-36, may be beneficial in the treatment of constipation.

Broide and colleagues [98] treated 17 children who had chronic constipation with five weekly placebo acupuncture sessions followed by 10 weekly true acupuncture sessions. Frequency of bowel movements improved from 1.4 per week at baseline to 4.4 per week in male subjects and from 1.4 per week at baseline to 5.6 per week in female subjects after the 10 true acupuncture sessions were completed. Basal panopioid levels were measured and were noted to be lower at baseline in constipated children but gradually increased to control levels after 10 true acupuncture sessions.

Homeopathy

Homeopathy is a therapeutic system developed in the nineteenth century by the German physician, Samuel Hahnemann. Homeopathy emphasizes a holistic approach with the individualization of treatment. The main tenet of homeopathy is the law of similars, which emphasizes the use of preparations of substances whose effects, when administered to healthy subjects, correspond to the manifestations of the disorder. For constipation, commonly used homeopathic remedies include alumina, bryonia, calcarea carb, and lycopodium [99]. The treatment is individualized to each person's presenting symptoms (eg, bryonia for hard, dry stools, nux vomica for incomplete evacuation, silica for large, hard stools, and sulfur for stool that is hard and painful to pass) [100]. Although there is evidence for the use of homeopathic approaches for other pediatric GI disorders, including acute infectious diarrhea [101], the authors could identify no studies that have examined the use of homeopathy for constipation and encopresis. It remains, however, a fairly popular and relatively safe approach.

Summary

Although the evidence base for conventional interventions for constipation and encopresis is strong and growing, not all children achieve complete symptom resolution from these treatments, and some experience side effects that limit their usefulness. An increasing number are seeking alternative treatments and are particularly open to less invasive nondrug options. An integrative approach to treatment of constipation and encopresis blends the best of conventional and alternative therapies in a personalized plan that best fits each child and family. Clearly, the heterogeneity of these disorders warrants individualized as well as holistic treatment. Because the extant research suggests a variety of subtypes of constipation and encopresis with multifactorial etiologies, satisfaction of existing diagnostic criteria does not, in itself, suggest a standard and optimal course of treatment for all children. It is authors' experience that optimal treatment of constipation and encopresis follows from a comprehensive evaluation of all potential physiologic and psychologic contributors as well as the child and family's values, beliefs, and culture. An understanding of these factors and processes allows the practitioner to develop a treatment plan that best fits the child's and family's needs. This plan may blend conventional treatment strategies, such as a high-fiber diet, stool softeners, and a bowel-training program, with complementary strategies like probiotics, biofeedback, and massage. Future treatments for children who have constipation/encopresis may be increasingly self-directed and even completed at home through the Internet [102]. As empirically informed practitioners, the authors believe that it is their responsibility to identify and recommend treatment strategies that have the greatest evidence base. As integrative and holistic practitioners, however, they encourage blending of alternative therapies for constipation and encopresis with empirically supported conventional approaches. When scientific evidence for a particular alternative treatment is limited, the authors place a priority on its safety, affordability, and congruence with patient values/beliefs [103]. If a treatment is safe, affordable, and acceptable to the patient (and family), the authors support its use in conjunction with more established treatment strategies. They expect that as more is learned about the efficacy and safety of certain alternative treatments for constipation and encopresis, the integration of these strategies and conventional treatments will become increasingly standard and best practice.

References

[1] Partin J, Hamill S, Fischel J, et al. Painful defecation and fecal soiling in children. Pediatrics 1992;89(6):107–9.
[2] Sonnenberg A, Koch T. Physician visits in the United States for constipation: 1958 to 1986. Dig Dis Sci 1989;34:606–11.
[3] Sonnenberg A, Koch T. Epidemiology of constipation in the United States. Dis Colon Rectum 1989;32:1–8.
[4] Loening-Baucke V. Constipation in early childhood: patient characteristics, treatment and long-term follow-up. Gut 1993;34:606–11.
[5] Rutter M. Helping troubled children. Harmonds-Worth (UK): Penguin Education; 1975.
[6] Levine M. Children with encopresis: a descriptive analysis. Pediatrics 1975;56:412–6.
[7] Loening-Baucke V. Biofeedback treatment for chronic constipation and encopresis in childhood: long-term outcome. Pediatrics 1995;96:105–10.

 [8] Youssef N, Langseder A, Verga B, et al. Chronic childhood constipation is associated with impaired quality of life: a case-controlled study. J Pediatr Gastroenterol Nutr 2005;41: 56–60.
 [9] Joinsen C, Heron J, Butler U, et al. Psychological differences between children with and without soiling problems. Pediatrics 2006;117(5):1575–84.
[10] Sikand A, Laken M. Pediatricians experience with and attitudes toward complementary/ alternative medicine. Arch Pediatr Adolesc Med 1998;152(11):1059–64.
[11] Sawni A, Thomas R. Pediatricians' attitudes, experience and referral patterns regarding complementary/alternative medicine: a national survey. BMC Complement Altern Med 2007;4:18.
[12] Kemper K, O'Connor K. Pediatricians' recommendations for complementary and alternative medical (CAM) therapies. Ambul Pediatr 2004;4(6):482–7.
[13] Heuschkel R, Afzal N, Wuerth A, et al. Complementary medicine use in children and young adults with inflammatory bowel disease. Am J Gastroenterol 2002;97(2):382–8.
[14] Day A, Whitten K, Bohane T. Use of complementary and alternative medicines by children and adolescents with inflammatory bowel disease. J Paediatr Child Health 2004;40(12): 681–4.
[15] Day A. Use of complementary therapies and probiotic agents by children attending gastroenterology outpatient clinics. J Paediatr Child Health 2002;38:343–6.
[16] Ernst E. Constipation. In: Ernst E, editor. The desktop guide to complementary and alternative medicine-an evidence based approach. St. Louis (MO): Mosby; 2001. p. 248–52.
[17] Koretz R, Rotblatt M. Complementary and alternative medicine in gastroenterology: the good, the bad and the ugly. Clin Gastroenterol Hepatol 2004;2(11):957–67.
[18] Tillisch K. Complementary and alternative medicine for functional gastrointestinal disorders. Gut 2006;55:593–9.
[19] Weaver L, Steiner H. The bowel habit of young children. Arch Dis Child 1984;59(7): 649–52.
[20] Corrazziari E, Cucchiara S, Staiano A, et al. Gastrointestinal transit time, frequency of defecation, and anorectal manometry in healthy and constipated children. J Pediatr 1985; 106(3):379–82.
[21] Read N, Timms J. Defecation and the pathophysiology of constipation. Clin Gastroenterol 1986;15(4):937–65.
[22] Wyman J, Heaton K, Manning A, et al. Variability of colonic function in healthy subjects. Gut 1978;19(2):146–50.
[23] Staiano A, Ciarla C. Pelvic floor syndromes: infant dyschezia, functional fecal retention, and nonretentive soiling. In: Hyman P, editor. Pediatric functional gastrointestinal disorders. New York: Academy Professional Information Services; 1999. p. 10.1–2.
[24] Diagnosis and statistical manual of mental disorders. Fourth edition. Washington, DC: American Psychological Association; 2000.
[25] Rasquin A, DiLorenzo C, Forbes D, et al. Childhood functional gastrointestinal disorders: child/adolescent. Gastroenterology 2006;130:1527–37.
[26] Cunningham C, Banez G. Pediatric gastrointestinal disorders. Biopsychosocial assessment and treatment. New York: Springer; 2006.
[27] Drossman D. The functional gastrointestinal disorders and the Rome II process. In: Drossman D, Corazziari N, Talley W, et al, editors. Rome II: the functional gastrointestinal disorders. Lawrence (KS): Allen Press; 2000. p. 1–29.
[28] Youssef N, DiLorenzo C. The role of mobility in functional abdominal disorders in children. Pediatr Ann 2001;30:24–30.
[29] McGrath M, Mellon M, Murphy L. Empirically supported treatments in pediatric psychology: constipation and encopresis. J Pediatr Psychol 2000;25:225–54.
[30] Blum N. Elimination disorders. In: Greydanus D, Patel D, Pratt H, editors. Behavioral pediatrics. 2nd edition. New York: iUniverse; 2006. p. 206–18.

[31] Thomson M, Jenkins H, Bisset W, et al. Polyethylene glycol 3350 plus electrolytes for chronic constipation in children: a double blind, placebo controlled trial. Arch Dis Child 2007;11:996–1000.

[32] Youssef N, DiLorenzo C. Treatment options for refractory childhood constipation. Curr Treat Options Gastroenterol 2002;5(5):377–87.

[33] National Center for Complementary and Alternative Medicine. Available at: www.nccam. nih.gov. Accessed September 1, 2007.

[34] Loening-Baucke V. Biofeedback training in children with functional constipation: a critical review. Dig Dis Sci 1996;41:65–71.

[35] Brooks R, Copen R, Cox D, et al. Review of the treatment literature for encopresis, functional constipation, and stool-toileting refusal. Ann Behav Med 2002;22(3):260–7.

[36] Loening-Baucke V. Modulation of abnormal defecation dynamics by biofeedback treatment in chronically constipated children with encopresis. J Pediatr 1990;116:214–22.

[37] Wald A, Chandra R, Gabel S, et al. Evaluation of biofeedback in childhood encopresis. J Pediatr Gastroenterol Nutr 1987;6:554–8.

[38] Cox D, Sutphen J, Ling W, et al. Additive benefits of laxative, toilet training, and biofeedback therapies in the treatment of pediatric encopresis. J Pediatr Psychol 1996;21:659–70.

[39] Cox D, Sutphen J, Borowitz S, et al. Contribution of behavior therapy and biofeedback to laxative therapy in the treatment of pediatric encopresis. Ann Behav Med 1998;20:70–6.

[40] Nolan T, Catto-Smith T, Coffey C, et al. Randomised controlled trial of biofeedback training in persistent encopresis with anismus. Arch Dis Child 1998;79:131–5.

[41] Van der Plas R, Benninga M, Buller H, et al. Biofeedback training in treatment of childhood constipation: a randomised controlled study. Lancet 1996;348:776–80.

[42] Olness K. Autohypnosis in functional megacolon in children. Am J Clin Hypn 1976;19: 28–32.

[43] Devroede G, Girard G, Bouchoucha M, et al. Idiopathic constipation by colonic dysfunction. Dig Dis Sci 1989;34(9):1428–33.

[44] Wald A, Hinds J, Caruana B. Psychological and physiological characteristics of patients with severe idiopathic constipation. Gastroenterology 1989;97:932–7.

[45] World Health Organization Technical Report Series 916. Diet, nutrition, and the prevention of chronic disease. Geneva (Switzerland): World Health Organization; 2003.

[46] Morais M, Vitolo M, Aquirre A, et al. Measurement of low dietary fiber intake as a risk factor for chronic constipation. J Pediatr Gastroenterol Nutr 1999;29(2):132–5.

[47] Mclung H. Constipation and dietary fiber intake in children. Pediatrics 1995;86:999–1001.

[48] Williams C. Children and fiber: how much is beneficial-how much is safe? Pediatric Basics 2006;2006:2–11.

[49] Cummings J. Constipation, dietary fiber and the control of large bowel function. Postgrad Med J 1984;60:811–9.

[50] Loening-Baucke V, Miele E, Staiano A. Fiber (glucomanna) is beneficial in the treatment of childhood constipation. Pediatrics 2004;113(3):e259–64.

[51] Castillejo G, Bullo M, Anguera A, et al. A controlled randomized double blind trial to evaluate the effect of a supplement of cocoa husk that is rich in dietary fiber on colonic transit in constipated pediatric patients. Pediatrics 2006;118:641–8.

[52] Turenen S, Karttunen T, Kokkonen J. Lymphoid nodular hyperplasia and cow's milk hypersensitivity in children with chronic constipation. J Pediatr 2004;145(5):606–11.

[53] Iacono G, Cavataio F, Montalto G, et al. Intolerance of cow's milk and chronic constipation in children. N Engl J Med 1998;339(16):1100–4.

[54] Ianoco G, Bonventure S, Scalici C, et al. Food intolerance and chronic constipation: manometry and histology study. Eur J Gastroenterol Hepatol 2006;18(2):143–50.

[55] Olness K, Tobin J. Chronic constipation in children: can it be managed by diet alone? Postgrad Med 1982;2(4):149–54.

[56] Young R. Pediatric constipation. Gastroenterol Nurs 1996;19:88–9.

[57] McLane A, McShane R. Nursing diagnosis: colonic constipation. In: Carroll-Johnson RM, editor. Classification of nursing diagnoses. Philadelphia: Lippincott; 1989. p. 431.

[58] Garcia-Careaga M, Kerner J. Gastrointestinal manifestations of food allergies in pediatric patients. Nutr Clin Pract 2005;20(5):526–35.

[59] Carroccio A, Iacono G. Chronic constipation and food hypersensitivity –an intriguing relationship. Aliment Pharmacol Ther 2006;24(9):1295–304.

[60] Williams C, Bollella M, Wynder E. A new recommendation for dietary fiber in childhood. Pediatrics 1995;96(5):S985–8.

[61] Hogstel M, Nelson M. Anticipation and early detection can reduce bowel elimination complications. Geriatr Nurs 1992;13(1):28–33.

[62] Whitehead W, Drinkwater D, Cheskin L, et al. Constipation in the elderly living at home. Definition, prevalence, and relationship to lifestyle and health status. J Am Geriatr Soc 1989;37(5):423–9.

[63] Stewart R, Moore M, Marks R, et al. Correlates of constipation in the ambulatory elderly population. Am J Gastroenterol 1992;7(7):859–64.

[64] Silverman A, Roy C. Pediatric clinical gastroenterology. St. Louis (MO): Mosby; 1983.

[65] Sikirov B. Primary constipation: an underlying mechanism. Med Hypotheses 1989;28(2): 71–3.

[66] Borowitz S, Cox D, Tam A, et al. Precipitants of constipation during early childhood. J Am Board Fam Pract 2003;16(6):213–8.

[67] Depaepe H, Renson C, Van Laeke E, et al. Pelvic-floor therapy and toilet training in young children with dysfunctional voiding and obstipation. BJU Int 2000;85:889–93.

[68] Hulme J. Bladder and bowel issues for kids. Missoula (MT): Phoenix Publishing; 2003. p. 63–8.

[69] Natural Medicines Comprehensive Database condition Search 2007. Constipation. Available at: www.naturaldatabase.com. Accessed September 1, 2007.

[70] Kline R, Kline J, Di Palma J, et al. Enteric-coated pH-dependent peppermint oil capsules for the treatment of irritable bowel syndrome in children. J Pediatr 2001;138(1):125–8.

[71] Iwai N, Kume Y, Kimura O, et al. Effects of herbal medicine dai-kenchu-to on anorectal function in children with sever constipation. Eur J Surgery 2007;17(2):115–8.

[72] Gardiner P, Kemper K. For GI complaints: which herbs and supplements spell relief? Contemp Pediatr 2005;22:50–5.

[73] Charrois T, Sandhu G, Vohra S. Probiotics. Pediatr Rev 2006;27(4):137–9.

[74] Penner R, Fedorak R, Madsen K. Probiotics and nutraceuticals: non-medicinal treatments of gastrointestinal disorders. Curr Opin Pharmacol 2005;5:596–603.

[75] Szajewska H, Setty M, Mrukowicz J, et al. Probiotics in gastrointestinal diseases in children: hard and not-so-hard evidence of efficacy. J Pediatr Gastroenterol Nutr 2006;42(5):454–75.

[76] Koebnick C, Wagner I, Leitzman P, et al. Probiotic beverage containing Lactobacillus casei Shirota improves gastrointestinal symptoms in patients with chronic constipation. Can J Gastroenterol 2003;17:655–9.

[77] Mollenbrink M, Bruckshen E. Treatment of chronic constipation with physiologic Escherichia coli bacteria. Results of a clinical study of the effectiveness and tolerance of microbiological therapy with the E. Coli Nissle 1917 strain (Mutaflor). Med Klin (Munich) 1994;89:587–93.

[78] Zoppi G, Cinquetti M, Luciano A, et al. The intestinal ecosystem in chronic functional constipation. Acta Paediatr 1998;87:836–41.

[79] Salminen S, Salminen E. Lactulose, lactic acid bacteria, intestinal microecology and mucosal protection. Scand J Gastroenterol 1997;2:45–8.

[80] Banaszkiewicz A, Szajewska H. Ineffectiveness of Lactobacillus GG as an adjunct to lactulose for the treatment of constipation in children: a double blind placebo controlled randomized trial. J Pediatr 2005;146:363–8.

[81] Moore N, Chao C, Yang L, et al. Effects of fructo-ologosaccharide-supplemented cereal: a double blind placebo controlled multinational study. Br J Nutr 2003;90:581–7.

[82] Jones D, editor. Textbook of functional medicine. Gig Harbor (WA): Institute for Functional Medicine; 2005.

[83] Lukaczer D. The 4R program. In: Jones D, editor. Textbook of functional medicine. Gig Harbor (WA): Institute for Functional Medicine; 2005. p. 462–9.

[84] Ernst E. Abdominal massage for chronic constipation: a systematic review of controlled clinical trails. Forsch Komplementarmed 1999;6:149–51.

[85] Preece J. Introducing abdominal massage in palliative care for the relief of constipation. Complement Ther Nurs Midwifery 2002;8:101–5.

[86] Ayas S, Leblebici B, Sozay S, et al. The effect of abdominal massage on bowel function in patients with spinal cord injury. Am J Phys Med Rehabil 2006;85(12):951–5.

[87] Reed-Gach M. Acupressure potent points. New York: Bantam books; 1990. p. 70.

[88] Quist D, Duray S. Resolution of symptoms of chronic constipation in an 8 yo male after chiropractic treatment. J Manipulative Physiol Ther 2007;30(1):65–8.

[89] Carreiro J. An osteopathic approach to children. London: Churchill Livingstone; 2003. p. 179–80.

[90] Chase J, Robertson V, Southwell B, et al. Pilot study using transcutaneous electrical nerve stimulation interferential current to treat chronic treatment-resistant constipation and soiling in children. J Gastroenterol Hepatol 2005;20(7):1054–61.

[91] Humphreys M, Vandersteen D, Slezak J, et al. Preliminary results of sacral neuromodulation in 23 children. J Urol 2006;176(5):2227–31.

[92] Bishop E, McKinnon E, Weir E, et al. Reflexology in the management of encopresis and chronic constipation. Paediatr Nurs 2003;15(3):20–1.

[93] Micozzi M. Fundamentals of complementary and integrative medicine. St Louis (MO): Saunders; 2006. p. 375–606.

[94] Yong F, Ng D, Chung-hong C, et al. Parental use of the term *hot qi* in their children in Hong Kong: a cross sectional survey of *hot qi* in children. J EthnoBiol Ethnomed 2006;2:2.

[95] Ouyang H, Chen J. Therapeutic roles of acupuncture in functional gastrointestinal disorders. Aliment Pharmacol Ther 2004;20:831–41.

[96] Takahashi T. Acupuncture for functional gastrointestinal disorders. J Gastroenterol 2006; 41:408–17.

[97] Loo M. Pediatric acupuncture. London: Churchill Livingstone; 2002. p. 200–7.

[98] Broide E, Pintov S, Portnoy S, et al. Effectiveness of acupuncture for treatment of childhood constipation. Dig Dis Sci 2001;46(6):1270–5.

[99] Ullman D. Homeopathic medicine for children and infants. New York: Tarcher/Putnam; 1992. p. 68–9.

[100] Mantle F. Complementary and alternative medicine for child and adolescent care. Edinburgh (Scotland): Butterworth Heinemann; 2004. p. 109–12.

[101] Jacobs J, Jonas W, Jimenez-Perez M, et al. Homeopathy for childhood diarrhea: combined results and meta-analysis from three randomized controlled clinical trials. Pediatr Infect Dis J 2003;22(3):229–34.

[102] Ritterband L, Cox D, Walker L, et al. An Internet intervention for pediatric encopresis. J Consult Clin Psychol 2003;71(5):910–7.

[103] Cohen M, Kemper K. Complementary therapies in pediatrics: a legal perspective. Pediatrics 2005;115:774–80.

ELSEVIER
SAUNDERS

PEDIATRIC CLINICS
OF NORTH AMERICA

Pediatr Clin N Am 54 (2007) 949–967

Probiotics in Children

Benjamin Kligler, MD, MPH[a,b,*], Patrick Hanaway, MD[c], Andreas Cohrssen, MD[a,d]

[a]Albert Einstein College of Medicine, 1300 Morris Park Avenue, Bronx, NY 10463, USA
[b]Continuum Center for Health and Healing, 245 Fifth Avenue, Second Floor, New York, NY 10016, USA
[c]Genova Diagnostics, 63 Zillicoa Street, Asheville, NC 28801, USA
[d]Beth Israel Residency Program in Urban Family Practice, 16 East 16th Street, New York, NY, USA

The gastrointestinal microflora has been a subject of interest in medical science since the early twentieth century when Nobel laureate Metchnikoff [1] proposed that many diseases were related to the action of gut bacteria and that consuming beneficial lactic acid–producing bacteria (by drinking fermented milk) was health promoting because it prevented growth of putrefactive bacteria in the gut. Recent scientific advances have reawakened interest in these clinical observations, highlighting the role of the gut flora in metabolism, protection, and immune regulation. The authors examine the development of this postnatal organ, review its role in health and disease, and discuss the clinical opportunities to modify its expression through the use of probiotics.

Gastrointestinal flora and probiotics: the development of a postnatal organ

At birth, the human body is sterile. Colonization of the mucosal membranes starts during delivery before the first breath and evolves quickly over the first days of life [2], but quantity and species vary markedly over the first 2 years of life [3]. There is a rapid succession of bacteria, depending on environmental influences including maternal flora, place of delivery, type of delivery (cesarean section or vaginal), age at birth, hygiene measures,

---

* Corresponding author. Continuum Center for Health and Healing, 245 Fifth Avenue, Second Floor, New York, NY 10016.
  E-mail address: bkligler@chpnet.org (B. Kligler).

antibiotics, birth order, and type of feeding. As the child moves to solid food, the gut flora becomes more adultlike in composition [4].

The variations in the gastrointestinal microbiota over the first 2 years of life have implications for the functional ability of gut flora to optimize its myriad activities in nutrition/metabolism, defense, and education of the immune system. Many species have evolved to peacefully coexist within the gastrointestinal tract. More than 500 species have been noted, each with numerous strains identified by molecular probes [5]. Overall, the number of bacteria present in the gastrointestinal lumen is tenfold the number of cells in the human body [2]. These species interact with the innate immune system and play a critical role in the dynamic education of the adaptive immune system, promoting balance and strength in the developing immune system.

The probiotic theory was championed by Metchnikoff [1], who recognized the value of fermented foods in promoting optimal digestive health. Today, the term *probiotics* (Greek, *pro*, "for," and *biosis*, "life") has been defined as nonpathogenic microorganisms that, when ingested, exert a positive influence on host health or physiology [6]. A probiotic must be of human origin, be resistant to destruction by gastric acid and bile, adhere to intestinal epithelial tissue, and be able to colonize the gastrointestinal tract (if only for a short period) [7]. Beneficial gut flora can also be stimulated by nondigestible foods, which are known as prebiotics [8]. Clinical studies show how these prebiotic and probiotic agents can be used to promote balance in the gut flora, creating benefit for a number of diseases.

Development of the gut flora

The child in utero is swimming in and drinking amniotic fluid, which is sterile. With delivery, environmental exposure to the maternal birth canal, fecal material, skin, and birthing assistants/nurses determines the initial make-up of facultative aerobic organisms that first colonize. This milieu rapidly gives way to *Enterobacter* and *Streptococcus* spp over the first few days of life and then to *Bifidobacterium* and *Bacteroides* spp by the end of the first week [9]. Factors that influence the succession of gut flora from that time forward include type of delivery [10], feeding habits [11], gestational age [10], hospitalization [3], and infant antibiotic use [12].

It is well established that the type of delivery has an impact on gut flora that goes beyond the first few days of life. Cesarean section is associated with a decrease in the beneficial obligate anaerobes *Bacteroides* and *Bifidobacterium*, along with an increase in *Clostridium* sp [13]. Of interest, these differences in gut flora are not found in developing countries where early colonization with enterobacteria is the norm in vaginal and in abdominal births [14].

Pronounced changes are again noted in differentiating gut flora in breast-fed versus bottle-fed infants [10]. Breast-fed infants derive benefit from the immunoregulatory nutrients present; they also benefit from the metabolic (essential fatty acid) and prebiotic (oligosaccharide) effects of breast milk. Bottle-fed infants have a higher amount of commensal flora overall, along with a broader and more heterogeneous distribution of gut flora, including coliforms, *Streptococcus* sp, *Clostridium difficile*, and other clostridial species. As many as 50% to 60% of bottle-fed infants have *Clostridium difficile* (versus 6%–20% of breast-fed control infants), but this bacteria does not have the same degree of pathogenicity in infants as it does in older children and adults. With age, the *Clostridium difficile* declines and the pattern of distribution becomes more adultlike.

Additional changes are noted independently with the use of antibiotics in infancy, although no clear relationship to intrapartum or prenatal maternal antibiotic use has been established. Infants receiving antibiotics change the succession by increasing *Klebsiella, Citrobacter,* and *Enterobacter;* by decreasing coliforms, *Bacteroides,* and *Bifidobacterium;* by decreasing short-chain fatty acids; and by increasing *Candida albicans* [15]. Antibiotics also disrupt individual species, leading to colonization resistance—an inability of beneficial flora to effectively colonize and competitively exclude less-desirable microbes. Other environmental factors, including more aggressive standards of hygiene, have led to a delayed development pattern and even the absence of certain groups of bacteria in the commensal flora of neonates [9].

Other factors influencing the succession of gut flora include gestational age and birth order. Preterm neonates have significantly altered microbiota, over and above that predicted by extensive hygiene, hospitalization, and antibiotic therapy. *Clostridium difficile* is present in most premature infants, and it takes over 6 months for the beneficial *Bifidobacterium* to reach normal values. The presence of an older sibling in the household helps to decrease the risk of altered gut flora by promoting an increase in *Bifidobacterium* [10].

Although the subspecies and quantities of bacteria vary over time, the families and species of commensal flora remain relatively constant within an individual over the course of a lifetime. Factors including weight gain [16], inflammation [17], and antibiotic use [18] cause disruptions in the balance of the gut flora through the remainder of childhood and into adulthood. Furthermore, in many cases, alterations in gut flora precede the development of illness, including atopic diseases [19]. The gastrointestinal microflora can be modified by diet and environmental factors to affect health [20].

Physiologic functions of the gut flora

Humans and bacteria have coevolved to offer mutual benefit. With more than 100 trillion bacteria present in the gastrointestinal tract, the necessity of a mutually beneficial relationship is clear [21]. The Intersection Human Genome Sequencing Consortium [22] identified 223 proteins from bacterial origin that have now been established as part of the human genome. The positive health contributions of these gut microflora are in the areas of nutrition, metabolism, protection, and immune regulation. Imbalances in the gut flora and alterations in the biologic terrain can have a deleterious effect on normal function in any of these areas.

Alterations in diet, including glycemic load, fiber content, essential fatty acid composition, pH balance, and macronutrient/micronutrient composition all have tremendous effects on the balance of commensal flora within the gastrointestinal tract [23]. The critical metabolic and nutritive functions of the gut flora include digestion, absorption, fermentation, vitamin synthesis, biotransformation, and energy production. This array of activities is required for normal human physiologic functioning. It is postulated that the short-chain fatty acid synthesis that provides energy to the gut epithelium may also be involved in the "cross-talk" that influences the development of humoral and cell-mediated portions of the mucosal immune system.

The "defense and protection" function of the microflora is mediated by a number of mechanisms, including competitive exclusion (competing for nutrients, space, and adherence); ensuring normal intestinal barrier function; stimulating immunoglobulin (Ig)A production; creating the mucoid bi-film layer; and producing antimicrobial substances such as bacteriocidins to actively stop infection [24]. Further trophic stimulation of the gut epithelium and modulation of intestinal permeability are also part of the inherent defense system.

Most important of the functions of the gut flora early in life are the development, education, and modulation of the mucosal immune system. New evidence is evolving that the persistent interactions between the host and its bacteria that take place in the gut may constantly reshape the immune system [5]. Nearly 70% of the human immune system is localized in the digestive tract. The mucosal surface of the gastrointestinal tract is 200 times the surface area of the skin. Defense against microbes is mediated by the early reactions of innate immunity, followed by the reaction of adaptive immunity. Innate immunity includes the skin, mucosal epithelia, cytokines, and phagocytes. These nonspecific defense mechanisms provide defense against common pathogens, but the innate immune response stimulates the adaptive immune system and influences the nature of the adaptive response [25]. The process of "oral tolerance" is an important example of this [26].

Through the process of coevolution, the body has developed a number of methods to identify microbes and modulate the adaptive immune system, based on the proper timing and presence of the bacterial stimuli. The body responds differentially to bacterial stimuli and responds to a variety of structural components on each bacterium.

The succession of gut flora, described earlier, offers early education to the innate immune system to begin to recognize "self." There are molecules of recognition—pattern recognition receptors, toll-like receptors, and pathogen-associated molecular patterns—that facilitate awareness of the bacterial environment and determine the release of stimulating or suppressive cytokines. Recent evidence demonstrates that immunostimulatory DNA [27] may derive from the copious amounts of bacterial DNA present in the gastrointestinal tract. The epithelial mucosa is equipped with pattern recognition receptors that recognize bacterial DNA from commensal bacteria and effectively modulate immune function [28]. Dendritic cells (DCs) also sample the gut milieu to define local antigens that induce IgA production. Pathogenic bacteria will up-regulate the adaptive immune system (by way of interleukin [IL]-12) within the Peyer's patches and the mesenteric lymph nodes, inducing nuclear factor-kappa β (NF-kB) activation of the inflammatory cascade. Conversely, the normal gut microflora promotes immune modulation (by way of IL-10) and has anti-inflammatory properties.

Oral tolerance is mediated by regulatory T (T_{reg}) cells, which have anti-inflammatory capabilities. Precursor T cells are transformed into T_{reg} cells when DCs have not been exposed to inflammation. Precursor T cells are transformed into $T_{effector}$ cells (T_H1 or T_H2) in the setting in which the DCs are mature (ie, activated by inflammatory signals) [29]. Gut flora (like *Lactobacillus*), however, can down-regulate DC maturation, thus preventing the activation of $T_{effector}$ cells [30]. Disruption of gut flora disrupts oral tolerance. Correction of gut flora improves oral tolerance. Thus, our immune system is dynamically educated by the presence of bacteria at the interface of the intestinal epithelium. The gut flora interacts with our innate immunity and influences the adaptive immune response in an important dialog between our immune system and the environment. Commensal bacteria are also able to modulate the expression of host genes involved in important intestinal functions including nutrient absorption, mucosal stimulation, xenobiotic metabolism, and intestinal maturation [31].

Different bacteria induce different immunologic responses. Nonpathogenic bacteria also elicit different cytokine responses from epithelial cells, inducing differential effects on the gut-associated lymphoid tissue (GALT) and on the adaptive immune system [32]. Because of this dynamic interplay between the gut flora and the GALT, the immunologic response system can be modified based on dietary change (in the form of prebiotics) and beneficial bacteria (in the form of probiotics) (Box 1).

Clinical applications

A wide range of probiotic strains and combinations of strains have been examined in clinical trials over the past 2 to 3 decades for indications ranging from prevention of antibiotic-associated diarrhea (AAD) to treatment of atopic dermatitis to infantile colic and irritable bowel syndrome. The most widely studied strains include *Lactobacillus* sp (including *L acidophilus, L rhamnosus, L bulgaricus, L reuteri,* and *L casei,* among others), *Bifidobacterium* sp, and *Saccharomyces boulardii,* a nonpathogenic yeast.

Prevention of antibiotic-associated diarrhea

There are a large number of clinical trials and several meta-analyses evaluating the effects of probiotics in preventing AAD. Many antibiotics

---

Box 1. "Hygiene hypothesis" versus "old friends"

In 1989, Strachan [33] described in the "hygiene hypothesis" that the increased prevalence of allergy and atopic illness in industrialized countries is a result of the decrease in exposure to common infections during early life, secondary to smaller family size. The theory tells us that there is a relative increase in T_H2 (humoral) activity due to the lack of T_H1 (cell-mediated) stimulation. Many have attempted to extend this hypothesis, based on epidemiologic evidence, to include the role of antibiotics, vaccines, and antimicrobial soaps, but their effects have not been proven [34]. Current research focuses on the role of nutrition, timing, and gut flora maturation on immunologic development [35].

More recent analyses have questioned the hygiene hypothesis' emphasis on T_H1/T_H2 imbalance, given the epidemic rises in allergic (T_H2) and autoimmune diseases (T_H1). Evolution has kept us in close contact with microorganisms including bacteria, viruses, parasites, and helminths. It appears that our innate immune system has evolved to recognize these "old friends" as harmless. Paradoxically, persons in affluent countries may not have the necessary "friends" present to consistently stimulate the maturation of T_{reg} cells. Thus, immunoregulation, as determined by the $T_{effector}/T_{reg}$ balance, may be more important than the T_H1/T_H2 balance [34].

Hooper and Gordon [36] highlighted the effects of imbalance within this complex ecosystem. The increasing prevalence of allergy and atopy is associated with alterations of intestinal colonization and decreased tolerance to common food proteins and inhaled allergens. Treatment with probiotics has helped to shift these symptoms back to normal [37]. Overall, we see that these critical environmental interactions highlight immunologic dysregulation arising from the combination of varied bacterial species (commensal and pathogenic), altered adaptive immune system activation, and multiple antigenic stimuli.

---

selectively eradicate lactobacilli and bifidobacteria, leaving enterotoxic *Escherichia coli* and *Clostridium difficile* to flourish. In some patients, this leads to an overgrowth of the more pathogenic bacteria and, subsequently, to diarrheal episodes [38,39]. Administration of probiotics is meant to reverse this overgrowth and rebalance the intestinal flora. Although there is still controversy regarding the optimal combination and dose of probiotic strains for this indication, there is consensus in the literature that a variety of probiotics, when started at or soon after the initiation of antibiotics, can reduce the incidence and the severity of AAD.

Kotowska and colleagues [40] studied 269 children in Poland aged 6 months to 14 years who were placed on antiobiotics in a double-blind, randomized placebo-controlled trial. These children received 250 mg of *Saccharomyces boulardii* or a placebo twice daily for the duration of antibiotic treatment. These investigators found a significantly reduced prevalence of diarrheal episodes (defined as three or more loose or watery stools per day for 48 hours or more, occurring during or up to 2 weeks after the antibiotic therapy) in children treated with *Saccharomyces boulardii* compared with controls subjects (9/119 [8%] versus 29/127 [23%]; relative risk [RR]: 0.3; 95% confidence interval [CI]: 0.2–0.7).

A smaller randomized controlled trial (RCT) in 157 patients from Brazil came to a similar conclusion. Correa and colleagues [41] gave infants aged 6 to 36 months a commercial formula containing *Bifidobacterium lactis* and *Streptococcus thermophilus* for a total of 15 days at the initiation of antibiotic therapy. They found substantially more diarrhea in the placebo-supplemented infants (32%) compared with the treatment group (16%). A Turkish study by Erdeve and colleagues [42] found similar benefits in 466 children aged 1 to 5 years randomized to receive sulbactam-ampicillin or azithromycin with placebo or *Saccharomyces boulardii*. AAD was observed in 42 of 222 patients (18.7%) in the placebo group versus only 4.7% in the probiotic group.

A meta-analysis by Szajewska and colleagues [43] in 2006 of six RCTs (n = 766) concluded that probiotics reduced the risk of AAD in children from 28.5% to 11.9% (RR: 0.44; 95% CI: 0.25–0.77) compared with placebo. The risk reduction was similar regardless of the type of probiotic used (*Lactobacillus* GG [LGG], *Saccharomyces boulardii*, or *Bifidobacterium lactis* plus *Streptococcus thermophilus*). These investigators concluded that for every seven patients who would develop diarrhea while being treated with antibiotics, one fewer would develop AAD if he or she also received probiotics. A second meta-analysis, by Johnston and colleagues [44], examined six RCTs (n = 707) and found that although a per-protocol analysis showed benefit for probiotics over placebo, a more sensitive intention-to-treat analysis did not show a significant benefit in reducing the incidence of AAD. The investigators attribute this lack of significant effect to excessive loss of subjects to follow-up in several of the trials. The investigators, however, found a significant benefit (RR: 0.36; 95% CI: 0.25–0.53) in a subgroup analysis of four studies that used at least 5 billion colony-forming units (CFUs) daily of LGG, *L sporogens*, or *Saccharomyces boulardii*, suggesting that inadequate dosing may be an important factor in the trials that do not show an effect.

In conclusion, the data to date support the use of probiotics in the prevention of AAD. Doses of 5 to 10 billion CFUs should be used, and various probiotic strains appear to be equally effective.

Treatment of acute diarrhea

Probiotics have also been extensively studied in the treatment of all-cause acute diarrhea in children. Many of these studies have methodological problems, and the heterogeneity in causes of acute diarrhea makes drawing definitive conclusions difficult. Nevertheless, it appears that probiotics may be effective in at least some cases of acute diarrhea.

For example, Sarker and colleagues [45], using *L paracasei* strain ST11 in 230 male infants and young children aged 4 to 24 months in Bangladesh, found a reduction of stool output (225 ± 218 mL/kg versus 381 ± 240 mL/kg), stool frequency (27.9 ± 17 versus 42.5 ± 26), and oral rehydration solution intake (180 ± 207 mL/kg versus 331 ± 236 mL/kg) in children who had moderate nonrotavirus diarrhea, but found no benefit in the treatment of severe rotaviral infection. Billoo and colleagues [46] studied 100 children aged 2 months to 12 years in Pakistan who received 250 mg of *Saccharomyces boulardii* for 5 days or placebo and found a reduction in diarrheal episodes to from 4.2/d (on day 3 of treatment) in the placebo group to 2.7/d in the probiotic group. This benefit was sustained for 2 follow-up months, with additional diarrheal episodes of 0.54 in the treatment group and 1.08 in the placebo group.

Szymanski and colleagues [47] randomized 87 infants and children aged 2 months to 6 years to *L rhamnosus* strains 573L/1 at a dosage of 12 billion CFUs twice daily for 5 days or to placebo. They found a nonsignificant trend in the nonrotavirus infection group (84 hours of diarrhea in the treatment group versus 96 hours in the placebo group), but a significant benefit in the outcome for the rotavirus infection group (duration of diarrhea 76 hours in the treatment group versus 115 hours in the placebo group). A Peruvian RCT by Salazar-Lindo and colleagues [48] in 179 infants and children aged 3 to 36 months did not find benefits of *L rhamnosus* LGG using an enriched milk formula compared with placebo. The investigators speculate that postdiarrheal lactose intolerance may have contributed to the lack of effect.

Several studies have looked at the impact of probiotics on duration of hospital stay in children who have acute diarrhea. For example, Krugol and Koturoglu [49] in Turkey published an RCT (n = 200) showing that 250 mg of *Saccharomyces boulardii* for 5 days reduced the length of the hospital stay from 3.9 days to 2.9 days.

One systematic review and one recent meta-analysis concluded that probiotics are probably effective in treatment of children who have acute diarrhea. In 2005, Allen and colleagues [50] examined 23 studies of probiotic use for acute diarrhea in adults and children (n = 1917). In a subset of 12 studies performed in infants and children, mean duration of diarrhea was reduced by 29.2 hours in subjects taking probiotics (95% CI: 25.1–33.2; $P < .00001$). Because a variety of probiotics were used in these trials, because the causes of diarrhea in these studies were so heterogeneous, and because the outcomes were often measured by parents rather than by the investigators, questions remain regarding the exact magnitude of the potential benefit. Nevertheless, the investigators concluded that probiotics "appear to be a useful adjunct to rehydration therapy in treating acute, infectious diarrhea in adults and children" [50].

Finally, Szajewska and colleagues [51] examined *Saccharomyces boulardii* in a meta-analysis for the treatment of acute gastroenteritis in children. These investigators combined data from four RCTs (n = 619) and found a significant reduction in duration of diarrhea (−1.1 days; 95% CI: −1.3 to −0.8) in children taking *Saccharomyces boulardii* compared with placebo. These investigators, however, qualified their conclusions with a caveat that their results should be interpreted with caution due to the methodological limitations of the included studies.

Given their wide margin of safety, probiotics should play a role in the treatment of acute infectious diarrhea despite the limitations of the literature to date. Some researchers further refine this observation and believe that LGG is the most effective strain for this indication and maintain that probiotics are most effective in treating rotaviral diarrhea [52]. These claims are not yet proven, and additional research is needed to clarify these questions. It is clear that probiotics should be started as early as possible in the course of the illness and that a dose of approximately 5 to 10 billion CFUs per day is probably appropriate.

Prevention of community-acquired diarrhea

Several studies have examined the utility of probiotics for preventing acute diarrheal episodes in the community setting. Given the facts that community-acquired diarrhea remains a major cause of death among children in the developing world and that probiotic-fortified formulas can be manufactured easily and cheaply, this research is of particular importance. For example, in a study of undernourished children aged 1 month to 2 years in Peru (n = 204), participants were randomized to LGG or placebo for 15 months. Children in the LGG group had significantly fewer diarrheal episodes (5.2 per child per year versus 6.0 in the placebo group, $P < .03$) [53].

Rio and colleagues [54] studied 135 children in Argentina to specifically examine the impact of underlying nutritional status on the effectiveness of probiotics. They compared undernourished children with well-nourished children, and used fermented milk, which provided *L acidophilus* and *L casei* ($1–10 \times 10^7$ CFUs/mL), versus regular milk (placebo). They found a reduced frequency of diarrheal episodes over a 3-month period in the well-nourished treated versus placebo groups (20 episodes in 35 actively treated patients versus 35 episodes in 27 patients in the placebo group). This difference was not seen in the undernourished treated group compared with the undernourished placebo group. Both treated groups, however, fared better in the prevention of protracted diarrhea than the placebo groups (0 episodes of diarrhea lasting over 14 days versus 12 episodes).

A number of studies have also been done in developed countries. Chouraqui and colleagues [55] studied 90 healthy children younger than 8 months living in residential or foster care settings in France and gave them acidified milk formula containing *Bifidobacterium lactis* BB12 or a conventional formula. They found a significant difference in the daily probability of diarrhea in the treated group (0.84) versus the placebo group (2.3). There was no significant difference, however, between the groups in terms of the overall prevalence of diarrhea during the study period.

Thibault and colleagues [56] examined the prevalence of diarrhea in a sample of over 900 healthy infants aged 4 to 6 months in child care settings given a formula enriched with *Bifidobacterium brevis* plus *Streptococcus thermophilus* 065 or standard formula. These investigators found no difference in incidence or duration of diarrheal episodes or hospital admissions but found that diarrheal episodes were less severe in the probiotic group, as measured by significantly fewer cases of dehydration, fewer formula changes, fewer prescriptions for oral rehydration salts, and fewer medical consultations.

Weizman and colleagues [57] studied 201 infants aged 4 to 8 months in 14 child care centers in Israel over a 12-week period. Children were randomized to a formula with *Bifidobacteriunm lactis* BB12 (1×10^7 CFUs/mL of formula), to a formula with *L reuteri* (1×10^7 CFUs/mL of formula), or to no probiotics. Infants on probiotics had significantly fewer febrile illnesses (0.27 versus 0.42) and fewer diarrheal episodes (0.13 versus 0.31) than the untreated controls. The effects were more prominent with *L reuteri*.

Sazawal and colleagues [58] published a meta-analysis of 34 RCTs examining probiotics of various types for prevention of acute diarrhea of all causes. In the 12 trials with data on children, Sazawal and colleagues [58] found an overall reduction in risk of developing diarrhea of 57% (95% CI: 35–71; $P < .001$). This analysis combined AAD with community and hospital-acquired diarrhea, making it difficult to evaluate the specific impact of probiotics on either of these relatively distinct clinical entities.

Finally, in another prevention-oriented study, Vendt and colleagues [59] examined the effect of probiotic supplementation on growth during the first 6 months of life. Infants up to age 2 months (n = 120) were randomized to LGG-enriched formula or to standard formula in a double-blind fashion. The treated group showed significantly greater height and weight than the standard formula group at age 6 months. As in the study by Weizman and colleagues [57], this effect was demonstrated in a well-nourished cohort in a developed country (Finland); if this finding could be replicated in a less well nourished group of children in a developing country, the implications for probiotics as a strategy for prevention and health promotion would be significant.

Prevention of necrotizing enterocolitis in premature children

Probiotics seem to hold substantial promise in the prevention of necrotizing enterocolitis (NEC) in premature infants. Bin-Nun and colleagues [60] randomized 155 premature infants having a birth weight lower than 1500 g to receive a probiotic-supplemented formula containing *Bifidobacterium infantis, Streptococcus thermophilus*, and *Bifidobacterium bifidus* or standard formula. The incidence of NEC was significantly reduced in the treatment group (4% versus 16.4%; $P = .03$). Three of 15 babies who developed NEC died, and all NEC-related deaths occurred in control infants.

A similar result was obtained by Lin and colleagues [61], who studied 367 very low birth weight infants (<1500 g) in China. These investigators added a mix of *L acidophilus* and *Bifidobacterium infantis* to breast milk. The risk of NEC was significantly reduced in the treatment group compared with the control group. The risk of death was 7 in 180 in the treatment group versus 14 in 187 in the control group, and the risk of NEC was 9 in 180 versus 24 in 187, respectively.

Irritable bowel syndrome and constipation

Although in clinical practice, probiotics are commonly used in the treatment of irritable bowel syndrome, to date, clinical trials have not shown substantial efficacy. An RCT by Bausserman and colleagues [62] (n = 50) in children fulfilling Rome II criteria for irritable bowel syndrome who were treated with LGG or placebo for 6 weeks found no significant benefit in the abdominal pain scale (44% response in the treatment group versus 40% response in placebo). There was, however, a significant effect on abdominal distention scores. Another study by Banaskiewicz and colleagues [63] in 84 children aged 2 to 16 years who had severe constipation examined LGG versus placebo as an adjunct to lactulose. The treatment group and the placebo group in this trial showed improvement in about two thirds of patients, making it difficult to draw definite conclusions.

Infantile colic

Recently, Savino and colleagues [64] compared the use of *L reuteri* with simethicone in the treatment of infantile colic. Simethicone, although not distinguishable in efficacy from placebo, has been the treatment of choice for colic for many years. Ten billion CFUs of probiotics were given daily to 41 breast-fed infants who met the clinical criteria for colic versus 60 mg of simethicone per day. Beneficial effects began to be noted in the probiotic group within 24 hours, and by 28 days, the average crying time was decreased by 65% in the probiotic group. In addition, 95% of all infants receiving probiotics responded positively compared with only 7% responders in the simethicone group.

Atopic dermatitis: treatment

Because of the apparent role of probiotics early in life in regulating systemic immunologic development, interest has recently developed in the impact of probiotics on atopic dermatitis in young children. In one placebo-controlled

RCT, for example, Weston and colleagues [65] treated 56 children (aged 6–18 months) who had moderate to severe atopic dermatitis with 1×10^9 CFUs of L $fermentum$ VRI-033 twice daily for 8 weeks. At the end of the study at 16 weeks, children in the probiotic group showed a significant reduction in the Severity Scoring of Atopic Dermatitis (SCORAD) index ($P = .03$) that was not seen in the placebo group. In this study, 92% of children in the treatment group had a SCORAD index that was better than baseline values at week 16 compared with 63% of children in the placebo group. This difference was also significant ($P = .01$). In an additional analysis of the children in the study, these investigators found that the probiotic group showed a significant increase over baseline in T_H1 cytokine interferon-γ responses at the end of the 8-week supplementation period. The placebo group showed no such change. Furthermore, this increase in interferon-γ responses was directly proportional to the decrease in the SCORAD index (r = -0.445; $P = .026$) during the intervention period, and the effect was still present 2 months after supplementation had ended [66].

Another study exploring possible mechanisms was performed by Rosenfeldt and colleagues [67]. In a double-blind, placebo-controlled crossover study (n = 41), these investigators used the lactulose/mannitol test—a validated measure of intestinal permeability—and found that improvement in atopic dermatitis was significantly correlated with decreased intestinal permeability ($P = .001$). These findings, according to the investigators, may suggest that "impairment of the intestinal mucosal barrier appears to be involved in the pathogenesis of atopic dermatitis."

Two other studies suggest that probiotics may be effective for atopic dermatitis only in children who have previous food sensitization. In a double-blind study of children who had suspected cow's milk allergy (n = 230), Viljanen and colleagues [68] found that LGG was only effective for atopic dermatitis in children who had documented IgE hypersensitivity.

A small randomized study (n = 59) from New Zealand, which treated children for 12 weeks with L $rhamnosus$ and $Bifidobacterium$ $lactis$, similarly showed an effect only in those who had documented food sensitization [69].

Finally, Passeron and colleagues [70] compared the effectiveness of a preparation containing only "prebiotics"—substances that "selectively stimulate the growth and/or the activity of a limited number of bacterial strains already established in the gut"—with a preparation containing prebiotics plus probiotics (L $rhamnosus$ Lcr35 1.2×10^9 three times daily) in a double-blind RCT of children aged 2 years and older who had atopic dermatitis (n = 48). After 3 months of treatment, both groups showed significant improvement in the SCORAD index, with no statistical difference between groups.

Atopic dermatitis: prevention

A Finnish RCT of infants at high risk for atopic disease based on family history (n = 132) examined the role of prenatal and postnatal administration of LGG in preventing the development of eczema. In the active group, mothers were given LGG (1×10^{10} CFUs daily) for 4 weeks prenatally and for 6 months postnatally if breastfeeding; babies who were not breastfeeding were given the same dose orally. At age 2 years, atopic eczema was diagnosed in 31 of 68 in the placebo group but only in 15 of 64 in the active group (RR: 0.51; 95% CI: 0.32–0.84) [71]. These beneficial effects persisted at 4 years without any additional treatment [37].

A recent Australian placebo-controlled RCT (n = 178) examined the effectiveness of L acidophilus LAVRI-A1 in preventing the onset of atopic dermatitis in newborns at high risk for this condition. In this study, newborns received 3×10^9 CFUs plus maltodextrin daily or maltodextrin alone from birth to 6 months; no difference in incidence of atopic dermatitis was found at age 6 months or 12 months [72]. Furthermore, subjects in the treatment group had a higher incidence of sensitization to milk protein at the end of the study than children in the placebo group. A potential confounder in this study was the use of maltodextrin as a placebo; because this substance is a prebiotic, it may exert its own beneficial effects. In addition, this study did not include a prenatal period of probiotic administration.

Other clinical indications

Probiotics have shown some promise for a number of other clinical indications in children, including acne [73], irritability in infants [74], and severe gingivitis (in a chewing gum preparation) [75]. LGG has also been examined as an adjunct to conventional therapy in children who have Crohn's disease and, although well tolerated, it did not change the time to relapse [76]. All these indications require further study before treatment recommendations can be made.

Safety considerations

Despite the extensive clinical trial literature described in this article, there are few reports of significant complications or adverse effects from the use of probiotics. Mild abdominal discomfort and flatulence are the only adverse effects reported regularly in most of the trials.

There have been concerns raised regarding the risk of septicemia from the use of probiotic supplementation. This can certainly occur, and there are case reports of bacteremia with probiotic species following oral administration. These cases are rare and without exception occurred in severely ill or immunocompromised hosts or in children who had short-gut syndrome or indwelling catheters. For example, De Groote and colleagues [77] reported a case of LGG bacteremia in a child who had short-gut syndrome and an indwelling Broviac catheter and gastrostomy tube. Alternately, Srinivasan and colleagues [78] examined the safety of L casei shirota in a group of critically ill children (n = 28) in a pediatric ICU and found no evidence of bacteremia. Likewise, the studies cited earlier using probiotics for the prevention of NEC in premature infants did not report any cases of bacteremia using the probiotic organisms. Given the potential benefits in this type of vulnerable patient and the awareness that there may be a risk of bacteremia, however small, it is advisable for decisions to be made on a case-by-case basis in children who are immunocompromised or have indwelling catheters.

In healthy children, it appears that the risk of bacteremia is almost nonexistent. Hammerman and colleagues [79] examined the safety of two specific strains—*L rhamnosus* GG and *Bifidobacterium* sp—in a recent systematic review and concluded that although case reports of sepsis do exist and deserve attention, the risk, at least with these two specific organisms, is extremely low. These investigators found no cases of sepsis reported in any prospective clinical trial. There are no reports of sepsis or other pathologic colonization in healthy patients.

Dosage

Given the wide range of types of probiotic combinations and dosages examined in the clinical trial literature to date, it is difficult to make definitive statements regarding specific choice of preparation and exact dosages. Doses ranging from several million CFUs per day to 600 billion CFUs (for chronic pouchitis) and 3.6 trillion CFUs (for remission of ulcerative colitis) have been used in published studies. Regarding *Saccharomyces boulardii*, the dose used in most studies is between 250 and 500 mg daily. Regarding LGG, *Bifidobacterium* sp, and combinations of other bacterial strains, it appears that, at least for the best-studied indications of prevention of AAD and prevention and treatment of acute infectious diarrhea, the minimum daily dose should be in the range of 5 to 10 billion CFUs regardless of the specific preparation. For example, the Canadian meta-analysis of AAD studies found strong evidence of effectiveness, even using intent-to-treat analysis, in the studies that used a dose of over 5 billion CFUs daily regardless of the specific strain. Given the wide safety margin of probiotics, in particular, and the lack of evidence that higher doses lead to any increase in risk, it is probably wise to err on the side of higher dosage ranges.

Regarding the less extensively studied indications such as atopic dermatitis, the optimal dose and preparation have not been clarified to date. Doses of 5 billion CFUs daily and higher are commonly used in clinical practice, even with very young infants, for these other indications.

Probiotics are available in a wide variety of preparations, including powders, capsules, and liquids. Although most studies use twice-daily dosing, there is no evidence to date that once-daily dosing is not adequate. Practitioners and patients should be aware that as with many other dietary supplements, the specific dose of active ingredient (in this case, CFUs per day) in a given amount of powder or liquid can vary tremendously between brands. Thus, careful reading of the label is paramount for parents, and practitioners should counsel on this point specifically. Quality is also a major issue in using probiotics in clinical practice. Many probiotic preparations do not contain the number of viable CFUs stated on the label. ConsumerLab.com, an independent laboratory that performs quality control assessments of dietary supplements, recently found in an analysis of probiotic products that 5 of 19 brands analyzed did not contain the number of live organisms claimed on the label [80]. Practitioners planning to use probiotics regularly in clinical practice should consult this site to familiarize themselves with several of the high-quality products available. Most probiotic preparations should be kept refrigerated, and in the case of prevention of AAD, probiotics should probably be taken at least 2 hours before or after the antibiotic, if possible.

Recently, a number of products have been developed to deliver probiotics in foods, most commonly yogurt. Conventional yogurt products generally contain only small amounts of live bacteria not adequate to deliver a therapeutic dose. This has led to the development of "therapeutic" yogurts, which can contain 1 billion or more CFUs, per 4-oz container. Although some of these products have been shown to decrease intestinal transit time [81]—suggesting that they may be helpful in treating constipation—none has been studied to date for a specific clinical problem.

The question of which strain or strains of probiotic to use for a given clinical situation is a challenging one. In the few cases in which a specific strain has been shown to be effective for a specific condition, there are likely few studies of other strains for the same indication. In the case of the best-studied indications—AAD and acute infectious diarrhea—meta-analyses show no significant difference in effectiveness among LGG, *Saccharomyces boulardii*, and a variety of combination products including *Bifidobacterium* sp and other strains. Thus, it appears that choosing the proper strain or combination of strains is less important than recommending a sufficiently high dose. Head-to-head trials comparing the effectiveness of specific probiotic strains or combinations for specific clinical indications will be needed to determine whether specific combinations are superior for specific situations. To date, few such trials have been published.

Summary

As should be obvious from this review, there is now an extensive body of medical literature on the use of probiotics in children. Several important points for the practicing clinician clearly emerge:

1. The gastrointestinal flora plays a complex and important role in the development of healthy immunologic and digestive function in young children. Understanding this role and assisting in the development of a healthy gastrointestinal flora (eg, by encouraging breastfeeding and minimizing the use of antibiotics whenever possible) is an important function for clinicians caring for young children.

2. Probiotics are extremely safe in healthy children, and even in immuno-compromised or seriously ill children, significant complications are rare.
3. Probiotics are almost certainly effective in reducing the risk of AAD and in reducing the duration of acute infectious diarrhea.
4. Probiotics may also be effective in preventing community-acquired diarrheal infections and in reducing the risk of NEC in premature infants. They may also be helpful in the prevention and treatment of atopic dermatitis.
5. The exact strain or combination of strains most effective for common clinical indications has yet to be determined; for now, the exact strain used seems less important than whether an adequate dose is used.
6. Doses in the range of 5 to 10 billion CFUs per day or higher are appropriate for most clinical indications in children.
7. There is a wide range in quality among products on the market; clinicians should familiarize themselves with several of the widely available high-quality products.

References

[1] Metchnikiff E. The prolongation of life. New York: Putman & Sons; 1908.
[2] Bengmark S. Ecological control of the gastrointestinal tract: the role of probiotic flora. Gut 1998;42:2–7.
[3] Bjorksten B. Effects of intestinal microflora and the environment on the development of asthma and allergy. Springer Semin Immunopathol 2004;25:257–70.
[4] Fanaro S, Chierici P, Vigi V. Intestinal microflora in early infancy: composition and development. Acta Paediatr Suppl 2003;441:48–55.
[5] Guarner F, Magdelena JR. Gut flora in health and disease. Lancet 2003;361:512–9.
[6] Schrezenemeir J, deVrese M. Prebiotics, probiotics, and synbiotics—approaching a definition. Am J Clin Nutr 2001;73:361S–4S.
[7] Isolauri E, Sutas Y, Kankaanpaa, et al. Probiotics: effects on immunity. Am J Clin Nutr 2001;73:444S–50S.
[8] Gibson GR, Roberfroid MB. Dietary modulation of the human colonic microbiota: introducing the concept of prebiotics. J Nutr 1995;125:1401–12.
[9] Mackie RI, Sghir A, Gaskins HR. Developmental microbial ecology of the neonatal gastrointestinal tract. Am J Clin Nutr 1999;69(Suppl):1035S–45S.
[10] Penders J, Thijs C, Vink C, et al. Factors influencing the composition of the intestinal microbiota in early infancy. Pediatrics 2006;118:511–21.
[11] Harmsen HJ, Wildeboer-Veloo AC, Raangs GC, et al. Analysis of intestinal flora development in breast-fed and formula-fed infants by using molecular identification and detection methods. J Pediatr Gastroenterol Nutr 2000;30:61–7.
[12] Teitelbaum JE, Walker WA. Nutritional impact of pre- and probiotics as protective gastrointestinal organisms. Annu Rev Nutr 2002;22:107–38.
[13] Gronlund MM, Lehtonen OP, Eerola E, et al. Fecal microflora in healthy infants born by different methods of delivery: permanent changes in intestinal flora after cesarean delivery. J Pediatr Gastroenterol Nutr 1999;28:19–25.
[14] Adlerberth I, Carlsson B, de Man P, et al. Intestinal colonization with Enterobaceriaceae in Pakistani and Swedish hospital-delivered infants. Acta Paediatr Scand 1991;80:602–10.
[15] Noverr MC, Huffnagle GB. Does the microbiota regulate immune responses outside the gut? Trends Microbiol 2004;12:562–8.

[16] Backhed F, Ding H, Wang T, et al. The gut microbiota as an environmental factor that regulates fat storage. Proc Natl Acad Sci U S A 2004;101:15718–23.

[17] Sartor RB. Probiotic therapy for intestinal inflammation and infection. Curr Opin Gastroenterol 2005;21:44–50.

[18] DeLa Cochetiere MF, Durand T, Lepage P, et al. Resilience of the dominant human fecal microbiota upon short-course antibiotic challenge. J Clin Microbiol 2005;43:5588–92.

[19] Kalliomaki M, Kirjavainen P, Eerola E, et al. Distinct patterns of neonatal gut microflora in infants in whom atopy was and was not developing. J Allergy Clin Immunol 2001;107: 129–34.

[20] Ley RE, Turnbaugh PJ, Klein S, et al. Microbial ecology. human gut microbes associated with obesity. Nature 2006;444:1022–3.

[21] Backhed F, Ley RE, Sonnenburg JL, et al. Host-bacterial mutualism in the human intestine. Science 2005;307:1915–20.

[22] International Human Genome Sequencing Consortium. Initial sequencing and analysis of the human genome. Nature 2001;409:860–921.

[23] Fioramonti J, Theodorou V, Bueno L. Probiotics: what are they? What are their effects on gut physiology? Best Pract Res Clin Gastroenterol 2003;17:711–24.

[24] Lievin-Le Moal V, Servin AL. The front line of enteric host defense against unwelcome intrusion of harmful microorganisms: mucins, antimicrobial peptides and microbiota. Clin Microbiol Rev 2006;19:315–37.

[25] Abbas AK, Lichtman AH, editors. Cellular and molecular immunology. 5th edition. Philadephia: Saunders; 2003.

[26] Brandtzaeg P. Current understanding of gastrointestinal immunoregulation and its relation to food allergy. Ann N Y Acad Sci 2002;964:13–45.

[27] Van Uden J, Rax E. Immunostimulatory DNA and applications to allergic disease. J Allergy Clin Immunol 1999;104:902–10.

[28] Jijon H, Backer J, Diaz H, et al. DNA from probiotic bacteria modulated murine and human epithelial and immune function. Gastroenterology 2004;126:1358–73.

[29] McGuirk P, Mills KH. Pathogen-specific regulatory T cells provoke a shift in the Th1/Th2 paradigm in immunity to infections diseases. Trends Immunol 2002;23:450–5.

[30] Christensen HR. Lactobacilli differentially modulated expression of cytokines and maturation surface markers in murine dendritic cells. J Immunol 2002;168:171–8.

[31] Hooper LV, Wong MH, Thelin A, et al. Molecular analysis of commensal host-microbial relationships in the intestine. Science 2001;291:881–4.

[32] Borruel N, Carol M, Casellas F, et al. Increased mucosal tumour necrosis factor alpha production in Crohn's disease can be downregulated ex vivo by probiotic bacteria. Gut 2002;51: 659–64.

[33] Strachan DP. Hay fever, hygiene, and household size. BMJ 1989;299:1259–60.

[34] Rook GAW, Brunet LR. Microbes, immunoregulation, and the gut. Gut 2005;54:317–20.

[35] Prescott SL. Allergy: the price we pay for cleaner living? Ann Allergy Asthma Immunol 2003; 90(Suppl 3):64–70.

[36] Hooper LV, Gordon JI. Commensal host-bacterial relationships in the gut. Science 2001; 292:1115–8.

[37] Kallomaki M, Salminen S, Poussa T, et al. Probiotics and prevention of atopic disease: 4-year follow-up of a randomised placebo-controlled trial. Lancet 2003;361:1869–71.

[38] Plummer S, Weaver MA, Harris JC, et al. Clostridium difficile pilot study: effects of probiotic supplementation on the incidence of C. difficile diarrhoea. Int Microbiol 2004;7(1): 59–62.

[39] Shimbo I, Yamaguchi T, Odaka T, et al. Effect of Clostridium butyricum on fecal flora in Helicobacter pylori eradication therapy. World J Gastroenterol 2005;11(47):7520–4.

[40] Kotowska M, Albrecht P, Szajewska H. Saccharomyces boulardii in the prevention of antibiotic-associated diarrhoea in children: a randomized double-blind placebo-controlled trial. Aliment Pharmacol Ther 2005;21(5):583–90.

[41] Correa NB, Peret Filho LA, Penna FJ, et al. A randomized formula controlled trial of *Bifidobacterium lactis* and *Streptococcus thermophilus* for prevention of antibiotic-associated diarrhea in infants. J Clin Gastroenterol 2005;39(5):385–9.

[42] Erdeve O, Tiras U, Dallar Y. The probiotic effect of *Saccharomyces boulardii* in a pediatric age group. J Trop Pediatr 2004;50(4):234–6.

[43] Szajewska H, Ruszczynski M, Radzikowski A. Probiotics in the prevention of antibiotic-associated diarrhea in children: a meta-analysis of randomized controlled trials. J Pediatr 2006; 149(3):367–72.

[44] Johnston BC, Supina AL, Vohra S. Probiotics for pediatric antibiotic-associated diarrhea: a meta-analysis of randomized placebo-controlled trials. CMAJ 2006;175(4):377–83 [Erratum in: CMAJ 2006;175(7):777].

[45] Sarker SA, Sultana S, Fuchs GJ, et al. *Lactobacillus paracasei* strain ST11 has no effect on rotavirus but ameliorates the outcome of nonrotavirus diarrhea in children from Bangladesh. Pediatrics 2005;116(2):e221–8.

[46] Billoo AG, Memon MA, Khaskheli SA, et al. Role of a probiotic (*Saccharomyces boulardii*) in management and prevention of diarrhoea. World J Gastroenterol 2006;12(28): 4557–60.

[47] Szymanski H, Pejcz J, Jawien M, et al. Treatment of acute infectious diarrhoea in infants and children with a mixture of three *Lactobacillus rhamnosus* strains—a randomized, double-blind, placebo-controlled trial. Aliment Pharmacol Ther 2006;23(2):247–53.

[48] Salazar-Lindo E, Miranda-Langschwager P, Campos-Sanchez M, et al. *Lactobacillus casei* strain GG in the treatment of infants with acute watery diarrhea: a randomized, double-blind, placebo controlled clinical trial. BMC Pediatr 2004;2:4–18.

[49] Kurugol Z, Koturoglu G. Effects of *Saccharomyces boulardii* in children with acute diarrhoea. Acta Paediatr 2005;94(1):44–7.

[50] Allen SJ, Okoko B, Martinez E, et al. Probiotics for treating infectious diarrhoea. Cochrane Database Syst Rev 2004;2:CD003084.

[51] Szajewska H, Skorka A, Dylag M. Meta-analysis: *Saccharomyces boulardii* for treating acute diarrhoea in children. Aliment Pharmacol Ther 2007;25(3):257–64.

[52] Guandalini S. Probiotics for children: use in diarrhea. J Clin Gastroenterol 2006;40:244–8.

[53] Oberhelman RA, Gilman RH, Sheen P, et al. A placebo-controlled trial of *Lactobacillus* GG to prevent diarrhea in undernourished Peruvian children. J Pediatr 1999;134:15–20.

[54] Rio ME, Zago LB, Garcia H, et al. [Influence of nutritional status on the effectiveness of a dietary supplement of live lactobacillus to prevent and cure diarrhoea in children]. Arch Latinoam Nutr 2004;54(3):287–92 [in Spanish].

[55] Chouraqui JP, Van Egroo LD, Fichot MC. Acidified milk formula supplemented with *Bifidobacterium lactis*: impact on infant diarrhea in residential care settings. J Pediatr Gastroenterol Nutr 2004;38(3):288–92.

[56] Thibault H, Aubert-Jacquin C, Goulet O. Effects of long-term consumption of a fermented infant formula (with *Bifidobacterium breve* c50 and *Streptococcus thermophilus* 065) on acute diarrhea in healthy infants. J Pediatr Gastroenterol Nutr 2004;39:147–52.

[57] Weizman Z, Asli G, Alsheikh A. Effect of a probiotic infant formula on infections in child care centers: comparison of two probiotic agents. Pediatrics 2005;115(1):5–9.

[58] Sazawal S, Hiremath G, Dhingra U, et al. Efficacy of probiotics in prevention of acute diarrhea: a meta-analysis of masked, randomized, placebo-controlled trials. Lancet Infect Dis 2006;6:374–82.

[59] Vendt N, Grunberg H, Tuure T, et al. Growth during the first six months of life in infants using formula enriched with *Lactobacillus rhamnosus* GG: double-blind, randomized trial. J Hum Nutr Diet 2006;19:51–8.

[60] Bin-Nun A, Bromiker R, Wilschanski M, et al. Oral probiotics prevent necrotizing enterocolitis in very low birth weight neonates. J Pediatr 2005;147(2):192–6.

[61] Lin HC, Su BH, Chen AC, et al. Oral probiotics reduce the incidence and severity of necrotizing enterocolitis in very low birth weight infants. Pediatrics 2005;115(1):1–4.

[62] Bausserman M, Michail S. The use of *Lactobacillus* GG in irritable bowel syndrome in children: a double-blind randomized control trial. J Pediatr 2005;147(2):197–201.

[63] Banaszkiewicz A, Szajewska H. Ineffectiveness of *Lactobacillus* GG as an adjunct to lactulose for the treatment of constipation in children: a double-blind, placebo-controlled randomized trial. J Pediatr 2005;146(3):364–9.

[64] Savino F, Pelle E, Palumeri E, et al. *Lactobacillus reuteri* (American Type Culture Collection Strain 55730) versus simethicone in the treatment of infantile colic: a prospective randomized study. Pediatrics 2007;119:124–30.

[65] Weston S, Halbert A, Richmond P, et al. Effects of probiotics on atopic dermatitis: a randomised controlled trial. Arch Dis Child 2005;90(9):892–7.

[66] Prescott SL, Dunstan JA, Hale J, et al. Clinical effects of probiotics are associated with increased interferon-gamma responses in very young children with atopic dermatitis. Clin Exp Allergy 2005;35(12):1557–64.

[67] Rosenfeldt V, Benfeldt E, Valerius NH, et al. Effect of probiotics on gastrointestinal symptoms and small intestinal permeability in children with atopic dermatitis. J Pediatr 2004;145(5):612–6.

[68] Viljanen M, Savilahti E, Haahtela T, et al. Probiotics in the treatment of atopic eczema/dermatitis syndrome in infants: a double-blind placebo-controlled trial. Allergy 2005;60(4): 494–500.

[69] Sistek D, Kelly R, Wickens K, et al. The effect of probiotics on atopic dermatitis confined to food sensitized children? Clin Exp Allergy 2006;36(5):629–33.

[70] Passeron T, Lacour JP, Fontas E, et al. Prebiotics and synbiotics: two promising approaches for the treatment of atopic dermatitis in children above 2 years. Allergy 2006;61:431–7.

[71] Kallomaki M, Salminen S, Arvilommi H, et al. Probiotics in primary prevention of atopic disease: a randomized placebo-controlled trial. Lancet 2001;357(9262):1076–9.

[72] Taylor AL, Dunstan JA, Prescott SL. Probiotic supplementation for the first six months of life fails to reduce the risk of atopic dermatitis and increases the risk of allergen sensitization in high-risk children: a randomized controlled trial. J Allergy Clin Immunol 2007;119(1): 184–91.

[73] Weber G, Adamczyk A, Freytag S. [Treatment of acne with a yeast preparation]. Fortschr Med 1989;107(26):563–6 [in German].

[74] Saavedra JM, Abi-Hanna A, Moore N, et al. Long-term consumption of infant formulas containing live probiotic bacteria: tolerance and safety. Am J Clin Nutr 2004;79(2):261–7.

[75] Krasse P, Carlsson B, Dahl C, et al. Decreased gum bleeding and reduced gingivitis by the probiotic *Lactobacillus reuteri*. Swed Dent J 2006;30(2):55–60.

[76] Bousvaros A, Guandalini S, Baldassano RN, et al. A randomized double-blind trial of *Lactobacillus* GG versus placebo in addition to standard maintenance therapy for children with Crohn's disease. Inflamm Bowel Dis 2005;11:833–9.

[77] DeGroote MA, Frank D, Dowell E, et al. *Lactobacillus rhamnosus* GG bacteremia associated with probiotic use in a child with short gut syndrome. Pediatr Infect Dis J 2005;24(3): 278–80.

[78] Srinivasan R, Meyer R, Padmanabhan R, et al. Clinical safety of *Lactobacillus casei* shirota as a probiotic in critically ill children. J Pediatr Gastroenterol Nutr 2006;42:171–3.

[79] Hammerman C, Kaplan M, Bin-Nun A. Safety of probiotics: comparison of two popular strains. BMJ 2006;333(7576):1006–8.

[80] ConsumerLab.com. Product review: probiotic supplements. Available at: http://www.consumerlab.com/results/probiotics.asp. Accessed May 1, 2007.

[81] Activia by Dannon: scientific Review for Health Professionals. Available at: http://www.activia.com/healthcare.asp. Accessed August 27, 2008.

ELSEVIER
SAUNDERS

PEDIATRIC CLINICS
OF NORTH AMERICA

Pediatr Clin N Am 54 (2007) 969–981

Integrative Approach to Obesity

Hilary H. McClafferty, MD, FAAP

*The Center for Children's Integrative Medicine, 55 Vilcom Circle,
Chapel Hill, NC 27514, USA*

Integrative medicine blends conventional and carefully evaluated complementary therapies and considers all aspects of a patient's lifestyle (physical, mental, and spiritual). Although a correlation between integrative medicine and pediatric obesity treatment may not seem immediately obvious, it is notable that several of the core themes of integrative medicine practice [1] have been independently identified as elements of successful pediatric and adult obesity treatment programs. These elements include the therapeutic use of nutrition, motivational interviewing, the use of the mind-body connection, exercise counseling, and a close partnership between patient and physician [2–6]. Education about integrative medicine practice may help pediatricians to increase their effectiveness in the treatment of pediatric obesity and to expand their treatment options for patients.

This article defines the diagnostic criteria for pediatric overweight and obesity, examines common elements of successful treatment strategies, and updates the practitioner on research in the use of several other integrative modalities as they relate to pediatric obesity treatment. The American Academy of Pediatrics (AAP) has excellent resources available on the current conventional medical diagnosis and treatment of pediatric obesity and its associated comorbidities, and recommends that a thorough medical screening be mandatory for every child who has overweight or obesity [7].

Background statistics

Pediatric obesity rates worldwide are continuing their alarming upward trend. Over the past 30 years, the obesity rate in United States has more than doubled for preschool children and adolescents and has more than tripled for children aged 6 to 11 years, a group that now numbers 9 million [8]. Overweight adolescents have a 70% chance of becoming overweight or obese adults, which increases to 80% if one or more parent is overweight

E-mail address: hmcclafferty@earthlink.net

or obese [9]. Based on a longitudinal population study noted in the 2005 Institute of Medicine report "Health in the Balance," 60% of obese children aged 5 to 10 years had at least one cardiovascular risk factor (elevated cholesterol, triglycerides, insulin, or blood pressure) and 25% had two or more risk factors [10]. A significant number of obese children have serious complications and comorbidities, ranging from life-threatening cardiomyopathy and pulmonary embolus to metabolic syndrome, type 2 diabetes mellitus, elevated cardiovascular risk factors, hypertension, nonalcoholic fatty liver disease, polycystic ovarian syndrome, pseudotumor cerebri, slipped capital femoral epiphysis, and obstructive sleep apnea syndrome [11].

The causes of obesity are multifactorial and include genetic predisposition, sedentary lifestyle, overeating, fast food diet, lack of adequate nutrition education, increasing portion size, family role modeling, school environment, and advertising and marketing of unhealthy foods. There are certain congenital medical syndromes and conditions associated with obesity in children, such as Prader-Willi syndrome, that are beyond the scope of this article [11].

The difficulty in preventing and reversing pediatric obesity has been well documented [12]. The recommendations for treatment seem straightforward: reduce energy intake while maintaining optimal nutrient intake to support growth and development, increase energy expenditure while reducing sedentary behaviors, actively engage parents and caretakers, and facilitate a supportive family environment [13]. Yet it is a sobering fact that only 21% of 64 preventative obesity programs for children reviewed in a recent meta-analysis resulted in even short-term weight loss in participants [14]. Pediatricians face a serious challenge in caring for children who have overweight or obesity and require new and effective options.

Body mass index

Body mass index (BMI; weight in kilograms divided by height in meters squared) has been demonstrated to correlate with direct measure of adiposity [15]. Development of adipose tissue differs in girls and boys and changes as children grow. These differences are reflected in the sex-specific BMI-for-age charts for children aged 2 to 18 years that have been developed and published by the Centers for Disease Control and Prevention (CDC). Easy-to-use BMI-for-age calculators are included within the CDC Web site [16,17].

Diagnostic criteria for overweight and obesity based on body mass index

Underweight: BMI-for-age <5th percentile
Normal: BMI-for-age 5th percentile to <85th percentile
At risk of overweight: BMI-for-age 85th percentile to <95th percentile
Overweight: BMI-for-age ≥95th percentile

Based on CDC recommendations, standard weight and height growth charts are used in children below age 2 years, and outliers in weight-to-length ratios should be identified for close observation. BMI may be artificially high in some very muscular athletes, for example, and such cases must be evaluated on an individual basis.

Predictive value of body mass index

BMI-for-age has been shown to be a reliable indicator for predicting risk of continuing overweight in children and shown to be predictive of obesity by age 12 years in children whose BMIs are elevated as early as age 24, 36, or 54 months [18]. The AAP currently recommends measurement of BMI-for-age at least once per year in all children aged 2 to 18 years [19]; however, recent studies evaluating the usefulness and efficacy of BMI screening in general pediatrician offices indicate that this tool is frequently underused [20]. The reasons most often cited for underuse of BMI screening by pediatricians in these studies included a lack of familiarity with the BMI graphs, doubt about their usefulness, time constraints, fear of offending parents, and the desire to not add to the nursing workload [21].

It may be beneficial for the pediatrician to consider introducing the BMI chart before age 24 months in preventative well visits, which would give the practitioner short, directed, and repeated opportunities to lay the groundwork in conveying the importance of obesity prevention and to make the parents aware of the developing research in this area for predicting overweight in children [22]. These interventions could potentially provide an important opportunity to clearly and factually state how normal weight relates directly to the child's health, longevity, and avoidance of serious chronic disease in the future.

Nutrition, inflammation, and integrative medicine

Nutrition, in its role in reducing inflammation, is a key element of an integrative medicine treatment plan [23]. Inflammation is especially relevant in obesity treatment because obesity has been strongly correlated with a proinflammatory state, as have cardiovascular disease and multiple other comorbidities such as hypertension, polycystic ovary syndrome, and obstructive sleep apnea syndrome [24–30]. Data demonstrating the elevation of cardiovascular risk factors, the early coronary atherosclerotic changes in children and adolescents [31], and the early imprinting of food preferences in preschoolers [32] highlight the importance of informed and timely nutritional counseling.

The anti-inflammatory diet

An anti-inflammatory diet places an emphasis on whole grains, daily multiple servings of a variety of fruits and vegetables, and legumes and nuts as main protein sources, with fish and lean poultry included weekly and red meat only sparingly. It emphasizes olive oil as its major source of fat and includes low-fat dairy or soy milk [33]. Phytochemicals, potent biologically active chemicals naturally present in plants, are an essential component of the anti-inflammatory diet. These compounds function as a natural defense system for plants and have multiple powerful anti-inflammatory and antioxidant effects when consumed [34]. Some examples of foods with the most potent protective effects are berries (especially raspberries, blackberries, and strawberries), tomatoes, orange and yellow fruits, and dark leafy green vegetables. Broccoli, cabbage, and cauliflower have strong protective effects against cancer. Plain dark chocolate, with a minimum content of 70% cocoa, is rich in phytochemicals, as are purple grape juice and tea (especially green tea), soy, and soy milk [33,35].

Data supporting the anti-inflammatory diet as being useful in the prevention of obesity and the reduction of cardiovascular risk factors are encouraging [23,36] and consistent with recommendations from the Healthy Children 2010 Objectives [37].

Omega-3 fatty acids and the pediatric diet

Omega-3 fatty acids are essential fatty acids shown to be highly protective in coronary artery disease and other inflammatory and autoimmune states associated with chronic disease [38]. There is a wealth of research available on their mechanism of action and effects on humans [39]. Omega-3 fatty acids are deficient in the typical pediatric diet in the United States [40]. Breast-fed infants receive some omega-3 fatty acids in breast milk, which is an especially good source of docosahexaenoic acid (DHA), and the AAP strongly advocates breastfeeding in the first year of life whenever possible [41]. The World Health Organization recommends that the weaning diet should provide levels of total fat and specific fatty acids similar to those found in breast milk until at least age 2 years, for the best protective effect [42]. Many infant formulas now have supplemental DHA to more closely resemble the amounts found in breast milk. The International Society for the Study of Fatty Acids and Lipids is currently (July 2007) revising their recommendations on dietary intake for infants; in the past, it has recommended 20 mg/kg/d of DHA for infants [43].

The US Government has not yet established a recommended amount for daily DHA intake in children. The American Heart Association currently recommends at least 1000 mg of fish oil daily for adults who have existing cardiovascular disease [44]. Although pediatric studies are lacking in this area, it seems likely that overweight or obese children may receive a protective benefit from daily omega-3 fatty acid supplementation. Some experienced pediatric practitioners begin omega-3 fatty acid supplementation in children using a dose of 15 mg/lb/d [45].

Although omega-3 fatty acids are found naturally in some fish (especially wild salmon), flaxseeds, and walnuts and in omega-3 fortified eggs, many children do not eat enough of these foods to satisfy minimum requirements.

Palatable high-quality supplements are commercially available for children in liquid and soft-gel tablet form.

Of note, omega-3 fatty acids should be stopped at least 2 weeks before any surgery to avoid any possible drug interaction or interference with platelet function because they inhibit thrombocytosis [46].

Carbohydrates, proteins, and fats

Current dietary guidelines from the AAP recommend that after age 2 years, 50% to 60% of calories should come from carbohydrates, about 20% to 30% from fats (with saturated fats making up no more than 10%), and 10% to 20% from protein. Fats used should mainly come from high-quality monounsaturated fats, which are associated with reduced risk of cardiovascular disease. Good sources of monounsaturated fats are olive oil, canola oil, nuts, (excluding peanuts, which are legumes), seeds, olives, and avocados. Trans fats should be avoided. Excellent resources are available that give detailed information on calorie requirements and age-appropriate serving sizes [11,24].

A call to action

Familiarity with the protective effects of the anti-inflammatory diet and omega-3 fatty acid supplementation, coupled with a working knowledge of age appropriate calorie requirements and portion size, may help pediatricians to more effectively impact health and longevity in their overweight and obese patients. Pediatricians can help educate families about the importance of food quality, encourage the use of organic foods whenever feasible, and become a stronger and more vocal force to counteract the aggressive food marketing and advertising campaigns that negatively impact the quality of children's nutrition in the United States.

Motivational interviewing and obesity

Counseling for prevention and treatment of obesity is perceived as difficult by pediatricians, of whom many have low perceived self-efficacy at this intervention [47]. Reasons frequently cited are lack of family involvement, lack of patient motivation, and lack of effective educational resources. Motivational interviewing, a technique used frequently in integrative medicine, may help pediatricians be more effective in coaching obese patients in behavior change. It is a directive style of counseling that [48], rather than focusing on negative behavior or issues, focuses on the patient's own perceptions and motivations, seeks to resolve ambivalence, strengthens the patient's reasons for positive behavior change, and therefore triggers change in a way that is consistent with the patient's goals and values. It is based on the assumption that people generally desire to be well [49] and, by extension, desire health and wellness for their children.

When motivational interviewing is effective, patients hear themselves presenting the argument in favor of the desired behavior change. It is a valuable technique, which can be applied in early preventative screening, preventative counseling, counseling of the already-obese child, or in the maintenance phase to help a patient maintain successful weight loss. Several studies have identified motivational interviewing as being a potentially useful tool in the treatment of pediatric obesity [13,50,51]. Motivational interviewing techniques can be learned and applied by a variety of health care professionals and are being introduced into some medical school curriculums as data accumulate about its usefulness [52,53].

The health coach model

A health coach model is one in which the physician and the health care team take an active role in patients' progress to help keep them on track with their health care goals. A caring and interested physician or other member of the clinical care team can have a powerful motivating effect on the patient and family by scheduling time during routine visits or by making follow-up phone calls to record progress, offer encouragement and support, and answer questions [54]. Skilled motivational interviewing can be a very useful tool in this setting. Successful pediatric and adult programs in obesity treatment and cardiovascular risk reduction programs emphasize the positive effects of this individualized model [4,55,56].

Mind-body medicine

Mind-body medicine is an approach to health that engages the power of thoughts and emotions to positively influence physical health. An extensive body of literature exists on the use of mind-body modalities combined with conventional treatments in people who have chronic illness [57]. The term *mind-body medicine* generally describes one or a combination of the following: mindfulness meditation, guided relaxation and imagery, clinical hypnosis, yoga, progressive muscle relaxation, biofeedback, cognitive behavior therapy, and spirituality as it relates to health. The use of these modalities can help children gain some feeling of control over their illness, which can be especially important in chronic disease.

Although specific studies on mind-body interventions in children who have obesity are few in number [58,59], mind-body medicine is widely used in children for the management of stress, depression, anxiety, low self-esteem, and coping—all of which have been shown to occur in children who have obesity [60,61]. Various mind-body modalities are gaining popularity as an adjunct to successful obesity treatment plans in adults [62], and more research is needed to explore these powerful modalities in the prevention and treatment of pediatric obesity.

The following mind-body techniques are some that have been integrated into academic pediatric centers with integrative medicine components [63]. These therapies are particularly helpful with the mental stress component of obesity. They may be used in combination and must be adapted to the patient's needs and developmental stage.

Yoga

Yoga is a gentle combination of breathing exercises and poses or postures used in many variations throughout the world to reduce stress, increase mindfulness, and improve fitness, flexibility, and mood. Although a few studies exist that have examined yoga specifically in children who have obesity, none have been published with sufficient sample size to conclude a positive effect [64]. There are, however, examples of yoga being successfully incorporated into pediatric obesity treatment programs [65]. The use of yoga in adults showed positive results in weight reduction and effective maintenance after weight loss in a large Vitamin and Lifestyle cohort study [66].

Mindfulness meditation

Meditation, including mindfulness-based stress reduction, has been used to promote feelings of well-being and to improve overall quality of life. Although meditation has been well studied in adult patients who have chronic illness [57,67], no controlled studies examining its specific use in pediatric obesity have been published. Simple focusing exercises (such as having children sit quietly, close their eyes, and breathe while thinking about a word or a calming idea) can be an effective introduction to meditation even in young children [68]. Meditation can be done seated or while walking, alone or in groups, and may be a useful adjunct to pediatric obesity treatment plans to help children experience relaxation and focus.

Spirituality

Although no studies are available on the specific use of spirituality in pediatric obesity treatment, research supports the importance and efficacy of addressing spirituality in the medical treatment plan if the patient and family so desire and resources are available to physicians on how to effectively include spirituality in the medical interview [69]. Studies have confirmed that patients value a discussion of spirituality as it relates to their health and may find inner resources of strength that can significantly contribute to healing or behavior change [70]. Discussion of spirituality may be a useful tool to assist patients and families in obesity treatment [71].

Biofeedback

Biofeedback is a technique in which people learn to control certain body functions such as heart rate, blood pressure, muscle tension, body temperature, or brain wave activity. It is especially powerful in children, with many clinical studies supporting its effectiveness in treating pain, stress, anxiety, and depression [57]. Patients are taught to use the information to gain control over their physiologic state. Physiologic changes are measured with simple equipment and displayed on monitors that give immediate feedback to the patient about the inner workings of their bodies. Biofeedback can give children powerful proof that they have the ability to exert some control over how their bodies react. Children can then go on to apply the learned relaxation skills in day-to-day situations. Biofeedback is used in many conditions and is often combined with relaxation therapies [72,73]. The effectiveness of biofeedback has been demonstrated in some small studies of children who have obesity [59].

Clinical hypnosis, visualization, and guided imagery

Clinical hypnosis, visualization, and guided imagery are closely related modalities that have been used for behavior modification, anxiety, depression, and sleep difficulties [57]. Practitioners of these disciplines should have specific training in clinical hypnosis or guided imagery, preferably with children. Children who have complex psychologic issues such as post-traumatic stress disorder or those who have a history of physical or sexual abuse should be treated by experienced pediatric specialists. Few studies on the use of medical hypnosis and guided imagery have been done specifically in obese children, although these modalities have shown benefit in the treatment of depression and anxiety that often accompany obesity [58]. Clinical hypnosis can be successfully learned by children as young as 3 years [74].

Mind-body therapies and surgery

Bariatric surgery procedures specifically aimed at assisting with weight loss are becoming more popular in adolescents [75]. A review of the literature did not identify any studies evaluating mind-body interventions specifically in pediatric bariatric surgery patients, but research supports the use of such interventions to assist children perioperatively [57,76].

Acupuncture and traditional Chinese medicine

Traditional Chinese medicine (TCM) is a complete medical system and dates back in written form to 200 BC. It is based on the philosophy that the flow of qi (vital energy or life force) must be in proper balance for optimum health. The practice of TCM includes acupuncture, herbal treatments, medicinal nutrition, therapeutic massage, and meditative exercise such as tai chi.

According to the National Center for Complementary and Alternative Medicine, acupuncture is the most familiar and well-studied TCM modality in the Western medical system [57]. Although the exact mechanism of its effect is not clear, it is suspected that acupuncture may work by effecting the release of endorphins that affect the brain's production of chemicals and neurotransmitters. It has been demonstrated that children are able to tolerate and benefit from acupuncture [77].

The small number of studies published on the use of acupuncture for treatment of adult obesity show encouraging results. There is evidence that stimulation of auricular acupuncture points stimulates the vagal nerve and raises serotonin levels. These physiologic events have been shown to increase tone in the smooth muscle of the stomach, thus suppressing appetite. Elevation of serotonin levels has been hypothesized to assist in depression and stress management in some patients [78–80].

Dietary supplements

There are no proven dietary supplements that promote weight loss in the pediatric population (although a plethora of herbal remedies and supplements is advertised for this purpose), and use of these products has increased markedly, especially in adolescents [81]. Few studies are available to guide physicians on the effectiveness and safety of these products in children, and incorrect labeling and identification of herbs or inclusion of contaminants such as lead can put children at serious risk for toxicity [82]. One striking example of an herb used for weigh loss that has shown potential for toxicity is ephedra, used as an appetite suppressant by adolescents. It has been associated with serious adverse consequences, including death, and in the United States, the legality of ephedra compounds is under close scrutiny [83]. Parents administering dietary supplements or herbal products to their children may not voluntarily discuss this practice with the child's health care provider, making it very important to routinely include questions about the use of any dietary supplement or herbal remedy in the medical history of a child being seen for obesity or overweight [82].

Summary

As primary advocates for children's health, pediatricians have a key role in educating families about nutrition and lifestyle issues that directly impact children's health, longevity, and risk for chronic disease. Obesity and its co-morbidities are increasingly prevalent and pose complex challenges for pediatric practitioners. Although more research is needed, an integrative medicine approach offers many potential advantages in the prevention and treatment of overweight and obesity in children. Promising therapeutic areas include nutritional modification and the anti-inflammatory diet, motivational interviewing and health coaching, and the incorporation of mind-body medicine therapies.

References

[1] Rakel D, Weil A. Philosophy of integrative medicine. In: Rakel D, editor. Integrative medicine. 2nd edition. Philadelphia: Saunders; 2007. p. 3–13.
[2] Flynn MA, McNeil DA, Maloff B, et al. Reducing obesity and related chronic disease risk in children and youth: a synthesis of evidence with 'best practice' recommendations. Obes Rev 2006;7(Suppl 1):7–66.

 [3] Perrin EM, Finkle JP, Benjamin JT. Obesity prevention and the primary care pediatrician's
     office. Curr Opin Pediatr 2007;19(3):354–61.
 [4] Savoye M, Shaw M, Dziura J, et al. Effects of a weight management program on body com-
     position and metabolic parameters in overweight children: a randomized controlled trial.
     JAMA 2007;297(24):2697–704.
 [5] Cullum-Dugan D, Saper R. Obesity. In: Rakel D, editor. Integrative medicine. 2nd edition.
     Philadelphia: Saunders; 2007. p. 435–6.
 [6] American Academy of Pediatrics. Promoting physical activity. Available at: www.aap.org/
     family/physicalactivity. Accessed July 28, 2007.
 [7] Hassink SG. Pediatric obesity: prevention, intervention, and treatment strategies for
     primary care. Elk Grove Village (IL): American Academy of Pediatrics; 2007.
 [8] Ogden CL, Carroll MD, Curtin LR, et al. Prevalence of overweight and obesity in the United
     States, 1999–2004. JAMA 2006;295:1549–55.
 [9] Whitaker RC, Wright JA, Pepe MS, et al. Predicting obesity in young adulthood from child-
     hood and parental obesity. N Engl J Med 1997;337:869–73.
[10] Institute of Medicine. Preventing childhood obesity: health in the balance, vol. 90. Washing-
     ton, DC: National Academies Press; 2005.
[11] Hassink SG. Childhood obesity: an overview. In: Pediatric obesity: prevention, intervention,
     and treatment strategies for primary care. Elk Grove Village (IL): American Academy of Pe-
     diatrics; 2007. p. 1–6, 22–5.
[12] Summerbell CD, Waters E, Edmunds LD, et al. Interventions for preventing obesity in
     children. Cochrane Database Syst Rev 2005;3:CD001871.
[13] Kirk S, Scott BJ, Daniels SR. Pediatric obesity epidemic: treatment options. J Am Diet Assoc
     2005;105(5 Suppl 1):S44–51.
[14] Stice E, Shaw H, Marti N. A meta-analytic review of obesity prevention programs for chil-
     dren and adolescents: the skinny on interventions that work. Psychol Bull 2006;132(5):
     667–91.
[15] Cole TJ, Bellizzi MC, Flegal KM, et al. Establishing a standard definition for child over-
     weight and obesity worldwide: international survey. BMJ 2000;320:11240–3.
[16] Centers for Disease Control and Prevention. Available at: www.cdc.gov/growthcharts.
     Accessed July 28, 2007.
[17] Centers for Disease Control and Prevention. Available at: www.cdc.gov/nccdphp/dnpa/
     bmi. Accessed July 28, 2007.
[18] Nader PR, O'Brien M, Houts R, et al. Identifying risk for obesity in early childhood.
     Pediatrics 2006;118(3):e594–601.
[19] Krebs NF, Jacobson MS, American Academy of Pediatrics Committee on Nutrition.
     Prevention of pediatric overweight and obesity. Pediatrics 2003;112:424–30.
[20] Perrin EM, Flower KB, Ammerman AS. Body mass index charts: useful yet underused.
     J Pediatr 2004;144(4):455–60.
[21] Flower KB, Perrin EM, Viadro CI, et al. Using BMI to identify overweight children: barriers
     and facilitators in primary care. Ambul Pediatr 2007;7(1):38–44.
[22] Gilbert MJ, Fleming MF. Use of enhanced body mass index charts during the pediatric
     health supervision visit increases physician recognition of overweight patients. Clin Pediatr
     (Phila) 2007;46(8):689–97.
[23] Rakel D, Rindfleisch JA. The anti-inflammatory diet. In: Rakel D, editor. Integrative
     medicine. 2nd edition. Philadelphia: Saunders; 2007. p. 961–9.
[24] Lucas BL. Nutrition in childhood. In: Mahan LK, Escott-Stump S, editors. Krause's: food,
     nutrition, diet therapy. 11th edition. Philadelphia: Elsevier; 2004. p. 259–83.
[25] Seaman DR. The diet-induced proinflamatory state: a cause of chronic pain and other degen-
     erative diseases? J Manipulative Physiol Ther 2002;25:168–79.
[26] Kapiotis S, Holzer G, Schaller G, et al. A pro-inflammatory state is detectable in obese
     children and is accompanied by functional and morphological vascular changes. Arterioscler
     Thromb Vasc Biol 2006;26(11):2541–6 [E pub September 14, 2006].

[27] Bastard JP, Maachi M, Lagathu C, et al. Recent advances in the relationship between obesity, inflammation, and insulin resistance. Eur Cytokine Netw 2006;17(1):4–12.

[28] Singer G, Granger N. Inflammatory responses underlying the microvasculature dysfunction associated with obesity and insulin resistance. Microcirculation 2007;14(4–5): 375–87.

[29] Khaodhiar L, Ling PR, Blackburn GL, et al. Serum levels of interleukin-6 and C-reactive protein correlate with body mass index across the broad range of obesity. JPEN J Parenter Enteral Nutr 2004;28(6):410–5.

[30] Reinehr T, de Sousa G, Toschke AM, et al. Long term follow up of cardiovascular risk factors in children after an obesity intervention. Am J Clin Nutr 2006;84(3):490–6.

[31] American Academy of Pediatrics, Committee on Nutrition: cholesterol in childhood. Pediatrics 1998;101:141.

[32] Wardle J, Guthrie C, Sanderson S, et al. Food and activity preferences in children of lean an obese parents. Int J Obes Relat Metab Disord 2001;25(7):971–7.

[33] Mathi K. Nutrition in the adult years. In: Mahan LK, Escott-Stump S, editors. Krause's food, nutrition & diet therapy. 11th edition. Philadelphia: Elsevier; 2004. p. 305–8.

[34] Lampe JW. Health effects of vegetables and fruit; assessing mechanisms of action in human experimental studies. Am J Clin Nutr 1999;7:475S–90S.

[35] Hasler CM, Blumberg JB. Phytochemicals: biochemistry and physiology. Introduction. J Nutr 1999;129:756S–7S.

[36] Lucas BL. The Mediterranean diet, pros and cons. In: Mahan LK, Escott-Stump S, editors. Krause's food, nutrition & diet therapy. 11th edition. Philadelphia: Elsevier; 2004. p. 279.

[37] Healthy Children 2010 Objectives. Available at: www.healthypeople.gov/documents/html/vol2/19nutrition.htm. Accessed July 28, 2007.

[38] Simopoulos AP, Leaf A, Salem N Jr. Statement on the essentiality of and recommended dietary intakes for omega-6 and omega-3 fatty acids. Prosteglandins Leukot Essent Fatty Acids 2000;63:119–21.

[39] Seo T, Blaner WS, Deckelbaum RJ. Omega-3 fatty acids: molecular approaches to optimal biological outcomes. Curr Opin Lipidol 2005;16:11–8 [Lipincot Williams & Wilkins].

[40] Devaney B, Ziegler P, Pac S, et al. Nutrient intake of infants and toddlers. J Am Diet Assoc 2004;104(Suppl 1):s14–21.

[41] Krebs N, Jacobsen M. American Academy of Pediatrics, policy statement: prevention of pediatric overweight and obesity. Pediatrics 2003;12(2):424–8.

[42] Institute of Medicine. Dietary intakes for energy, carbohydrate, fiber, fat, fatty acids, cholesterol, protein and amino acids. Washington, DC: The National Academy Press; 2005.

[43] The International Society for the Study of Fatty Acids and Lipids (ISSFAL). Available at: www.issfal.org.uk/pufa-recommendations.html. Accessed July 28, 2007.

[44] American Heart Association. Fish and omega-3 fatty acids. American Heart Association Recommendations. Available at: http://www.americanheart.org/. Accessed July 28, 2007.

[45] Newmark S. Autism. In: Rakel D, editor. Integrative medicine. 2nd edition. Philadelphia: Saunders; 2007. p. 126.

[46] Ettinger S. Macronutrients: carbohydrates, proteins, and lipids. In: Mahan LK, Escott-Stump S, editors. Krause's food, nutrition & diet therapy. 11th edition. Philadelphia: Elsevier; 2004. p. 58.

[47] Perrin EM, Flower KB, Ammerman AS. Pediatricians' own weight: self-perception, misclassification, and ease of counseling. Obes Res 2005;13(2):326–32.

[48] Brown RL. Motivational interviewing. In: Rakel D, editor. Integrative medicine. 2nd edition. Philadelphia: Saunders; 2007. p. 1065–71.

[49] Miller WR. Motivational interviewing in service to health promotion. The Art of Health Promotion, supplement to the American Journal of Health Promotion. 2004 Jan-Feb.

[50] Resnicow K, Davis R, Rollnick S. Motivational interviewing for pediatric obesity: conceptual issues and evidence review. J Am Diet Asoc 2006;106(12):2024–33.

[51] Schwartz RP, Hamre R, Dietz WH, et al. Office based motivational interviewing to prevent childhood obesity: a feasibility study. Arch Pediatr Adolesc Med 2007;161(5):495–501.

[52] Conroy MB, Delichatsios HK, Hafler JP, et al. Impact of a preventative medicine and nutrition curriculum for medical students. Am J Prev Med 2004;27(1):77–80.

[53] Martino S, Haeseler F, Belitsky R, et al. Teaching brief motivational interviewing to year three medical students. Med Educ 2007;41(2):160–7.

[54] Teutsch C. Patient-doctor communication. Med Clin North Am 2003;7(5):1115–45.

[55] Vale MJ, Jelinek MV, Best JD, et al. Coaching patients with coronary heart disease to achieve the target cholesterol: a method to bridge the gap between evidence-based medicine and the "real-world"—randomized controlled trial. J Clin Epidemiol 2002;55(3):245–52.

[56] Vale MJ, Jelinek MV, Best JD, et al. COACH study group. Coaching patients on achieving cardiovascular health (COACH): a multi-center randomized trial in patients with coronary heart disease. Arch Intern Med 2003;163(22):2775–83.

[57] National Center for Complementary and Alternative Medicine. Available at: www.nccam.nih.gov. Accessed July 28, 2007.

[58] Kohen DP, Olness KN, Colwell SO, et al. The use of relaxation-mental imagery (self-hypnosis) in the management of 505 pediatric behavioral encounters. J Dev Behav Pediatr 1984; 5(1):21–5.

[59] Pop-Jordanova N. Psychological characteristics and biofeedback mitigation in preadolescents with eating disorders. Pediatr Int 2000;42(1):76–81.

[60] Strauss RS. Childhood obesity and self-esteem. Pediatrics 2000;105(1):e15.

[61] Lowry KW, Sallinen BJ, Janicke DM. The effects of weight management on self-esteem in pediatric overweight populations. J Pediatr Psychol 2007;9 [E pub ahead of print].

[62] Shaw H, O'Rouke P, Del Mar C, et al. Psychological interventions for overweight or obesity. Cochrane Database Syst Rev 2005;2:CD003818.

[63] Lin YC, Lee AC, Kemper KJ, et al. Use of complementary and alternative medicine in pediatric pain management service: a survey. Pain Med 2005;6(6):452–8.

[64] Larun L, Nordheim LV, Ekeland E. Exercise in prevention and treatment of anxiety and depression among children and young people. Cochrane Database Syst Rev 2006;3:CD004691.

[65] Slawta J, Bently J, Smith J, et al. Promoting healthy lifestyles in children: a pilot program of Be a Fit Kid. Health Promot Pract 2006 [E pub ahead of print].

[66] Kristal AR, Littman AJ, Benitez D, et al. Yoga practice is associated with attenuated weight gain in healthy, middle aged men and women. Altern Ther Health Med 2005;11(4):28–33.

[67] Majumdar M, Grossman P, Kersigs S. Does mindfulness meditation contribute to health? Outcome evaluation of a German sample. J Altern Complement Med 2002;8(6):719–30.

[68] Ditchek S, Greenfield RH. Mind body medicine for children in healthy child, whole child. NewYork: HarperCollins; 2001. p. 182–3.

[69] Anandarajah G, Hight E. Spirituality and medical practice using the HOPE questions as a practical tool for spiritual assessment. Am Fam Physician 2001;63:81–8.

[70] McBride JL, et al. The relationship between a patient's spirituality and health experiences. Fam Med 1998;30(2):122–6.

[71] Waldfogel S. Spirituality in medicine. Prim Care 1997;24(4):963–76.

[72] Duckro PN, Cantwell-Simmons E. A review of studies evaluating biofeedback and relaxation training in the management of pediatric headache. Headache 1989;29:19–27.

[73] Zastowny TR, Kirschenbaum DS, Meng AI. Coping skills training for children: effects on distress before, during and after hospitalization for surgery. Health Psychol 1986;5:231–47.

[74] Butler LD, Symons BK. Henderson SL hypnosis reduces distress and duration of an invasive medical procedure for children. Pediatrics 2005;115(1):e77–85.

[75] Tsai WS, Inge TH, Burd RS. Bariatric surgery in adolescents: recent national trends in use and in hospital outcome. Arch Pediatr Adolesc Med 2007;161(3):217–21.

[76] Astin J. Mind-body therapies for the management of pain. Clin J Pain 2004;20(1):27–32.

[77] Kemper KJ, Sarah R, Silver-Highfield E, et al. On pins and needles? Pediatric pain patients' experience with acupuncture. Pediatrics 2000;105:941–7.

[78] Cabyoglu MT, Ergene N, Tan U. The treatment of obesity by acupuncture. Int J Neurosci 2006;116(2):165–75.

[79] Lacey JM, Tershakovec AM, Foster GD. Acupuncture for the treatment of obesity: a review of the evidence. Int J Obes Relat Metab Disord 2003;27(4):419–27.

[80] Richards D, Marley J. Stimulation of auricular acupuncture points in weight loss. Aust Fam Physician 1998;27(Suppl 2):S73–7.

[81] Pittler MH, Ernst E. Dietary supplements for body-weight reduction: a systematic review. Am J Clin Nutr 2004;79(4):529–36.

[82] Gardiner P. Dietary supplement use in children: concerns of efficacy and safety. Am Fam Physician 2005;71.1068, 1071.

[83] Henry KL, Edwards RW, Oetting ER. Use of ephedra among rural dwelling U.S. adolescents. Subst Use Misuse 2007;42(6):949–59.

PEDIATRIC CLINICS
OF NORTH AMERICA

ELSEVIER
SAUNDERS

Pediatr Clin N Am 54 (2007) 983–1006

Complementary and Alternative Medical Therapies for Attention-Deficit/Hyperactivity Disorder and Autism

Wendy Weber, ND, MPH[a],*, Sanford Newmark, MD[b,c]

[a]School of Naturopathic Medicine, Bastyr University, 14500 Juanita Drive NE,
Kenmore, WA 98021, USA
[b]Center for Pediatric Integrative Medicine, 310 North Wilmot, Suite 307,
Tucson, AZ 85711, USA
[c]Program in Integrative Medicine, University of Arizona, Tucson, AZ, USA

This article addresses the common use of complementary and alternative medicine (CAM) therapies used for the treatment of attention-deficit/hyperactivity disorder (ADHD) and autism in children and adolescents. The article first discusses the prevalence and standard treatment of ADHD and summarizes the current evidence on CAM therapies for the treatment of ADHD. The treatments for ADHD include nutritional interventions, biofeedback, herbal and natural products, vitamins and minerals, homeopathy, massage and yoga, the beneficial impact of playing in green spaces, and the detriment of neurotoxicants. The article then describes the prevalence and likely causes of autism and the CAM approaches to working with children who have autism. CAM therapies for autism include addressing metabolic disorders; gastrointestinal (GI) problems, including dysbiosis, "leaky gut," food sensitivities, and autoimmunity; heavy metal toxicities; and providing nutritional interventions and supplements with potential benefit for children who have autism.

Prevalence of attention-deficit/hyperactivity disorder and standard treatment

ADHD is estimated to affect 3% to 12% of school-aged children [1,2]. The *Diagnostic and Statistical Manual of Mental Disorders, Fourth Edition,*

This work was supported by Grant No. AT000929 from the National Center for Complementary and Alternative Medicine of the National Institutes of Health.
* Corresponding author.
E-mail address: wendyw@bastyr.edu (W. Weber).

doi:10.1016/j.pcl.2007.09.006   *pediatric.theclinics.com* criteria for diagnosis of ADHD requires a minimum of six of nine inattentive or hyperactive/impulsive symptoms for a minimum of 6 months, and the symptoms must be developmentally inconsistent and cause problems in more than one location (home and school) [3]. The most common treatments offered to these children are stimulant medications, such as methylphenidate and dextroamphetamine, and slow-release stimulants, such as amphetamine-dextroamphetamine and methylphenidate extended-release tablets [4]. The stimulant medications have a 30-year history of efficacy and safety in children and adolescents who have ADHD [4]. Up to 30% of patients on stimulant medications, however, may experience side effects, such as decreased appetite, insomnia, and abdominal pain, with as many as 10.9% of children experiencing a serious adverse event [4]. Stimulants are classified as schedule 2 controlled substances, which limits the prescription to a 30-day supply. Many physicians consider this burdensome [5]. Nonstimulant treatment options for ADHD include atomoxetine, and, in some cases, bupropion and clonidine are used as second-line treatment options. Only atomoxetine is approved by the Food and Drug Administration to treat ADHD in children, however. Even these nonstimulant medications have potential side effects, including increased heart rate, increased diastolic blood pressure, decreased appetite, vomiting, nausea, fatigue, liver toxicity, insomnia, or increased risk for suicidal ideation and seizures [6–9].

In the United States, an estimated 2.5 million children take stimulants [10]. Despite the evidence of efficacy for the stimulant treatments, many parents seek alternatives to stimulant medication for their children because of their concern about giving their child a controlled substance or because of the changes in personality some parents report when their child is on stimulant medications. Some parents worry that their child will develop drug abuse problems after using stimulants for ADHD, despite clear evidence to the contrary [11]. Parents and the medical and lay communities often express concern about the number of children prescribed these controlled substances and question the possibility of misdiagnosis or over-diagnosis of ADHD [12]. Further studies are needed to better understand the long-term effects of stimulant medications on the developing brain and the neuronal imprinting effects of these medications [13].

Pathophysiology of attention-deficit/hyperactivity disorder

Research is ongoing to determine the cause of ADHD, including studies on genetic risk factors, environmental risk factors, and structural and physiologic alterations in brain function [2]. Twin studies have estimated the heritability of ADHD to be 0.76 [2]. Dopamine receptors are the focus of genetic study, and the dopamine D4 receptor, which is found in the frontal-subcortical networks, functions poorly in individuals who have ADHD [14]. Dopamine and norepinephrine neural pathways are believed the likely site of pathophysiologic dysfunction of ADHD because animals that have dysregulation of these pathways exhibit symptoms similar to ADHD [2,15]. Stimulants block the reuptake of norepinephrine and dopamine by their transporters and enhance the release of these neurotransmitters, and some inhibit monoamine oxidase [15]. Imaging studies have noted differences in the activity of the dorsolateral prefrontal cortex, ventrolateral prefrontal cortex, dorsal anterior cingulate cortex, and striatum (caudate and putamen) [16]. The dorsal anterior cingulated cortex plays an important role in attention motor control and reward-based decision making, and the striatum is the location of the dopamine transporter and dopaminergic abnormalities [16,17]. More recent reviews of the neurophysiology of ADHD conclude that there unlikely is a single dysfunction underlying this disorder, and that it is more likely that the various forms of ADHD are the result of a combination of risk factors, including genetic, biologic, environmental, and psychosocial [2,18].

Complementary and alternative medicine therapies for attention-deficit/hyperactivity disorder

The frequency of CAM use in children who have ADHD ranges between 12% and 64%, with the lower estimates likely the result of a narrow definition of CAM [12,19–21]. One report documents that nutritional changes were the most common CAM therapy used by children who had ADHD [12]. When parents of children and adolescents who had ADHD were surveyed in community mental health centers, a 19.6% lifetime prevalence of herbal therapy use was found and a 15% prevalence of herbal therapy use was found in the year preceding the survey [22]. A majority (83%) of caregivers noted that the herbal therapy was the main source of drug treatment when it was used [22]. The parents of children who had ADHD referred for care at a tertiary outpatient clinic at a children's hospital were more likely to indicate CAM use if they rated natural therapy or "control over treatment" as important in making therapeutic decisions [21]. A search on the Internet for ADHD treatment provides hundreds of links to over-the-counter products and treatments that are a "definitive cure" for ADHD. The majority of these products and treatments have little if any research documenting their safety let alone their efficacy. The remainder of this article highlights the CAM evidence available on natural treatments of ADHD.

Nutritional interventions

Feingold diet

Much attention was given to the effect of diet on the symptoms of ADHD after Dr. Feingold [23] published his findings that 50% of his patients who had ADHD improved with the elimination of all food additives and naturally occurring salicylates. The Feingold diet eliminates nearly all processed

foods and a large proportion of fruits and vegetables, which are high in salicylates, a drastic change for most children. The extensive restriction on dietary intake required by the Feingold diet has made replicating the findings
of Dr. Feingold difficult [24]. Complete control of a child's diet is difficult
unless children are admitted to a clinical research center for the entire trial.
The evaluation of symptoms in the contrived circumstances of a clinical research center, however, may not replicate the real world situations in which
these children demonstrate their inattentive or hyperactive/impulsive symptoms. A review by Wender [25] provides an excellent summary of the origins
of the Feingold diet and a summary of the clinical trials evaluating the efficacy of this dietary intervention. Although initial studies seemed to show
a benefit with the diet, replication of these studies found no benefit with
the Feingold diet. In the few studies that did find benefit, the blinding of
the placebo intervention has been called into question because improvement
was seen only when the Feingold diet was the second intervention in the
crossover trials. Wender concludes that a small percentage of children
who have ADHD may benefit from the Feingold diet. The expense of providing food for all participants in these trials often limits the size of the
study; the largest trial included only 40 participants, decreasing the power
to detect more modest effects of the dietary intervention. It is possible
that a large, well-designed trial with careful controls for the intervention
may find benefit for a portion of children who have ADHD symptoms. A
recent double-blind, placebo-controlled study examined the effects of artificial food coloring and additives (AFCAs) on hyperactive behavior in 3- to 4-
year-old and 8- to 9-year-old children from the general population [26]. All
children had AFCAs removed from their diet for the 6-week trial and then
consumed one of the matched study drinks containing either one of two
mixes of AFCAs or placebo in random order during weeks 2, 4, and 6.
The investigators reported increased global hyperactivity in the 3 to 4
year olds and the 8 to 9 year olds after consuming the AFCAs [26].

Food sensitivities

   Food sensitivities are a speculated cause of ADHD symptoms and several
laboratories offer serum tests for specific antibodies to a variety of foods.
The specificity of these laboratory measures is not good enough to rely
solely on the results [27]. Two clinical trials have examined the effect of multiple eliminations from the diet (foods, dyes, and preservatives) in an open-
label manner followed by a double-blind, placebo-controlled challenge of
the eliminated items [28,29]. In both trials, those who improved during
the elimination phase demonstrated a greater frequency of reaction to
some of the eliminated item challenges than to the placebo challenges.
Only those children who responded favorably to the elimination were challenged in a double-blind manor, which would bias toward detecting a beneficial effect. The results of these studies are promising, yet clinicians need to

keep in mind the importance of challenging the eliminated foods, rather than just restricting a child's diet. Families could work with a child's teacher to evaluate the child's behavior in a blinded manner when the foods are being challenged to decrease the expectancy effect of the challenge situation.

Sugar avoidance

Many parents note a change in their child's behavior when they reduce the amount of sugar in the child's diet. Wolraich and colleagues [30] conducted a complex 9-week intervention, supplying all food for participants, to examine the effect of three different diets: high sucrose, high aspartame, and saccharin sweetener diet. No differences in behavioral or cognitive measures were found among children believed to be sensitive to sugar by their parents while on the different diets, yet these children were not diagnosed with ADHD. None of the diets, however, eliminated other sources of sugar, such as fruit or unsweetened fruit juices. A revealing study by Hoover and Milich [31] found that parental expectation of aggravation resulting from sugar ingestion may play a significant role in the perceptions of parents. In this trial, half of the mothers were told their child received a large dose of sugar and half of the mothers were told that their child received a placebo. In reality, all of the children believed to be sugar sensitive by their parents received an aspartame sweetened snack. Mothers who were told their child received a large amount of sugar rated their child's behavior as more hyperactive and were more critical of their child than the mothers who were told their child had a low sugar snack. An excellent review of the effects of diet on ADHD concludes that clinical trials do not support a link between sucrose consumption and hyperactivity [32]. No studies have examined the link between hyperactivity and the glycemic index of the diet, which may be a better measure of the amount of simple sugars consumed in the diet. Dr. David Ludwig of Boston's Children Hospital states, "A child eats a breakfast that has no fat, no protein, and a high glycemic index—let's say a bagel with fat-free cream cheese. His blood sugar goes up, but pretty soon it crashes, which triggers the release of stress hormones like adrenaline. What you're left with, at around 10 AM, is a kid with low blood sugar and lots of adrenaline circulating in his bloodstream. He's jittery and fidgety and not paying attention. That's going to look an awful lot like ADHD to his teacher" [33]. Although the results of clinical trials do not consistently demonstrate a negative effect of high sugar diets on behavior, recommending moderate consumption of sugar intake seems most appropriate given the growing epidemics of obesity and diabetes.

Essential fatty acids

Some of the most important fats used by the human body and brain for development and function must be supplied from the diet or supplementation because of the inability of the human body to synthesize these fats. These polyunsaturated fatty acids are known as essential fatty acids (EFAs). EFAs include the omega-3 fatty acids, eicosapentaenoic acid (EPA) and docosahexaenoic acid (DHA), and the omega-6 fatty acid, arachidonic acid. A growing body of evidence suggests that individuals who have ADHD may have low levels of these EFAs, specifically DHA and arachidonic acid [34]. The standard American diet is not abundant in dietary sources of omega-3 fats, which include flax, cold water fish, and certain nuts (brazil nuts, cashews, and walnuts). Children are at particular risk for low concentrations of these omega-3 fatty acids because of the recommendations that children not consume fish on a frequent basis because of its high mercury content.

Richardson [35] published a recent review of the effects of omega-3 fatty acids in ADHD, including information on the clinical trials performed in children who have ADHD. A few of the randomized controlled trials have examined the efficacy of EFAs for the treatment of disruptive behavioral disorders or learning disabilities rather than ADHD. Few studies have examined the effect of EFAs in children who have ADHD specifically and used a randomized controlled study design. Voigt and colleagues [36] randomized children who had ADHD to receive DHA (345 mg) or placebo and found no beneficial effect on computer or parental ratings of ADHD symptoms. All of the children enrolled in this trial had their symptoms managed effectively by stimulant medication during the trial, which makes detecting the impact of the EFAs more difficult. Parental and computer assessments of symptoms were done after a 24-hour withdrawal of medication. Stevens and colleagues [37] randomized children to a blended EFA supplement containing omega-3 and omega-6 fatty acids or an olive oil placebo. In children who were taking the EFA supplement in addition to pharmacotherapy, 2 of 16 measures showed improvement including conduct problems, as rated by parents, and attention symptoms, as rated by teachers. Sinn and Bryan [38] randomized children not on stimulant medication to a blended EFA (fish oil and evening primrose oil) with or without a multivitamin or to placebo (palm oil). In the per protocol analysis, the participants on the EFA showed improvements in the Conners' Parent Rating Scale scores over 15 weeks compared with the placebo group. This study excluded 21% of participants who dropped out before 15 weeks or did not complete the required questionnaires or take required study medicine. Exclusion of such a large portion of the participants eliminates the benefits of randomization because of differences in the patients who dropped out early (worse ADHD symptoms) and biases the results toward finding a positive effect. Other studies of a blended EFA supplement have found benefit in the treatment of dyslexia with ADHD features and developmental coordination disorder (DCD) [35]. The growing body of evidence supports the use of an EFA supplement for children who have ADHD.

Electroencephalographic biofeedback

The field of electroencephalographic (EEG) biofeedback is a growing area of research for the treatment of ADHD. This form of treatment is based on the finding that children who have ADHD demonstrate abnormal quantitative EEG findings in a pattern of underactivity in the majority of cases or hyperarousal in some patients [39]. EEG biofeedback uses a series of sessions (more than 30) over several weeks to teach patients how to alter their quantitative EEG activity to a more balanced level by rewarding children when their activity is sustained in the level desired. Monastra and colleagues [40] provide an extensive review of the theory behind EEG biofeedback, the protocols developed, and the results of case studies and controlled trials. A few controlled studies have been conducted comparing EEG biofeedback to stimulant treatment or a wait list control, and these trials demonstrate improvement in ADHD symptoms and improved quantitative EEG activity [41]. Nearly all of the controlled clinical trials of EEG biofeedback allowed the participants to self-select to EEG biofeedback treatment; thus, the findings are subject to substantial selection bias. In addition, several of the trials used an active control (stimulants), yet the studies were not powered to detect noninferiority to the stimulants, which would require a large sample size. Small sample sizes favor not detecting a difference between the active control and the EEG biofeedback intervention. To evaluate the potential benefits for EEG, future studies need to randomize participants to treatment allocation, and ideally a "placebo" form of EEG biofeedback should be used as the control to account for the nonspecific effects of multiple treatment sessions over a short time period.

Herbal and natural health products

The use of herbal treatments in children often is based on use in adults, yet little is known about the safety or appropriate dosing of these herbal treatments in children. Despite the common use of herbal treatments by children who have ADHD, only one study has examined the effect of an herbal product containing *Ginkgo biloba* and *Panax quinquefolius* (American ginseng) in pediatric patients who have ADHD [42]. Ginsengs and ginkgo are believed to have nootropic effects to improve memory and facilitate learning. The study found improvement in ADHD symptoms over the 4-week intervention, but no comparison group was studied so efficacy could not be determined. Fourteen of the 36 participants were allowed to continue on medications that were not controlling their symptoms before starting the trial and two of 36 participants experienced increased symptoms of hyperactivity or impulsivity. A sufficiently powered randomized controlled study is needed to determine the efficacy and side effects of this herbal combination.

One study has examined the effects of L-carnitine for the treatment of ADHD in a placebo-controlled crossover study and found that 50% of the participants responded to the carnitine treatment [43]. The investigators, however, do not present baseline and follow-up data for all participants in each treatment period, making it difficult to interpret the efficacy of carnitine. L-Carnitine is a necessary component of fatty acid metabolism and ATP synthesis, although how this translates specifically into improvement in ADHD symptoms is unknown. Another randomized controlled study examined the efficacy of pycnogenol (1 mg/kg per day) for the treatment of ADHD and found improvements in teacher and parent ratings of symptom severity compared with a placebo intervention [44]. The study treatment had a short duration of 4 weeks, so future studies need to examine if the effects seen continue over a longer treatment period. The pycnogenol used in this study was a standardized extract from the bark of the French maritime pine tree (*Pinus pinaster*). The proposed mechanism of action of pycnogenol is that it increases production of nitric oxide, which regulates dopamine and norepinephrine release and intake. Dopamine and norepinephrine are the targets of standard pharmacotherapy.

Massage and yoga

A small controlled trial to study the effect of yoga enrolled children who had ADHD whose symptoms were stable on medication. The investigators reported improvement in ADHD symptoms in the yoga group on some of the measures of Conners' Parent Rating Scale, but the limited sample size made between group comparisons underpowered to detect an effect [45]. In another study, when adolescents who had ADHD were randomized to massage therapy or relaxation treatment, the adolescents in the massage group were rated by their teachers to have decreased symptoms of hyperactivity, anxiety, and inattention but the difference was not statistically better than the improvement seen in the relaxation group [46]. The lack of difference between the groups may be the result of potential benefit from the relaxation treatment or a result of the small sample size enrolled in the study. The positive trend in the findings do support further research into the efficacy of yoga and massage for ADHD symptoms.

Vitamins and minerals

Several individual vitamins and minerals are proposed as possible treatments for ADHD, yet there are few randomized controlled trials evaluating the efficacy of these treatments. Zinc reduced symptoms of hyperactivity, impulsivity, and socialization difficulties in children and adolescents who had ADHD, but it did not improve symptoms of inattention [47]. This study used a high dosage of zinc for a period of 12 weeks and more than 50% of both groups dropped out of the study. Even though benefit was seen from zinc treatment, full therapeutic response was seen in only 29% of the zinc group versus 20% of the placebo group. Replication of these findings in another study with better retention is needed. Another study examined the effects of zinc with and without methylphenidate in a randomized controlled trial. The investigators found an improvement in parent and teacher ratings of ADHD symptoms for both groups, but those on zinc and methylphenidate had greater improvement than those on methylphenidate alone [48]. Konofal and colleagues [49] reported that children who have ADHD have lower serum ferritin levels than children who do not have ADHD symptoms and that the severity of symptoms correlates with low ferritin levels. In an open-label study, iron supplementation was found to improve symptoms of ADHD in nonanemic children, yet no controlled studies have evaluated its efficacy [50]. One small study examined the effectiveness of megavitamin therapy in a controlled trial and concluded no benefit was detected, and increased disruptive behavior and elevated serum transaminase levels were seen in the group on the megavitamin treatment [51]. If using doses of vitamins or minerals higher than the recommended daily allowance, it is important to monitor serum or cell membrane levels of these nutrients and liver enzymes to prevent toxicity.

Homeopathy

Homeopathy is a medical practice based on the belief that "like treats like" and that the energetics of a small amount of a substance can have healing effects on individuals. At least three randomized controlled trials have evaluated the efficacy of homeopathy for the treatment of ADHD with mixed results [52]. Strauss [53] reported improvements on the Conners' Parent Symptom Questionnaire for children treated with homeopathy for 2 months, although no data on the other outcomes examined were provided, making the overall effect of homeopathy difficult to interpret. The second study enrolled patients who responded to a homeopathic treatment and randomized them into a crossover discontinuation study [54]. It found improvement of ADHD symptoms on the Conners' Global Index, but the lack of a washout period before randomization resulted in all patients worsening in the first treatment period regardless of group assignment. In the final trial, all participants experienced the same interaction with the homeopath, who was allowed to change the remedy and potency used over the 18-week trial [55]. Participants were randomized to receive the active homeopathic remedy prescribed by the homeopath or a placebo homeopathic remedy. Both groups improved over the course of the trial, but no differences were detected in the magnitude of improvement between the placebo and active homeopathy groups. These findings led the investigators to conclude that the effectiveness of homeopathy may be the result of the nonspecific effects of the interaction with the homeopath and not the actual remedy given, and future research should explore this possibility. Homeopathy offers potential as a possibly effective treatment option for ADHD, but it is unclear if this efficacy is the result of the interaction with the homeopath or the actual homeopathic remedy.

Environmental issues

Several investigators have discussed the symptoms of ADHD as a physical and mental manifestation of nature deficit disorder [56,57]. In his book, *Last Child in the Woods: Saving our Children from Nature-Deficit Disorder*, Louv [56] provides anecdotal evidence of how the loss of green spaces and creative play outdoors is correlated with the increase in childhood mental health disorders, including ADHD. Kuo has started evaluating this theory with rigorously designed research studies. In a national online survey of parents of children who have ADHD, Kuo and Taylor [57] reported improvement in ADHD symptoms with green outdoor play compared with indoor and "built outdoor" play. This cross-sectional survey provides some evidence of the benefit of green spaces for ADHD; only two of the 339 reasons parents gave as to why the activity might reduce symptoms related to being in an outdoor setting decreases the likelihood that the results are biased. The investigators suggest rigorously designed randomized controlled trials to differing play experiences to determine the effects on ADHD as rated by a blinded evaluator. Many parents have always known that a connection to nature is beneficial to children; we are now on the cusp of having documented efficacy of the beneficial effect of nature for children who have ADHD.

The environment contains a variety of chemicals and toxins, many of which are linked to neurodevelopmental disorders. The toxic effects of mercury and lead are well known, and the symptoms of these toxicities resemble the symptoms of ADHD and even autism [58,59]. The effects of heavy metals, pesticides, polychlorinated biphenyls, and polybrominated diphenyl ethers on the human brain are just being elucidated [59]. Environmental advocates and researchers are pushing for more research into the effect of even low doses of these chemicals on the developing brain in utero and during childhood [59]. The elucidation of the effects of these chemicals is more difficult when taking into consideration the large number of exposures individuals have to the thousands of chemicals in the environment and the unique susceptibility of individuals from genomics [59]. The health implications of neurotoxicants are of concern in the development of ADHD but many are concerned that these compounds may be the cause of autism (heavy metal toxicity in autism is discussed later).

Autism

Autism is a neurodevelopmental disorder characterized by deficits in social interaction, language development, and a restricted or stereotypical pattern of interests and activities. Formerly a rare condition well out of the public eye, the prevalence of autism has increased more than tenfold in the past 20 years, from an estimated prevalence of approximately 5 to 6 per 10,000 children to 65 per 10,000 in more recent studies [60]. There is no scientific agreement as to the cause of this rapid increase in prevalence, often referred to as an "epidemic" in the media. The three most likely possibilities are (1) there is a true increase in the prevalence of the disorder; (2) there is increased case-finding resulting from increased awareness of the disorder on the part of the public and medical and other professionals; and (3) there has been a loosening of the definition of autism so that more children are being diagnosed.

To complicate matter, other diagnostic categories, such as autism spectrum disorder, pervasive developmental disorder, and Asperger's syndrome have been added to the mix, including children who have some features of autism but do not meet the full criteria. The Brick Township study separated autism from autism spectrum disorder and Asperger's syndrome, however, and still recorded a prevalence of 40 per 10,000 of autism itself [61]. A recent study in Minnesota, in which autism is separated out from these other categories, gives a striking picture of the rapidity of the increase in the prevalence of this disorder [62].

Regressive autism

Regressive autism refers to children who have normal development until the age of 1 to 2 years, after which there is a loss of language, social interaction, and other developmental milestones. It is this type of autism that has caused the widespread public concern over the influence of the measles, mumps, and rubella vaccine and mercury-containing vaccines on the development of autism. The available studies indicate, however, that regressive autism accounts for only 30% of autism, although there is surprisingly sparse research on this question.

Etiology

Currently it is believed that autism is a genetically based disorder requiring an environmental trigger to manifest. This is supported by the 90% concordance rate in identical twins as opposed to the 30% concordance rate in fraternal twins [63]. There are many gene loci associated with autism, but no single gene or group of genes has been linked definitively to this disorder [64]. There is little scientific research concerning which environmental factors may trigger the expression of this disease. Many patients and physicians interested in alternative treatment of autism, however, are concerned about the role of mercury, immunizations, and other environmental toxins in triggering the development of autism.

Complementary and alternative medical therapies for autism

CAM therapies are used with great frequency in the treatment of autism. A study in 2006 showed that overall, an astonishing 74% of families of children who had autism spectrum disorder were using some type of CAM therapy. Although these included the full spectrum of CAM therapies, the highest frequency of use (more than 54% of families) involved what were termed, "biologically based" therapies, including modified diets, vitamins and minerals, and other nutritional supplements [65]. Several other studies have demonstrated similarly high frequency of use, from 30% in a regional referral center to 92% in two primary care practices [66–68]. This reflects the high acceptance, among families and many physicians, of what is commonly referred to as a "biomedical" approach to autism. The basis of this approach is that autism is a genetics-based syndrome triggered by certain fetal, neonatal, and early childhood stimuli, and that this syndrome is associated with a variety of nutritional, GI, metabolic, and autoimmune abnormalities that can be corrected partially or fully. Most of the remainder of this article is devoted to a discussion of this approach.

The gastrointestinal system

One of the most common problems seen in children who have autism is a variety of GI symptoms and clear GI pathology. The incidence of GI problems in autism varies by study but seems to be approximately 30% to 40% of children. Symptomatically, the most common reports are of chronic constipation or diarrhea and chronic abdominal pain.

GI pathology is common and widespread. One study of children who had autism and GI symptoms showed that 69.4% of subjects had reflux esophagitis, 42% had chronic gastritis, and 67% had chronic duodenitis [69]. Many of these children are nonverbal and cannot express GI discomfort; thus, these children may react to pain by exhibiting behaviors not obviously referable to the GI system, such as self-stimulation or temper tantrums.

There are several studies demonstrating definite pathology of the small and large bowels. Torrente and colleagues [70] performed biopsies of 25 children who had autism and found duodenitis in almost all of the children. He described increased lymphocytic proliferation in the epithelium and lamina propria. Horvath and colleagues [69] also documented significant dissacharidase deficiencies in a population of children who had autism and GI symptoms.

Dysbiosis

Dysbiosis, or abnormalities of GI microflora, also is believed a common problem. Rosseneu [71] analyzed 80 children who had autism and GI symptoms and found that 61% had growth of abnormal aerobic gram-negative, endotoxin-producing bacteria. These aerobic gram-negative bacteria are producers of endotoxin, which could cause ongoing bowel damage. Fifty-five percent had overgrowth of *Staphylococcus aureus* and 95% had overgrowth of pathogenic *Escherichia coli*. There were no abnormal amounts of yeast noted in this study. In a fascinating pilot study, 11 of these children were treated with a nonabsorbable antibiotic and not only did the abnormal flora disappear but also GI symptoms and autistic behaviors decreased significantly. This study did not have a control group, and after 2 months the abnormal bacteria returned to pretreatment levels. In another study, vancomycin treatment of children who had regressive autism and diarrhea resulted in decreased autistic behaviors as measured by blinded observers [72].

An overgrowth of yeast is widely believed part of dysbiosis and responsible for many GI and behavioral symptoms of autism, and many children are treated with antifungal agents as part of their "bowel detoxification" protocol. The evidence for this yeast overgrowth is limited. As discussed previously, Rosseneu's study failed to identify any yeast among the abnormal bacteria, and there have been no good controlled studies evaluating yeast overgrowth in autism. Some research shows the presence of urine organic acids suggestive of yeast overgrowth in children who have autism, but the significance of these byproducts is unclear. There is widespread use of antifungals, such as nystatin, fluconazole, and ketoconazole, with much anecdotal evidence of positive results but no controlled studies.

"Leaky gut"

Another GI abnormality commonly attributed to children who have autism is called the "leaky gut" phenomena, related to a theorized increased intestinal permeability. In a study by D'Eufemia and colleagues [73], examination of 21 autistic children who had no known intestinal disorders confirmed increased intestinal permeability in 43%, as opposed to zero controls. Horvath and Perman [74] examined 25 children who had autism and GI symptoms using lactulose/mannitol testing and found 76% had altered intestinal permeability.

Food sensitivities/allergies

Food sensitivities or allergies also are believed to play an important role in the pathophysiology of autism. The evidence for this is indirect but suggestive. In one study, 36 children who had autism were compared with healthy controls and had significantly higher levels of IgA, IgG, and IgM antigen-specific antibodies for specific food proteins, such as lactoglobulin, casein, and β-lactoglobulin, than did controls [75]. Also, a study by Jyonouchi and colleagues [76] showed that children who had autism had higher intestinal levels of inflammatory ctytokines directed against specific dietary proteins than did controls.

Some researchers believe that gluten and casein that pass through a leaky gut barrier can form gluteomorphins and caseomorphins, which then have important central nervous system effects; however, the research in this area is inconsistent. These putative food protein sensitivities do not show up as immediate hypersensitivity on standard skin testing or IgE radioallergosorbent testing, leading to the question of whether or not children who have autism have true food allergies or food sensitivities that are not IgE mediated.

Autoimmunity

There are several studies that suggest that autoimmune abnormalities are common in children who have autism. Some of these can be linked directly to the central nervous system. Connolly and colleagues [77] examined the sera of children who had autism for antibrain antibodies. IgG antibrain antibodies were present in the sera of 27% of children and only 2% of controls. IgM antibodies were present in 36% of the sera of autistic children and in 0% of controls. Singh and colleagues [78] evaluated the prevalence of antibodies to various brain structures in 68 autistic children and 30 controls. Of the autistic children, 49% had serum antibodies to the caudate nucleus as opposed to 0% of controls. Antibodies to the cerebral cortex and cerebellum were 18% and 9%, respectively, again with 0% of controls having these antibodies. Most recently, Cabanlit and colleagues [79] described a significantly increased incidence of brain-specific (thalamic and hypothalamic) autoantibodies in the plasma of children who had autism compared with controls. It is not clear if these antibodies cause neurologic problems or merely are a byproduct of central nervous system damage caused by other factors (eg, viral infections).

Metabolic disorders

There are several studies that demonstrate some abnormalities in the metabolic functioning of children who have autism with defects in areas such as glutathione synthesis, sulfation deficits, and folate metabolism. For instance, a study in the *American Journal of Clinical Nutrition* demonstrated that relative to the control children, the children who had autism had significantly lower baseline plasma concentrations of methionine, S-adenosyl methionine (SAM), homocysteine, cystathionine, cysteine, and total glutathione and significantly higher concentrations of S-adenosyl homocysteine (SAH), adenosine, and oxidized glutathione [80]. This metabolic profile is consistent with impaired capacity for methylation (significantly lower ratio of SAM to SAH) and increased oxidative stress. In another study, activities of erythrocyte superoxide dismutase and erythrocyte and plasma glutathione peroxidase in autistic children were significantly lower than in children who did not have autism [81]. These results indicate that autistic children have low levels of activity of blood antioxidant enzyme systems.

A review article by McGinnis [82] documents several positive markers of oxidative stress in children who have autism. Among other factors, he cites indirect markers for greater oxidative stress, such as (1) lower endogenous antioxidant enzymes and glulathione; (2) lower antioxidant nutrients; (3) higher organic toxins and heavy metals; (4) higher xanthine oxidase and cytokines; and (5) higher production of nitric oxide, a toxic free radical.

Heavy metal toxicity

It is a widespread belief among many clinicians and families involved in the alternative treatment of autism that increased body levels of heavy metals, especially mercury, are an important part of the pathophysiology of autism. A study in Texas showed that there was a direct correlation between the incidence of autism and the amount of mercury expelled from industrial pollution [83]. For each 1000 pounds of environmentally released mercury, there was a 43% increase in the rate of special education services and a 61% increase in the rate of autism. This is a correlation only and does not prove causation but nevertheless is concerning, especially as environmental mercury pollution continues to rise.

The concern about mercury is linked to the assumption that the thimerosal contained in (later withdrawn from) infant immunizations is a major factor in the rise in autism prevalence. Because children who have autism likely are not exposed to more mercury or other heavy metals than other children, it is postulated that these children have impaired abilities to detoxify or excrete mercury and other heavy metals. This is believed the result of various methylation, sulfation, and antioxidant deficiencies (discussed previously).

What is the evidence that there is an increased body burden of mercury and other heavy metals in children who have autism? There is surprisingly little. One of the problems in discussing heavy metal toxicity is that there are no simple tests for determining body levels of heavy metals. Blood tests for mercury are not useful because mercury remains in the tissues and not the circulation. Hair analysis has been used, but it is not clear that these tests adequately reflect body burdens of mercury. In conventional medicine, mercury toxicity is measured by giving a dose of a chelating agent, such as ethylene diamine tetraacetic acid (EDTA) or 2,3-dimercaptosuccinic acid (DMSA), and then measuring urine mercury levels. There is no significant body of data using this procedure to compare autistic children and controls. One study compared blood and hair levels of autistic children with those of controls and found no significant differences. It did not examine, however, urine levels after chelation [84]. A study by Adams and colleagues [85] did show that children who had autism had significantly higher levels of mercury in their baby teeth than typically developing children. Bradstreet and colleagues [86] performed a retrospective analysis of 221 children and 18 controls who had been treated with three doses of DMSA. Heavy metal concentrations in the urine were analyzed showing urinary concentrations of mercury were significantly higher in 221 autistic children than in the 18 controls. Limitations of this study were that it was a retrospective study with nonrandom selection of controls and that the imbalance between the number of cases and the control group was large. Selection bias is a concern for controls and autistic children. Also it is unknown if the control group was representative of all children (the general pediatric population), because it was such a small sample size and the way they were selected was not delineated.

In summary, although it is clear that mercury is a potent neurotoxin, especially in the developing brain, the idea that mercury exposure is a significant cause of autism is at this point largely is unproved. There is a need for a prospective study comparing postchelation urinary heavy metal levels in autistic children compared with controls. In addition, chelation therapy is recommended widely by biomedical practitioners for children who have autism, based on the assumption that removing these metals will result in improvement in autistic symptoms. There is no scientific support for this contention at this time. There are possible electrolyte imbalances that could accompany chelation therapy and, if used at all, should be done carefully under the direction of an experienced practitioner.

Nutritional deficiencies, including omega-3 fatty acids

It is a tenet of the biomedical approach that nutritional deficiencies are widespread and important in autism. It is believed these are linked mainly to poor digestion and absorption of nutrients resulting from GI problems (discussed previously) and abnormalities in the metabolic processing of nutrients. The evidence for these nutritional deficiencies, however, is uneven and rarely complete.

Vancassel and colleagues [87] evaluated levels of omega-3 fatty acids and other polyunsaturated fatty acids in the serum of children who had autism compared with controls. Children who had autism had 23% lower levels of plasma omega-3 fatty acids than did controls. Autistic children also had 20% lower levels of plasma polyunsaturated fatty acids than did controls. The reason for this is unclear. Do children who have autism have different levels of omega-3 fat intake than control children? Perhaps children who have autism have differences in how they use and metabolize these fats. More research is needed to elucidate the mechanisms responsible for these observed differences.

Integrative therapies for autism

Conventional behavioral approaches

Speech therapy is recommended almost universally to deal with the language deficits of children who have autism. Anecdotally, it is believed effective by almost all parents and most professionals. There is little solid research supporting the efficacy of speech therapy for autism. Although several studies show specific areas of language improvement, all of these involve few subjects and none have been randomized or controlled. Considering the almost universal use of speech therapy in the treatment of autism, this is an area with surprisingly inadequate research.

Intensive behavioral therapy is another therapy commonly used for children who have autism. Direct behavioral intervention by trained facilitators occurs in home and school settings from 20 to 40 hours a week. There are several specific methods, such as Lovaas, Floortime, and applied behavior analysis. Intervention is directed at increasing appropriate social and language behavior while decreasing self-stimulatory activities. Overall, there is reasonable evidence as to the effectiveness of this modality. A 2003 review in the *Canadian Journal of Psychiatry* concludes, "delivering interventions for more than 20 hours weekly that are individualized, well planned, and target language development and other areas of skill development significantly increases children's developmental rates, especially in language, compared with no or minimal treatment" [88].

Alternative behavioral approaches

Another modality used commonly in children who have autism is sensory integration therapy. Children who have autism have significant sensory issues. They often do not enjoy touching, can be upset by noisy environments, and exhibit other sensory difficulties. To modify these deficits, sensory integration therapy often is recommended. This usually involves a variety of sensory stimuli administered under controlled conditions. As with the therapies described previously, there is only anecdotal evidence of effectiveness. There are several small studies but any evidence of efficacy is preliminary at best.

A second alternative behavioral modality is auditory integration therapy. This is based on the idea that a hypersensitivity to certain sounds can cause behavioral and emotional difficulties in autistic children. Essentially, auditory integration therapy attempts to reprogram and "integrate" the auditory system by sending randomized sound frequencies through earphones worn by an autistic child. This usually is done in 20- to 30-minute sessions over a period of approximately 10 days. There are many anecdotal reports of efficacy, but studies so far are uncontrolled or limited to small numbers. A systematic review of the few controlled studies showed equivocal results and found insufficient evidence to support its use [89].

Nutrition

Dietary interventions

The most common alternative biomedical intervention used with autistic children is the gluten-free casein-free (GFCF) diet. This is based on the theory (discussed previously) that food sensitivities, especially to gluten and casein, can produce not only GI symptoms but also, in association with gut inflammation and increased gut permeability (leaky gut), can lead to many of the neurologic manifestations of autism. In general, for the GFCF diet, parents are advised to strictly avoid all foods containing gluten or casein for periods of 60 days or more.

The anecdotal evidence for the efficacy is abundant. In various support groups, chat groups, and other situations bringing together parents of children who have autism, the GFCF diet often is described as promoting significant and positive changes in GI symptoms, language, socialization, and other autistic behaviors.

What about the evidence? There are only two controlled studies concerning the efficacy of the GFCF diet in the treatment of autism, but both show positive results. In the first study, by Knivsberg and colleagues [90], 10 matched pairs of children who had autism were randomized to a GFCF diet or a placebo control for 1 full year. Behaviors then were evaluated by blinded observers using the DIPAB, a Danish instrument for measuring autistic traits. Post intervention, the diet group had a mean DIPAB rating of 5.60, significantly ($P = .001$) better than the control group rating of 11.20. Specifically, social contact increased in 10 of 15 of the treated children, whereas ritualistic behaviors in that group decreased in 8 of 11 children. In the second study, by Lucarelli and colleagues [75], autistic children were found to have decreased behavioral symptoms after 8 weeks on a dairy elimination diet. Too often in clinical practice, the GFCF diet is started in conjunction with nutritional supplements and other interventions, making it difficult to know if behavioral or other improvements can be attributed to the diet.

Supplements

There are many nutritional supplements used in the treatment of autism, including omega-3 fatty acids, probiotics, zinc, vitamin B_6, and other multivitamin and mineral supplements.

Omega-3 fatty acids

Omega-3 fatty acids are used widely in the treatment of autism. The research on this is preliminary but encouraging. In a pilot study, 18 children were given an omega-3 fatty acid supplement (with 247 mg of omega-3s and 40 mg of omega-6s) for 3 months [91]. Their language skills were measured at baseline and after the 3-month trial. There was a highly significant increase in language skills over a variety of measures. A double-blind, placebo-controlled study evaluated the effects of 1.5 mg total omega-3 fatty acids on children who have autistic disorders accompanied by severe tantrums, aggression, or self-injurious behavior [92]. It was a small study, with only 22 children, but it did show significant advantages of omega-3s over placebo.

Another study of relevance concerned the use of omega-3 fatty acids in DCD [93]. Although not part of the autistic spectrum, DCD is relevant because children who have this disorder present with some of the features of autism spectrum disorders. In this double-blind, controlled trial, 117 children were given an omega-3 fatty acid supplement or placebo for 3 months.

Treated children made startling gains in reading, spelling, and mathematic skills compared with the placebo group. For example, the average reading scores in the treatment group advanced 9.5 months in 3 months as opposed to an increase of 3.5 months in the placebo group ($P = .004$). There are no clearly accepted guidelines for the dosage or ratio of omega-3 fatty acids in autism treatment. Further research is needed.

Probiotics

Probiotics are used frequently in the biomedical treatment of autism. As discussed previously, it is speculated that children who have autism have abnormal gut flora and increased intestinal permeability. Treatment with antibiotics for presumed bowel bacterial overgrowth seems to result in only temporary changes in bowel flora, however, leading to the conclusion that ongoing use of probiotics might be necessary to ensure normal bowel flora. Despite widespread use and anecdotal reports of efficacy, there are no well-designed studies concerning the impact of probiotic treatment on the treatment of autism.

Zinc

Zinc is one of the single minerals recommended most widely for children who have autism. Its use stems from research by Dr. William Walsh [94], of the Pfeiffer Institute in Chicago, who found that copper-to-zinc ratios were increased in more than 85% of children who have autism. He also found that a dysfunction of metallothionein, a protein involved in the regulation of these and other metals, was present in 99% of 503 autistic children. This research was published by the Pfeiffer Institute only, however, and not in any peer-reviewed journals. There are no controlled studies indicating the efficacy and safety of zinc supplementation in the treatment of autism.

Metabolic interventions

There are several metabolic interventions intended to provide support based on the theory that autistic children have defects in methylation and sulfation. These include the use of methylcobolamin, folic acid derivatives (eg, folinic acid), and trimethylglycine or dimethylglycine. Based on the work by James and colleagues [80], biomedical practitioners often recommend the use of injectable subcutaneous methyl B-12 and oral supplementation of folinic acid and other methylating agents to increase language and social functioning. Although James' study did demonstrate correction of laboratory values of metabolic factors in autistic children, there are no published randomized controlled trials to date demonstrating safety and efficacy of these interventions. This is an area ripe for well-designed intervention trials, especially considering that children who have autism and their families may have an increased frequency compared with the general population of single nucleotide polymorphisms in the methylenetetrahydrofolate reductase and other methylation genes [95].

Other complementary and alternative medical therapies

Complementary therapies, such as homeopathy, craniosacral therapy and other manipulative therapies, Reiki and other energy medicine modalities, biofeedback, and traditional Chinese medicine all are used. There are scattered anecdotal reports of efficacy, but no research evidence exists to support their use in the treatment of autism.

Summary

The repeating theme of all of the natural treatments for ADHD and autism is the large gap between high use rate and the low number of well-controlled, large, randomized trials. It is essential for researchers to include a comparison group when studying natural treatments for these conditions, which often are based on parental or teacher reports. The beneficial effects demonstrated in uncontrolled trials could be explained by the regression to the mean phenomenon in a condition with symptoms that wax and wane. Without a control group, it is impossible to determine if the improvement seen in a trial is the result of the natural course of the symptoms. Effective CAM treatments for ADHD are highly desired by parents who seek alternatives to stimulant medications. This also is true for parents of children who have autism who actively seek out any therapeutic option with potential for benefit. More well-conducted, controlled, clinical trials are needed to determine the safety and efficacy of these natural therapeutic options.

References

[1] Clinical practice guideline: diagnosis and evaluation of the child with attention-deficit/hyperactivity disorder. American Academy of Pediatrics. Pediatrics 2000;105(5):1158–70.
[2] Biederman J, Faraone SV. Attention-deficit hyperactivity disorder. Lancet 2005;366(9481): 237–48.
[3] American Psychiatric Association. Diagnostic and statistical manual of mental disorders. Fourth edition. Washington, DC: APA; 1995.
[4] Schachter HM, Pham B, King J, et al. How efficacious and safe is short-acting methylphenidate for the treatment of attention-deficit disorder in children and adolescents? A meta-analysis. CMAJ 2001;165(11):1475–88.
[5] Stockl KM, Hughes TE, Jarrar MA, et al. Physician perceptions of the use of medications for attention deficit hyperactivity disorder. J Manag Care Pharm 2003;9(5):416–23.
[6] Michelson D, Allen AJ, Busner J, et al. Once-daily atomoxetine treatment for children and adolescents with attention deficit hyperactivity disorder: a randomized, placebo-controlled study. Am J Psychiatry 2002;159(11):1896–901.
[7] New warning about ADHD drug. FDA Consum 2005;39(2):3.
[8] Miller MC. What is the significance of the new warnings about suicide risk with Strattera? Harv Ment Health Lett 2005;22(6):8.

[9] Nissen D, editor. Mosby's drug consult 2003. 13th edition. St. Louis (MD): Mosby; 2003.

[10] Nissen SE. ADHD drugs and cardiovascular risk. N Engl J Med 2006;354(14):1445–8.

[11] Dosreis S, Zito JM, Safer DJ, et al. Parental perceptions and satisfaction with stimulant medication for attention-deficit hyperactivity disorder. J Dev Behav Pediatr 2003;24(3): 155–62.

[12] Stubberfield T, Parry T. Utilization of alternative therapies in attention-deficit hyperactivity disorder. J Paediatr Child Health 1999;35(5):450–3.

[13] Andersen SL, Navalta CP. Altering the course of neurodevelopment: a framework for understanding the enduring effects of psychotropic drugs. Int J Dev Neurosci 2004;22(5–6): 423–40.

[14] Faraone SV, Biederman J, Weber W, et al. Psychiatric, neuropsychological, and psychosocial features of DSM-IV subtypes of attention-deficit/hyperactivity disorder: results from a clinically referred sample. J Am Acad Child Adolesc Psychiatry 1998;37(2):185–93.

[15] Seeman P, Madras BK. Anti-hyperactivity medication: methylphenidate and amphetamine. Mol Psychiatry 1998;3(5):386–96.

[16] Bush G, Valera EM, Seidman LJ. Functional neuroimaging of attention-deficit/hyperactivity disorder: a review and suggested future directions. Biol Psychiatry 2005;57(11):1273–84.

[17] Spencer TJ, Biederman J, Madras BK, et al. In vivo neuroreceptor imaging in attention-deficit/hyperactivity disorder: a focus on the dopamine transporter. Biol Psychiatry 2005; 57(11):1293–300.

[18] di Michele F, Prichep L, John ER, et al. The neurophysiology of attention-deficit/hyperactivity disorder. Int J Psychophysiol 2005;58(1):81–93.

[19] Bussing R, Zima BT, Gary FA, et al. Use of complementary and alternative medicine for symptoms of attention-deficit hyperactivity disorder. Psychiatr Serv 2002;53(9):1096–102.

[20] Chan E. The role of complementary and alternative medicine in attention-deficit hyperactivity disorder. J Dev Behav Pediatr 2002;23(1 Suppl):S37–45.

[21] Chan E, Rappaport LA, Kemper KJ. Complementary and alternative therapies in childhood attention and hyperactivity problems. J Dev Behav Pediatr 2003;24(1):4–8.

[22] Cala S, Crismon ML, Baumgartner J. A survey of herbal use in children with attention-deficit-hyperactivity disorder or depression. Pharmacotherapy 2003;23(2):222–30.

[23] Feingold B. Why your child is hyperactive. New York: Random House; 1975.

[24] Mattes JA, Gittelman R. Effects of artificial food colorings in children with hyperactive symptoms. A critical review and results of a controlled study. Arch Gen Psychiatry 1981; 38(6):714–8.

[25] Wender EH. The food additive-free diet in the treatment of behavior disorders: a review. J Dev Behav Pediatr 1986;7(1):35–42.

[26] McCann D, Barrett A, Cooper A, et al. Food additives and hyperactive behaviour in 3-year-old and 8/9-year-old children in the community: a randomised, double-blinded, placebo-controlled trial. Lancet 2007;5:5.

[27] Ricci G, Capelli M, Miniero R, et al. A comparison of different allergometric tests, skin prick test, Pharmacia UniCAP and ADVIA Centaur, for diagnosis of allergic diseases in children. Allergy 2003;58(1):38–45.

[28] Boris M, Mandel FS. Foods and additives are common causes of the attention deficit hyperactive disorder in children. Ann Allergy 1994;72(5):462–8.

[29] Egger J, Carter CM, Graham PJ, et al. Controlled trial of oligoantigenic treatment in the hyperkinetic syndrome. Lancet 1985;1(8428):540–5.

[30] Wolraich ML, Lindgren SD, Stumbo PJ, et al. Effects of diets high in sucrose or aspartame on the behavior and cognitive performance of children. N Engl J Med 1994;330(5):301–7.

[31] Hoover DW, Milich R. Effects of sugar ingestion expectancies on mother-child interactions. J Abnorm Child Psychol 1994;22(4):501–15.

[32] Schnoll R, Burshteyn D, Cea-Aravena J. Nutrition in the treatment of attention-deficit hyperactivity disorder: a neglected but important aspect. Appl Psychophysiol Biofeedback 2003;28(1):63–75.

[33] Scholastic Parent & Child. Turn off the TV to fight fat—and ADHD: television commercials can affect your child's diet, and in turn, his learning. Scholastic Inc 2007 [online article]. Available at http://content.scholastic.com/browse/article.jsp?id=1441. Accessed September 5, 2007.

[34] Burgess JR, Stevens L, Zhang W, et al. Long-chain polyunsaturated fatty acids in children with attention-deficit hyperactivity disorder. Am J Clin Nutr 2000;71(1 Suppl):327S–30S.

[35] Richardson AJ. Omega-3 fatty acids in ADHD and related neurodevelopmental disorders. Int Rev Psychiatry 2006;18(2):155–72.

[36] Voigt RG, Llorente AM, Jensen CL, et al. A randomized, double-blind, placebo-controlled trial of docosahexaenoic acid supplementation in children with attention-deficit/hyperactivity disorder. J Pediatr 2001;139(2):189–96.

[37] Stevens LJ, Zentall SS, Deck JL, et al. Essential fatty acid metabolism in boys with attention-deficit hyperactivity disorder. Am J Clin Nutr 1995;62(4):761–8.

[38] Sinn N, Bryan J. Effect of supplementation with polyunsaturated fatty acids and micronutrients on learning and behavior problems associated with child ADHD. J Dev Behav Pediatr 2007;28(2):82–91.

[39] Butnik SM. Neurofeedback in adolescents and adults with attention deficit hyperactivity disorder. J Clin Psychol 2005;61(5):621–5.

[40] Monastra VJ, Monastra DM, George S. The effects of stimulant therapy, EEG biofeedback, and parenting style on the primary symptoms of attention-deficit/hyperactivity disorder. Appl Psychophysiol Biofeedback 2002;27(4):231–49.

[41] Fuchs T, Birbaumer N, Lutzenberger W, et al. Neurofeedback treatment for attention-deficit/hyperactivity disorder in children: a comparison with methylphenidate. Appl Psychophysiol Biofeedback 2003;28(1):1–12.

[42] Lyon MR, Cline JC, Totosy de Zepetnek J, et al. Effect of the herbal extract combination Panax quinquefolium and Ginkgo biloba on attention-deficit hyperactivity disorder: a pilot study. J Psychiatry Neurosci 2001;26(3):221–8.

[43] Van Oudheusden LJ, Scholte HR. Efficacy of carnitine in the treatment of children with attention-deficit hyperactivity disorder. Prostaglandins Leukot Essent Fatty Acids 2002;67(1): 33–8.

[44] Trebaticka J, Kopasova S, Hradecna Z, et al. Treatment of ADHD with French maritime pine bark extract, Pycnogenol. Eur Child Adolesc Psychiatry 2006;15(6):329–35.

[45] Jensen PS, Kenny DT. The effects of yoga on the attention and behavior of boys with Attention-Deficit/hyperactivity Disorder (ADHD). J Atten Disord 2004;7(4):205–16.

[46] Khilnani S, Field T, Hernandez-Reif M, et al. Massage therapy improves mood and behavior of students with attention-deficit/hyperactivity disorder. Adolescence 2003;38(152):623–38.

[47] Bilici M, Yildirim F, Kandil S, et al. Double-blind, placebo-controlled study of zinc sulfate in the treatment of attention deficit hyperactivity disorder. Prog Neuropsychopharmacol Biol Psychiatry 2004;28(1):181–90.

[48] Akhondzadeh S, Mohammadi MR, Khademi M. Zinc sulfate as an adjunct to methylphenidate for the treatment of attention deficit hyperactivity disorder in children: a double blind and randomized trial [ISRCTN64132371]. BMC Psychiatry 2004;4(1):9.

[49] Konofal E, Lecendreux M, Arnulf I, et al. Iron deficiency in children with attention-deficit/hyperactivity disorder. Arch Pediatr Adolesc Med 2004;158(12):1113–5.

[50] Sever Y, Ashkenazi A, Tyano S, et al. Iron treatment in children with attention deficit hyperactivity disorder. A preliminary report. Neuropsychobiology 1997;35(4):178–80.

[51] Haslam RH, Dalby JT, Rademaker AW. Effects of megavitamin therapy on children with attention deficit disorders. Pediatrics 1984;74(1):103–11.

[52] Altunc U, Pittler MH, Ernst E. Homeopathy for childhood and adolescence ailments: systematic review of randomized clinical trials. Mayo Clin Proc 2007;82(1):69–75.

[53] Strauss L. The efficacy of a homeopathic preparation in the management of attention deficit hyperactivity disorder. Journal of Biomedical Therapy 2000;18(2):197–201.

[54] Frei H, Everts R, von Ammon K, et al. Homeopathic treatment of children with attention deficit hyperactivity disorder: a randomised, double blind, placebo controlled crossover trial. Eur J Pediatr 2005;164(12):758–67.

[55] Jacobs J, Williams AL, Girard C, et al. Homeopathy for attention-deficit/hyperactivity disorder: a pilot randomized-controlled trial. J Altern Complement Med 2005;11(5): 799–806.

[56] Louv R. Last child in the woods: saving our children from nature-deficit disorder. New York: Algonquin Books of Chapel Hill; 2005.

[57] Kuo FE, Taylor AF. A potential natural treatment for attention-deficit/hyperactivity disorder: evidence from a national study. Am J Public Health 2004;94(9):1580–6.

[58] Braun JM, Kahn RS, Froehlich T, et al. Exposures to environmental toxicants and attention deficit hyperactivity disorder in U.S. children. Environ Health Perspect 2006;114(12): 1904–9.

[59] Szpir M. New thinking on neurodevelopment. Environ Health Perspect 2006;114(2): A100–7.

[60] Center for Disease Control and Prevention. Prevalence of the autism spectrum disorders in multiple areas of the United States surveillance years 2000 and 2002. National Center on Birth Defects and Developmental Disabilities. 2007; [website] Available at: http://www. cdc.gov/ncbddd/dd/addmprevalence.htm. Accessed September 17,2007.

[61] Bertrand J, Mars A, Boyle C, et al. Prevalence of autism in a United States population: the Brick Township, New Jersey, investigation. Pediatrics 2001;108(5):1155–61.

[62] Gurney JG, Fritz MS, Ness KK, et al. Analysis of prevalence trends of autism spectrum disorder in Minnesota. Arch Pediatr Adolesc Med 2003;157(7):622–7.

[63] Muhle R, Trentacoste SV, Rapin I. The genetics of autism. Pediatrics 2004;113(5):E472–86.

[64] Shastry BS. Molecular genetics of autism spectrum disorders. J Hum Genet 2003;48(10): 495–501.

[65] Hanson E, Kalish LA, Bunce E, et al. Use of complementary and alternative medicine among children diagnosed with autism spectrum disorder. J Autism Dev Disord 2007;37(4):628–36.

[66] Harrington JW, Rosen L, Garnecho A, et al. Parental perceptions and use of complementary and alternative medicine practices for children with autistic spectrum disorders in private practice. J Dev Behav Pediatr 2006;27(2 Suppl):S156–61.

[67] Levy SE, Mandell DS, Merhar S, et al. Use of complementary and alternative medicine among children recently diagnosed with autistic spectrum disorder. J Dev Behav Pediatr 2003;24(6):418–23.

[68] Wong HH, Smith RG. Patterns of complementary and alternative medical therapy use in children diagnosed with autism spectrum disorders. J Autism Dev Disord 2006;36(7): 901–9.

[69] Horvath K, Papadimitriou JC, Rabsztyn A, et al. Gastrointestinal abnormalities in children with autistic disorder. J Pediatr 1999;135(5):559–63.

[70] Torrente F, Ashwood P, Day R, et al. Small intestinal enteropathy with epithelial IgG and complement deposition in children with regressive autism. Mol Psychiatry 2002;7(4):375–82, 334.

[71] Rosseneu S. Aerobic gut flora in children with autism specturm disorder and gastrointestinal symptoms. Presented at: Defeat Autism Now Conference. San Diego (CA), October 3, 2003.

[72] Sandler RH, Finegold SM, Bolte ER, et al. Short-term benefit from oral vancomycin treatment of regressive-onset autism. J Child Neurol 2000;15(7):429–35.

[73] D'Eufemia P, Celli M, Finocchiaro R, et al. Abnormal intestinal permeability in children with autism. Acta Paediatr 1996;85(9):1076–9.

[74] Horvath K, Perman JA. Autism and gastrointestinal symptoms. Curr Gastroenterol Rep 2002;4(3):251–8.

[75] Lucarelli S, Frediani T, Zingoni AM, et al. Food allergy and infantile autism. Panminerva Med 1995;37(3):137–41.

[76] Jyonouchi H, Sun S, Itokazu N. Innate immunity associated with inflammatory responses and cytokine production against common dietary proteins in patients with autism spectrum disorder. Neuropsychobiology 2002;46(2):76–84.

[77] Connolly AM, Chez MG, Pestronk A, et al. Serum autoantibodies to brain in Landau-Kleffner variant, autism, and other neurologic disorders. J Pediatr 1999;134(5):607–13.

[78] Singh VK, Warren R, Averett R, et al. Circulating autoantibodies to neuronal and glial filament proteins in autism. Pediatr Neurol 1997;17(1):88–90.

[79] Cabanlit M, Wills S, Goines P, et al. Brain-specific autoantibodies in the plasma of subjects with autistic spectrum disorder. Ann N Y Acad Sci 2007;1107:92–103.

[80] James SJ, Cutler P, Melnyk S, et al. Metabolic biomarkers of increased oxidative stress and impaired methylation capacity in children with autism. Am J Clin Nutr 2004;80(6):1611–7.

[81] Yorbik O, Sayal A, Akay C, et al. Investigation of antioxidant enzymes in children with autistic disorder. Prostaglandins Leukot Essent Fatty Acids 2002;67(5):341–3.

[82] McGinnis WR. Oxidative stress in autism. Altern Ther Health Med 2004;10(6):22–36, quiz 37, 92.

[83] Palmer RF, Blanchard S, Stein Z, et al. Environmental mercury release, special education rates, and autism disorder: an ecological study of Texas. Health Place 2006;12(2):203–9.

[84] Ip P, Wong V, Ho M, et al. Mercury exposure in children with autistic spectrum disorder: case-control study. J Child Neurol 2004;19(6):431–4.

[85] Adams JB, Romdalvik J, Ramanujam VM, et al. Mercury, lead, and zinc in baby teeth of children with autism versus controls. J Toxicol Environ Health A 2007;70(12):1046–51.

[86] Bradstreet J, Geier D, DKartzinel J, et al. A case-control study of mercury burden in children with autistic spectrum disorders. Journal of American Physicians and Surgeons 2003;8(3): 76–9.

[87] Vancassel S, Durand G, Barthelemy C, et al. Plasma fatty acid levels in autistic children. Prostaglandins Leukot Essent Fatty Acids 2001;65(1):1–7.

[88] Bryson SE, Rogers SJ, Fombonne E. Autism spectrum disorders: early detection, intervention, education, and psychopharmacological management. Can J Psychiatry 2003;48(8): 506–16.

[89] Sinha Y, Silove N, Wheeler D, et al. Auditory integration training and other sound therapies for autism spectrum disorders: a systematic review. Arch Dis Child 2006;91(12):1018–22.

[90] Knivsberg AM, Reichelt KL, Hoien T, et al. A randomised, controlled study of dietary intervention in autistic syndromes. Nutr Neurosci 2002;5(4):251–61.

[91] Patrick L, Salik R. The effect of essential fatty acid supplementation on language development and learning skills in autism and asperger's syndrome. Autism-Asperger's Digest 2005;36–7.

[92] Amminger GP, Berger GE, Schafer MR, et al. Omega-3 fatty acids supplementation in children with autism: a double-blind randomized, placebo-controlled pilot study. Biol Psychiatry 2007;61(4):551–3.

[93] Richardson AJ, Montgomery P. The Oxford-Durham study: a randomized, controlled trial of dietary supplementation with fatty acids in children with developmental coordination disorder. Pediatrics 2005;115(5):1360–6.

[94] Walsh W. Metallothionein and autism. Presented at: Defeat Autism Now Conference. San Diego (CA), October 3, 2003.

[95] James SJ, Melnyk S, Jernigan S, et al. Metabolic endophenotype and related genotypes are associated with oxidative stress in children with autism. Am J Med Genet B Neuropsychiatr Genet 2006;141(8):947–56.

ELSEVIER
SAUNDERS

PEDIATRIC CLINICS
OF NORTH AMERICA

Pediatr Clin N Am 54 (2007) 1007–1023

Integrative Medicine and Asthma

John D. Mark, MD

*Pediatric Pulmonary Medicine, Lucile Packard Children's Hospital, Stanford University
Medical Center, 770 Welch Road, Suite 350, Palo Alto, CA 94305, USA*

Mechanism of asthma

Asthma is a complex and heterogeneous disease with many phenotypic expressions; often it is difficult even to make the diagnosis, especially in young children who may wheeze as infants, outgrowing it after 6 years of age [1]. It is a multifactorial disease and almost always represents an interaction between a genetically determined predisposition to allergic diseases and environmental factors that serve to enhance inflammation. Genetic factors include regulation of cytokines that control the production of IgE along with polymorphisms in genes that regulate airway tone and repair mechanisms for acute injuries [2]. Several studies [3,4] show that environmental factors, especially exposures in early infancy, may play a major role in the development of the immune system. Such exposures include microbial products, food and aeroallergens, stress, and infections, such as respiratory syncytial virus and rhinovirus. These exposures may help the immune system to mature so that allergies are less likely to occur. If asthma or allergies already are present, however, then a respiratory infection may cause damage to the lungs and increase inflammatory responses in the lower airway, which then may promote the development of asthma. With all the factors involved in such a process, with even the diagnosis at times uncertain, many nonmedical approaches to asthma and asthma-like conditions, including prevention or attenuation, have been promoted.

Complementary and alternative medicine (CAM) and associated therapies are popular approaches used by parents in the treatment of asthma and encompasses many therapies, including nutritional and dietary supplements, herbal medications, traditional Chinese medicine (including acupuncture), homeopathy, mind-body techniques, and manual therapies. CAM is a group of diverse medical and health care systems, practices, and products that often are not integrated with conventional medicine.

E-mail address: jmark@stanford.edu

doi:10.1016/j.pcl.2007.09.005
pediatric.theclinics.com

CAM also is described, however, as a broad domain of healing resources that encompasses all health systems, modalities, and practices and their accompanying theories and beliefs other than those intrinsic to the politically dominant health system of a particular society or culture in a given historical period [5]. What is considered CAM in one country may be considered as part of standard treatment in another country or region.

There have been attempts to determine the prevalence of CAM therapies in the treatment of asthma, because few patients volunteer information about CAM use unless questioned directly by their health care practitioner. Many studies trying to determine CAM use in asthma have used different definitions of CAM, making the prevalence rates variable. A recent review of the literature of CAM use in asthma [6] found 17 studies—seven of adults, seven of children, one of adolescents, and two of children and adults. This review found the level of use for adults ranged from 4% to 79% and for children from 33% to 89%. The most commonly used CAM therapies in children were herbal products, including vitamins and minerals; breathing techniques; massage; homeopathy; and prayer. In one study [7], 71% of the caregivers said they would consider using CAM for their child in the future.

Given the common use of CAM therapies in children who have asthma, the variable disclosure to health care providers, and the potential life-threatening nature of the disease, it is important to know which factors might predict CAM use in children. In a review of questionnaire studies in children, however, there was no association between children's age, duration or severity of asthma, and the presence of concurrent illness [8]. Other pediatric studies have found increased CAM use in those classified as having mild or moderate persistent asthma; those receiving high-dose inhaled steroids; and those patients who had poor symptom control or frequent physician visits, including going to the emergency room [9–12]. A more recent survey of 228 families found CAM use among children 5 to 12 years old who had asthma (as reported by their parents) at 65%. Usage was highest among families who were black, poorer, and less educated. CAM use was not limited by asthma severity and was 78%, 75%, and 81% among children who had mild, moderate, or severe persistent classification, respectively. Types of CAM differed by poverty and a trend for differences by race and education emerged. As an example, black and Hispanic families used mind-body therapies (most common therapy being prayer) more often then did white families, who used more biologically based therapies. Of the biologically based therapies used, 77% were over-the-counter medications, including decongestants and cough syrups. The survey concluded that because of the high prevalence of CAM use in pediatric asthma, health care providers should educate themselves about these CAM therapies so they might better discuss the implications of using these therapies and potentially improve adherence to the prescribed medication regimen [13].

The symptoms associated with asthma range from mild to severe and often begin in infancy; the severity of asthma is believed in part the result of genetic predisposition and environmental exposures. The ability to modify a child's genetic heritage is limited, but certain environmental factors more likely are amenable to a variety of interventions. For this reason, CAM therapies, from diet to herbal medications to breathing exercises and yoga, are becoming popular in treating asthma. There have been some high-quality studies of CAM therapies that have demonstrated evidence for safety and efficacy. Some CAM therapies do not lend themselves to evidence-based medical research for a variety of reasons, ranging from patient preference to highly individualized approaches. Health care providers should consider balancing risks and benefits of CAM therapies as they would with conventional therapies, such as the use of inhaled corticosteroids (ICS). Using conventional and CAM therapies may obtain the best control of asthma. This integrative medicine approach may result in improved overall adherence, because, as shown in at least one study of adult patients, 79% believed that using a combination of conventional and CAM therapies was better then using either one alone [14]. Because CAM therapies generally are perceived as safe and effective by patients, it is important for health care providers to know what has been studied and some of the potential interactions between CAM therapies and conventional medical care.

Conventional therapies

Although there are no evidence-based guidelines for the pharmacologic treatments of infants and preschool children, there are classifications for severity of asthma and suggested therapies for older children and adults from the National Asthma and Education Program through the National Institutes of Health (NIH). These therapies are not discussed in this article but can be found in a recent excellent review by Milgrom [15]. The use of controller medications, such as ICS, which is the mainstay of chronic asthma in children and adults, has made a tremendous difference in the severity and frequency of children who have chronic asthma. Patients and families are aware of the potential side effects and complications of chronic steroids use, however, and often withhold this type of medication in favor of non-pharmacologic treatments. This reluctance, in addition to the potential overuse of short-acting inhaled β_2-agonists, may lead to the undertreatment of children who have asthma. By using conventional and CAM therapies, the integrative approach may lead to better adherence and control of asthma in children; this has yet to be studied.

Nutrition

The role of nutrition in the development of asthma is believed important. Because diet is the major source of antioxidants, suboptimal intake during airway growth may lead to airway damage and reduced airway compliance. It is hypothesized that in industrialized countries there has been a decrease in vegetable and fruit consumption in addition to an increase in environmental risk factors, such as atmospheric pollution and cigarette smoke. This decrease in the consumption of fruit and vegetable may lead to a diet deficient in antioxidants and, therefore, an increased susceptibility to oxidant damage [16]. This reduced consumption of foods rich in antioxidants has been accompanied by the decrease in dietary intake of oily fish (tuna, herring, mackerel, trout, and salmon) and fish oil (cod liver oil), which are high in n-3 polyunsaturated fatty acids (PUFAs), eicosapentaenoic acid (EPA), and docosahexaenoic acid (DHA). This reduction in n-3 PUFAs was observed at the same time as an increase in the intake of n-6 PUFAs, which are present in margarine, vegetable oils, and trans fatty acids. It is hypothesized that the consequence of increasing n-6 and decreasing n-3 PUFA intakes may result in increased arachidonic acid and prostaglandin E2 production with consequent increase in atopic type 2 helper T-cell sensitization, asthma, and atopic disease [17]. This most likely is an oversimplification in that n-3 and n-6 PUFAs can modulate T-cell function [18].

There are epidemiologic studies showing the beneficial association between fruits, vegetables, and other antioxidant-rich foods. One study, using a 58-item food frequency questionnaire, investigated 690 children taking in a traditional Mediterranean diet, which is characterized by an increase in plant foods, such as fruits and vegetables, bread and cereals, and legumes and nuts (all sources of dietary antioxidants), and in which the primary oil was olive oil. Eighty percent of these children were eating fresh fruit and 68% were eating vegetables twice a day. This diet was found protective for wheezing and atopy when compared to children who had similar allergies that were documented by skin testing [19]. The Children's Health Study (a 10-year longitudinal study of respiratory health in more than 2000 school children living in and near Los Angeles, California) used a cross-sectional analysis of dietary intake data to look at the effect of antioxidant vitamin intake on lung function comparing low intake with high intake [20]. Fruit and vegetable intake was monitored using servings per day. This study showed that low intake of antioxidant vitamins had adverse effects on pulmonary function with lower forced vital capacity (FVC), forced expiratory volume in 1 second (FEV_1) and forced expiratory flow ($FEF_{25\%-75\%}$) in boys and girls. The effects of vitamins A, C, and E seemed independent of asthma status. The deficits found in this study were believed clinically significant.

Another study [21] examined the association of diet (fruit, vegetables, vitamin C, vitamin E, β-carotene, retinol, and n-3 PUFAs) with lung health in 2112 high school students in the United States and Canada. It was hypothesized that fruits, antioxidants, and other micronutrients may prevent or limit the inflammatory response of the respiratory system by reducing reactive oxygen species and inhibiting lipid peroxidation. Because adolescents often have poor dietary habits, this group of children may have had lower lung function and decreased pulmonary function. In reviewing completed questionnaires, it was found that dietary fruit and vegetables, vitamin E, vitamin A, β-carotene, and n-3 PUFAs were low in one third or more of the students. Low fruit intake was associated with lower FEV_1 compared with a higher intake and increased report of chronic bronchitic symptoms and asthma. Low vitamin E intake was associated with an increased report of asthma, and low dietary n-3 PUFAs had an increased report in chronic bronchitic symptoms, wheeze, and asthma compared with higher intake. The investigators conclude that lower pulmonary function, chronic cough, and wheeze were found more often in adolescents who had low dietary micronutrient intake. The promoting of fruit and fish consumption in addition to vitamin supplementation may be important to ensure adequate intake of antioxidants and n-3 PUFAs in this group of rapidly growing children.

The relationship between dietary antioxidant deficiency and lung health, however, has not been established in interventional studies using asthma as the disease model. A *Cochrane Database of Systemic Review* meta-analysis of nine randomized controlled trials conducted in adults and children who had established asthma concluded that there was no consistent effect of n-3 PUFA supplementation on asthma symptoms, asthma medication use, lung function, or bronchial hyper-responsiveness [22]. There was some evidence that fish oil supplementation may have a protective effect on exercise-induced bronchoconstriction (EIB) attributable to its anti-inflammatory properties. In a pilot study of 16 young adult patients who were asthmatic and who had documented EIB, one group (n = 8) received fish oil supplementation (3.2 g of EPA and 2.0 g of DHA) and the other group (n = 8) was given placebo. Pre-exercise and postexercise measurements were assessed and the fish oil diet improved pulmonary function to below the diagnostic EIB threshold with a concurrent reduction in bronchodilator use. Biomarkers of inflammation, using induced sputum and activated polymorphonuclear leukocytes for eicosanoid metabolites, prostaglandin D2, and cytokines, were reduced in the subjects on the fish oil diet. It was believed that fish oil supplementation may represent a potentially beneficial intervention for asthmatic subjects who have EIB [23].

It may be that dietary intervention, such as increased antioxidant intake, is important particularly during pregnancy and early childhood. This is not yet verified. In the Childhood Asthma Prevention Study, 616 children were randomized to an active diet intervention and received fish oil supplements high in n-3 PUFA and minimized n-6 PUFA intake. Of the 189 children who completed all parts of the study, there was no association between plasma levels of n-3 or n-6 PUFAs at 10 months, 3 years, and 5 years and the prevalence of asthma or wheezing illness, eczema, or atopy at 5 years, even though the active dietary intervention group had high levels of n-3 PUFAs and lower levels of n-6 PUFAs at 5 years of age [24]. Further research of dietary manipulation as a public health measure is needed to evaluate its role in reducing the risk for asthma. Even though there is evidence of antioxidant vitamins' and other dietary immunomodulators' role in asthma, it is insufficient at this time to allow recommendations for the treatment of asthma. Nutritional and dietary interventions may be important especially in combination with other therapies (breast feeding and avoidance of environmental tobacco smoke and air pollution) in improving overall lung health but the evidence is not clear in children as to which ones are most efficacious and how much to take.

Herbal supplements

Herbal medications are classified as dietary supplements and are derived from plants. They be taken orally as pills, freeze dried capsules, or powders; used as tinctures or syrups; brewed in teas or decoction; or "applied" as salves, ointments, or poultices to the skin or mucous membranes. In survey studies, herbal supplements are often the most common CAM therapy reportedly used for the treatment of asthma. In a review of 17 studies, including seven in pediatric populations, one in adolescents, and two including adults and children, the use of dietary supplements ranged from 12% to 53% of patients surveyed (therapies used included herbs, minerals, vitamins, naturopathic medicines, and Ayurvedic therapies) [6]. The use of herbal or "medicinal" supplements may be even higher in certain ethnic groups. In one study of patients living in the Caribbean, 30.4% of patients reported using herbal remedies for symptomatic relief and almost 60% stated they obtained herbs from their backyards or the supermarket with only 24.1% obtaining herbs from an herbalist or pharmacy. Relatives and friends were the most common source of information in this group of 191 patients who had asthma [25].

This has caused concern, because herbs may have interactions with conventional medications and even other herbal supplements. In the United States, herbal and other dietary supplements are regulated by the Food and Drug Administration (FDA) as foods as outlined by the Dietary Supplement Health and Education Act of 1994 [26], and they do not have to meet the same standards as pharmaceutic medications for proof of safety and effectiveness. Also, in many herbal supplements, the plant itself may not be characterized adequately, active ingredients and standardization may not be clear, and there may be many chemical compounds present in any given herbal supplement. This makes the conventional scientific understanding of how herbal supplements might affect the body in conditions, such as asthma, difficult. Safety is a concern and there are reports of some supplements being contaminated with metals, unlabeled prescription drugs, microorganisms, and other substances [27]. In June of 2007, the FDA announced new regulations for good manufacturing practices. These new rules ensure that dietary supplements are produced in a reliable manner, do not contain contaminants or impurities, and are labeled accurately.

There has been research regarding herbal supplements in the treatment of asthma, including several in children. One study investigated the use of

Butterbur (*Petasites hybridus*) in children and adults who had asthma. Butterbur is a perennial shrub traditionally used for such things as urinary problems, back pain, wound healing, and asthma. In this study, 64 adults and 16 children were studied in a prospective nonrandomized open trial in subjects who had mild to moderate asthma. The subjects took Butterbur for 8 weeks in addition to their regular asthma medications and by the end of the study the number and duration of asthma exacerbations had decreased by 48% and 75%, respectively. There also was a reported reduction in the dose of ICS (42.9%), reduction in the use of short-acting β_2-agonists (48.3%), and improvement in FEV_1 and peak flow (70.6 and 83.9%, respectively). The Butterbur was well tolerated but with 11 adverse events in seven subjects who had such complaints as abdominal pain, allergic-type symptoms (sneezing and rhinitis), and halitosis [28]. Although this seems promising, the study was limited by the lack of blinding and small sample size.

There have been recent attempts to improve the study design for herbal supplements and asthma in children. In a randomized, placebo-controlled, double-blind study involving 60 subjects ages 6 to18 years, Pycnogenol (a proprietary mixture of water-soluble bioflavonoids extracted from French maritime pine) was studied in mild to moderate asthma [29]. Using peak flow monitoring, symptom diaries, medication use, changes in oral medications (zafirlukast), and urine samples for leukotrienes C4, D4, and E4, the group who took Pycnogenol for 3 months had significant improvement in pulmonary function and asthma scores along with reduction in urinary leukotrienes. The Pyconogenol group also was able to reduce or discontinue their use of rescue inhalers (primarily albuterol) more often then the placebo group, including 18 of 30 subjects in the Pyconogenol group who did not use their albuterol inhaler during the third month. To be included in the study, the subjects had FEV_1 between 50% and 85% predicted and showed a 12% or more increase after two puffs of rescue medication, suggesting inadequate control of asthma before beginning the study. There was no repeat of spirometry during or after the study but only peak flow monitoring was used to assess lung function. Nevertheless, this herbal supplement, which is believed to have potent anti-inflammatory properties, may be useful as an adjunctive therapy for children who have asthma. Another small, double-blind, placebo-controlled, 6-week study in 40 adults who had asthma using *Boswellia serrata* gum (believed to inhibit leukotriene synthesis) showed that the group taking the gum resin had a 70% decrease in dyspnea, number of asthmatic attacks, and improvement in FVC, FEV_1, and peak expiratory flow rate. They also demonstrated a decrease in eosinophilia in peripheral blood and lower erythrocyte sedimentation rate [30].

Many of the studies of herbal supplementation include antioxidants, such as vitamin C and selenium. Antioxidants may help limit oxidative stress, which is believed to play a role in the pathogenesis of asthma. These studies primarily are in adults who have asthma but because many children are given these types of supplements, they are discussed briefly. Vitamin C is an antioxidant vitamin that has been promoted as a supplement that may help asthma control and even decrease asthma attacks. It is shown to be low in children and adults who have asthma, in particular subjects who have a low intake of fruits and vegetables (discussed previously). In a Cochrane review of vitamin C supplementation for asthma [31], 71 abstracts and titles were analyzed and eight studies selected for inclusion. Of the eight studies, one involved children only and one involved children and adults. All studies were placebo controlled and randomized. The conclusion was that from these randomized controlled trials, there was insufficient evidence to recommend a specific role for vitamin C in the treatment of asthma. Another antioxidant that may suppress asthma inflammation by increasing glutathione peroxidase in the airway epithelial lining fluid is selenium [32]. In a randomized, double-blind, placebo-controlled trial using selenium in 197 adults who had asthma, there was no significant improvement in asthma-related quality-of-life scores, lung function, asthma symptom scores, peak flow measurements, or bronchodilator usage [33]. At this time, there is insufficient evidence to suggest the routine addition of vitamin C and selenium improves asthma or prevents exacerbations.

Magnesium is a supplement that long has been known to be a potent bronchodilator. It is found in the diet in whole seeds, grains, nuts, and vegetables, but the United States Department of Agriculture survey in 1990 showed that children's mean intakes of some vitamins and minerals, including magnesium, were below the recommended daily allowance. Epidemiologic data shows that low magnesium intake is associated with airway hyper-reactivity and self-reported wheezing [34,35]. Magnesium often is promoted as a routine supplement for asthma by providers of alternative health care and is an ingredient of many herbal supplements for improving lung health. A recent study [36] investigated the effects of oral magnesium supplementation on clinical symptoms, bronchial reactivity, lung function, and allergen-induced skin responses in children who had moderate persistent asthma. This randomized, placebo-controlled study in 37 subjects, ages 7 to 19, in which both groups were taking ICS (fluticasone), showed that after 2 months of therapy, the magnesium group had a decrease in airway reactivity using methacholine challenge, had a decrease in skin responses to known allergens, had fewer asthma exacerbations, and used less rescue medication (salbutamol) compared with the control group. The pulmonary lung function (FVC, FEV_1, $FEF_{25\%-75\%}$, and FEV_1/FVC) was similar in both groups. The role of magnesium in the general treatment of asthma in children needs to be studied further.

Asian medicine, including acupuncture

Traditional Chinese medicine (TCM) is the form of Asian medicine encountered most commonly in the United States, and its origins date back several thousand years. At its core it strives to understand the connections between body, mind, and spirit in health and disease. The belief in an unseen vital energy that affects patients' health and how this energy, or qi (chi), flows through the appropriate channels forms the basis for the practice of Asian medicine. Practitioners can affect this flow or intensity by manipulating its balance using acupuncture, Asian herbs, diet, and physical therapy.

Combination herbal supplements commonly are used for asthma in TCM and are a component, along with acupuncture, of the practice of Asian medicine in the United States. Asthma has been recognized in Asian medicine for centuries and there are traditional herbal formulas used in the everyday practice of TCM. The classic Asian herbal remedy used for breathing disorders, such as asthma, contains, among other ingredients, ephedra (also known as Ma huang or *Ephedra sinica*). The pharmaceutic, ephedrine, derived from Ma huang, was used in asthma therapy until the advent of more specific β_2-agonists medications. Ma huang may be present in many combinations of other botanicals for respiratory problems, including licorice. Most recently, it has been available in combinations with other stimulant herbal supplements, such as caffeine and caffeine-related products (primarily promoted for weight loss and energy), and there are reported deaths associated with its use. Central nervous system problems, such as nausea, vomiting, sweating, and nervousness, along with heart palpitations, tachycardia, hypertension, anxiety, and even myocardial infarction, all are reported [37]. For this reason, ephedra is not recommended in the treatment of asthma because of the warnings from the FDA and reports of serious side effects, even though those warnings come from the use of ephedra in doses that are much larger than those used for the treatment of asthma in TCM.

In TCM, herbal supplements commonly are prepared as a combination of many herbs tailored for individual patients. The herbal combination then is decocted (concentrated by boiling) by a practitioner or patient for use. There usually are one or two main herbal supplements that target the asthma symptoms particular to a patient and there are several others added to adjust the formula to achieve balance (yin/yang) for a patient's condition. The balance and interaction of the ingredients are believed as important as the effect of the individual ingredients. It is believed that the complex interaction between the various herbs in the formulation produces synergistic effects and may help reduce potential side effects of some of the individual herbs [38]. In the past several years, there have been several double-blind, placebo-controlled, clinical studies investigating the safety and efficacy of Asian herbal supplements in the treatment and the mechanism of asthma. Although few studies have been reported using these herbal supplements in children who have asthma, a recent review presented an update on some of the more promising Asian herbal remedies for asthma [39]. The asthma herbal medicine intervention, a three-herb asthma formulation, was compared with prednisone in a study of 91 adults who had asthma. This study showed significant reduction in clinical symptoms, airway reactivity, and biomarkers of airway inflammation [40]. Three other Asian formulations, modified Mai Men Dong Tang (five herbs), Ding Chuan Tan (nine herbs), and *Sophora flavescens* Ait all showed potential as safe alternatives or complements to conventional therapies for asthma.

STA-1 is another Asian herbal mix studied in 120 children ages 5 to 20, seen in a clinic in the Oriental Medical Center in Taiwan, who had mild to moderate asthma and frequent respiratory symptoms. This randomized, double-blind, placebo-controlled study took place over 6 months using two different formulations and showed that pulmonary function (FEV_1) and clinical symptoms improved in the STA-1 group over placebo and STA-2 combination group, especially in those children who had dust mite allergy and asthma [41]. The role of these various Asian herbal mixtures in the control of asthma still is to be determined but there are promising studies primarily in adults who have asthma.

The other modality used commonly as a TCM therapy for asthma is acupuncture. Although the NIH 1997 Consensus Development Conference on Acupuncture [42] did recommend acupuncture for many conditions, including asthma, studies have not supported the use of acupuncture in children or adults for chronic or acute therapy. A review by the Cochrane collaboration of 11 studies for acupuncture and asthma concluded that there is not enough evidence to make recommendations about the value of acupuncture in asthma treatment. The review goes on to recommend further research considering the complexities and different types of acupuncture [43]. Until recently, most studies were small and uncontrolled and there were methodologic problems with blinding, lack of standardization, and developing controls, such as sham acupuncture. Recently, using techniques, such as laser acupuncture, some of these methodologic problems have been addressed. In a double-blind, placebo-controlled, crossover study, laser acupuncture was studied in 44 children who had known exercise-induced asthma. Laser acupuncture was performed on real and placebo points, and lung function was measured before and after cold air challenge using isocapnic hyperventilation. There was no significant difference in the FEV_1 or other lung function parameters between the two groups [44]. Another study in 17 children who had asthma investigated whether or not a 10-week course of acupuncture using a laser pen and 7 weeks of using probiotic drops (*Enterococcus faecalis*) offered better asthma control then did a control group, who were given a non-laser pen and placebo drops instead of probiotics. This pilot study was randomized, placebo-controlled, and double-blinded but the numbers were small (eight and nine patients in each group). Measurement of asthma control included peak flow variability, FEV_1, and quality of life using a standard questionnaire. The laser acupuncture and probiotics decreased peak flow variability significantly. There was no significant effect on FEV_1, quality-of-life criteria, or need for additional medication [45].

Even though research methods are improving for evaluating acupuncture and asthma, there is insufficient evidence at this time to recommend acupuncture in the treatment of acute or chronic asthma. There is some research and speculation, however, about the lack of positive findings in acupuncture and asthma studies being, in part, due to model of research used [46]. Attempts to isolate the effect of a specific therapy, or "needling," may interfere with the positive outcomes that are not part of the study design, because TCM is a holistic approach to a chronic problem and acupuncture only one part of the therapeutic relationship, which may include an individualized herbal remedy prescription.

Homeopathy

Homeopathy has become popular in the treatment of acute and chronic health problems and globally is among the five most widely used CAM therapies. In India there are more than 200,000 registered practitioners, 182 colleges, and more than 300 homeopathic hospitals [5]. It is classified as a drug therapy in the United States by the FDA and in some countries integrated into the national health care systems. There are national homeopathic pharmacopoeias in Brazil, France, Germany, India, and the United States. In the United States, the qualifications of practitioners vary. Some are trained exclusively in homeopathy; others are trained in homeopathy after professional qualification as a medical doctor, dentist, naturopath, or osteopath.

Homeopathy is a therapeutic method using specific preparations of substances whose effects, when administered to healthy subjects, correspond to the manifestations of a disorder (symptoms, clinical signs, and pathologic states) in individual patients. It is believed that the effect is to stimulate a healing response in patients. A second principle in homeopathy is individualization of treatment. This may be at the whole person level or at a more clinical level, especially in the treatment of acute conditions, such as acute asthmatic exacerbations. The doses used in homeopathy range from those that are similar in concentration to those of some conventional medicines to high dilutions containing no material trace of the starting substance. There currently is no understood way that substances that have no material trace could have a specific physiologic effect, and this is the primary source of skepticism about the claimed results of clinical trials in homeopathy.

Homeopathy is an increasingly popular CAM modality used to treat asthma. In a Cochrane review, six trials for treating asthma with homeopathy were analyzed and found to have variable quality of methodology in the treatment of chronic asthma. Because homeopathy treatments tend to be individualized, no quantitative pooling of results was possible. There was no significant effect when measuring lung function and the investigators concluded that there is further need for observational data to document the different methods of homeopathic prescribing and patient response, because, like TCM, this individualistic type of therapy is difficult to monitor using conventional randomized control trials [47]. In a randomized, double-blind, placebo-controlled trial, individualized homeopathic remedies were added as adjunctive therapies and compared with placebo homeopathic remedies in 96 children who had mild to moderate asthma. The study used a childhood asthma questionnaire as the primary outcome measure in addition to peak flow measurement, medication use, symptoms scores, days missed from school, asthma events, and adverse reactions. The study found no evidence that using classical homeopathic remedies (individualized for each subject) were effective and no evidence of improvement in the quality of life or a decrease in asthma exacerbations [48]. There have been several randomized, double-blind, controlled studies using homeopathic medications for hay fever and allergic rhinitis [49–52]. One study showed a statistically significant drop in symptom severity score compared with the placebo group and a significant reduction in antihistamine use over a 4-week time period. Another study evaluating homeopathic immunotherapy showed a significant improvement in allergic rhinitis accompanied by trends in improvement in respiratory function and bronchial reactivity. This was supported further in a study demonstrating improved nasal airflow in subjects who had seasonal allergic rhinitis using homeopathic medications compared with placebo.

At this time, there is not sufficient evidence available to recommend specific homeopathic treatments in the treatment of chronic or acute asthma; however, further studies may show benefit as in allergic rhinitis and hay fever. Homeopathic medications in the United States (and Europe) are regulated as drugs according to section 201(g)(l) of the Food, Drug, and Cosmetic Act and must comply with the labeling provisions of the FDA for over-the-counter drugs. They must be manufactured according to good manufacturing practices and are regulated by the FDA. Even though homeopathic medications are well regulated for production, the rapidly growing use of homeopathic products and the increasing practice of self-medication raise inevitable questions about effectiveness of these products [53].

Mind-body therapies

Mind-body therapies have been used in the treatment of asthma in various ways. They also are referred to as cognitive behavioral therapies and encompass several approaches. Research in this area started in the early 1960s, and approaches have included relaxation therapy, breathing exercises, biofeedback, and hypnosis and guided imagery. The theory behind using mind-body therapies is based on improving the inflammatory process that can be triggered by the autonomic nervous system through emotions. It has been reported that stress, particularly in children who have asthma and are from lower socioeconomic levels, is associated with higher morbidity and cytokine levels attributed to airway inflammation [54]. In addition to anxiety, stress is shown to influence the immune response and may promote increased sympathetic activity, augment IgE production, shift from a helper T-cell type 1 to type 2 allergic type response, and promote airway inflammation without overt symptoms [55]. Studies also show that using different types of cognitive behavioral therapies, such as relaxation, story telling, and self-hypnosis, may decrease symptoms and medication use [56–58]. This can be accomplished by a team approach and referral to specialist, such as a psychologist. During a 3-year period, one pediatric pulmonary center reported instructing 72 children (average age 11.6 years) in self-hypnosis and 82% reported improvement or resolution in symptoms, such as anxiety, asthma, chest pain, dyspnea, habitual cough, sighing, and vocal cord dysfunction [59].

The use of breathing exercises may be considered a type of mind-body therapy. Since the 1960s, dysfunctional breathing has been known to be associated with asthma symptoms. The use of breathing exercises in controlling asthma symptoms has been taught and promoted by the American Lung Association and the Centers for Disease and Prevention through the Open Airways for Schools, and belly breathing (diaphragmatic breathing) is taught as one of the lessons for doing well at school. Other types of breathing exercises and breathing retraining are used in the management of asthma. One specific form of breathing therapy, known as the Buteyko breathing technique, is believed to help asthma by decreasing the respiratory rate, allowing carbon dioxide to increase, resulting in bronchodilation. There are several studies suggesting that this breathing technique may be beneficial, but the studies have been small and the actual P_{CO_2} has not been measured [60]. In one study in which adults who had asthma were taught Buteyko breathing, there was a reduction in symptoms and medication use but not in lung function or airway reactivity [61]. A Cochrane review concluded that breathing exercises for asthma, such as Buteyko, yoga, and diaphragmatic breathing, led to decreased use of short-acting β_2-agonists and a trend toward improvement in quality of life but not in decreasing the amount of anti-inflammatory medications, reducing airway reactivity, or improving lung function [62]. In a subsequent double-blind, randomized, controlled study of two breathing techniques in 57 adults who had asthma, one group tried to reduce tidal volume and rate and encourage nasal breathing (Buteyko style) whereas the other group used nonspecific upper body mobility exercises. The study found both groups were able to reduce the use of their reliever medication and reduce their dose of ICS. Although there were no significant changes in lung function and airway reactivity measurements (FEV_1 and response to mannitol), the groups did not have any increased problem with disease control [63]. The use of mind-body therapies also has included prayer in many CAM questionnaire studies. Prayer has not been studied in asthma in children or adults as a therapy. Most investigators believe that if used with conventional therapies, various mind-body modalities seem safe and possibly efficacious in treating chronic asthma.

Manual therapies

Manual therapies encompass a variety of techniques that frequently are used as part of CAM in the treatment of asthma and other chronic conditions. These include massage therapy, chiropractic manipulation, osteopathic manipulation (including cranial osteopathy), chest percussion, and vibrational therapy. Chiropractic physicians have used chiropractic spinal manipulation as a standard of care for asthma for the past several years. A randomized controlled trial of chiropractic manipulation in 91 children who had mild to moderate asthma did not show any significant difference in peak flow monitoring and there was no difference between quality-of-life scores and use of rescue medications [64]. In a smaller study, 36 subjects ages 6 to 17 who had mild to moderate asthma were given chiropractic spinal manipulative therapy (SMT) in addition to their medical management. Outcome measures included pulmonary function tests, quality-of-life questionnaires, asthma severity, peak flow measurements, and symptom diaries. The subjects received 3 months of active SMT or sham SMT. At the end of the study, the quality-of-life measurements improved and asthma severity was lower in the treatment group [65].

A Cochrane review of a variety of manual therapies in the treatment of asthma was undertaken, because a similar biologic mechanism of action has been postulated. From more than 473 citations, three randomized control trials met inclusion criteria. Two were chiropractic manipulation studies and one compared massage therapy with relaxation. The conclusion was there is insufficient evidence to support the use of manual therapies in the treatment of asthma. As is common in other CAM research, the many studies in the literature are small in number of subjects and have poor methodology in regard to controls, and blinding and future trials should be designed to account for these weaknesses in study designs [66].

Summary

CAM and conventional medicine often are used in combination in the treatment of asthma in children. These integrative medicine approaches may have success in reaching the objectives of asthma therapy: reducing symptoms, preventing exacerbations, and promoting a healthy lifestyle with minimal adverse effects from the therapies used. There is no consensus, however, on which type of CAM therapies should be combined with conventional ones, which CAM therapies have advantages over others, and which CAM therapies may cause harm. With the multiple and complex interaction of genetic influences and environmental exposures playing a role in asthma, further studies using CAM therapies with conventional treatments in the treatment of asthma in children are warranted.

References

[1] Martinez F, Wright A, Taussig L, et al. Asthma and wheezing in the first six years of life. The Group Health Medical Associates. N Engl J Med 1995;332(3):133–8.

[2] Gern J, Lemanske R. Infectious triggers of pediatric asthma. Pediatr Clin North Am 2003; 50(3):555–75.

[3] Taussig L, Wright A, Holberg C, et al. Tucson children's respiratory study: 1980 to present. J Allergy Clin Immunol 2003;11:661–75.

[4] Bisgaard H. The Copenhagen Prospective Study on Asthma in Childhood (COPSAC): design, rationale, and baseline data from a longitudinal birth cohort study. Ann Allergy Asthma Immunol 2004;93:381–9.

[5] Vickers A, Zollman C. ABC of complementary medicine: homeopathy. BMJ 1999;319: 1115–8.

[6] Slader C, Reddel H, Jenkins C, et al. Complementary and alternative medicine use in asthma: who is using what? Respirology 2006;11:373–87.

[7] Ernst E. Use of complementary therapies in childhood asthma. Pediatr Asthma Allergy Immunol 1998;12:29–32.

[8] Andrews L, Lokuge S, Sawyer M, et al. The use of alternative therapies by children with asthma: a brief report. J Paediatr Child Health 1998;34:13–4.

[9] Braganza S, Ozuah P, Sharif I. The use of complementary therapies in inner-city asthmatic children. J Asthma 2003;40:823–7.

[10] Orhan F, Sekerel B, Kocabas C, et al. Complementary and alternative medicine in children with asthma. Ann Allergy Asthma Immunol 2003;90:611–5.

[11] Shenfield G, Lim E, Allen H. Survey of the use of complementary medicine and therapies in children with asthma. J Paediatr Child Health 2002;38:252–7.

[12] Reznik M, Ozuah P, Franco K, et al. Use of complementary therapy by adolescents with asthma. Arch Pediatr Adolesc Med 2002;156:1042–4.

[13] Sidora-Arcoleo K, Yoos L, McMullen A, et al. Complementary and alternative medicine use in children with asthma: prevalence and sociodemographic profile of users. J Asthma 2007; 44(3):169–75.

[14] Eisenberg D, Kessler R, Von Rompay M, et al. Perceptions about complementary therapies relative to conventional therapies among adult who use both: results from a national survey. Ann Intern Med 2001;135:344–51.

[15] Milgrom H. Childhood asthma: breakthroughs and challenges. Adv Pediatr 2006;53: 55–100.

[16] Devereux G, Seaton A. Diet as a risk factor for atopy and asthma. J Allergy Clin Immunol 2005;115:1107–17.

[17] Black P, Sharpe S. Dietary fat and asthma: is there a connection? Eur Respir J 1997;10:6–12.

[18] Calder P, Yaqoob P, Thies F, et al. Fatty acids and lymphocyte functions. Br J Nutr 2002; 87(Suppl):S31–48.

[19] Chatzi L, Apostolaki G, Bibakis I, et al. Protective effect of fruits, vegetables and the Mediterranean diet on asthma and allergies among children in Crete. Thorax 2007;62:677–83.

[20] Gilliland F, Berhane K, Li YF, et al. Children's lung function and antioxidant vitamin, fruit, juice, and vegetable intake. Am J Epidemiol 2003;158:576–84.

[21] Burns J, Dockery D, Neas L, et al. Low dietary nutrient intakes and respiratory health in adolescents. Chest 2007;132:238–45.

[22] Woods R, Thien F, Abramson J. Dietary marine fatty acids (fish oil) for asthma in adults and children. Cochrane Database Syst Rev 2002:CD001283.

[23] Mickleborough T, Lindley M, Ionescu A, et al. Protective effect of fish oil supplementation on exercise-induced bronchoconstriction in asthma. Chest 2006;129:39–49.

[24] Almqvist C, Garden F, Xuan W, et al. Omega-3 and omega-6 fatty acid exposure from early life does not affect atopy and asthma at age 5 years. J Allergy Clin Immunol 2007;119: 1438–44.

[25] Clement Y, William A, Aranda D, et al. Medicinal herb use among asthmatic patients attending a specialty care facility in Trinidad. BMC Complement Altern Med 2005;5:1–8.

[26] US Food and Drug Administration. Dietary Supplement Health and Education Act of 1994. Available at: http://www.fda.gov/opacom/laws/dshea.html. Accessed October 23, 2007.

[27] Woolf A. Herbal remedies and children: do they work? Are they harmful? Pediatrics 2003;
     112:240–6.
[28] Danesch U. Petasites hybridus (Butterbur root) extract in the treatment of asthma-an open
     trial. Altern Med Rev 2004;9:54–62.
[29] Lau B, Riesen S, Truong K, et al. Pycnogenol as an adjunct in the management of childhood
     asthma. J Asthma 2004;41:825–32.
[30] Gupta I, Gupta V, Parihar A, et al. Effects of Boswellia serrata gum resin in patients with
     bronchial asthma: results of a double-blind, placebo-controlled, 6-week clinical study. Eur
     J Med Res 1998;3:511–4.
[31] Ram F, Rowe B, Kaur B. Vitamin C supplementation for asthma. Cochrane Database Syst
     Rev 2004;3:CD00093.
[32] Kelly F, Mudway I, Blomberg A, et al. Altered lung antioxidant status in patients with mild
     asthma. Lancet 1999;354:482–3.
[33] Shaheen S, Newson R, Rayman M, et al. Randomised, double blind, placebo-controlled trial
     of selenium supplementation in adult asthma. Thorax 2007;62:483–90.
[34] Britton J, Pavord I, Richards K, et al. Dietary magnesium, lung function, wheezing and air-
     way hyperreactivity in a random population sample. Lancet 1994;344:357–62.
[35] Soutar A, Seaton A, Brown D. Bronchial reactivity and dietary antioxidants. Thorax 1997;
     52:166–70.
[36] Gontijo-Amaral C, Ribeiro M, Gontijo L, et al. Oral magnesium supplementation in asth-
     matic children: a double-blind randomized placebo-controlled trial. Eur J Clin Nutr 2007;61:
     54–60.
[37] Haller C, Benowitz N. Adverse cardiovascular and central nervous system events associ-
     ated with dietary supplements containing ephedra alkaloids. N Engl J Med 2000;343:
     1833–8.
[38] Bensky D, Clavey S, Stoger F, et al. Chinese herbal medicine: materia medica. 3rd edition.
     Seattle (WA): Eastland Press; 2004.
[39] Li X. Traditional Chinese herbal remedies for asthma and food allergy. J Allergy Clin Immu-
     nol 2007;120:25–31.
[40] Wen M, Wei C, Hu Z, et al. Efficacy and tolerability of anti-asthma herbal medicine inter-
     ventions in adult patients with moderate-severe allergic asthma. J Allergy Clin Immunol
     2005;116:517–24.
[41] Chang T, Huan C, Hsu C. Clinical evaluation of the Chinese herbal medicine formula STA-1
     in the treatment of allergic asthma. Phytother Res 2006;20:342–7.
[42] National Institutes of Health. Acupuncture. NIH Consensus Statement 1997;15(5):1–34.
[43] McCarney R, Brinkhaus B, Lasserson T, et al. Acupuncture for chronic asthma. Cochrane
     Database Syst Rev 2004;1:CD000008.
[44] Gruber W, Eber E, Malle-Scheid D, et al. Laser acupuncture in children and adolescents with
     exercise induced asthma. Thorax 2002;57:222–5.
[45] Stockert K, Schneider B, Porenta G, et al. Laser acupuncture and probiotics in school age
     children with asthma: a randomized placebo-controlled pilot study of therapy guided by
     principles of Traditional Chinese Medicine. Pediatr Allergy Immunol 2007;18:160–6.
[46] Paterson C, Britten N. Acupuncture as a complex intervention: a holistic model. J Altern
     Complement Med 2004;10:791–801.
[47] McCarney R, Linde K, Lasserson T. Homeopathy for chronic asthma. Cochrane Database
     Syst Rev 2004;1:CD000353.
[48] White A, Slade P, Hunt C, et al. Individualised homeopathy as an adjunct in the treatment of
     childhood asthma: a randomised placebo controlled trial. Thorax 2003;58:317–21.
[49] Reilly D, Taylor M. Potent placebo or potency? A proposed study model with intitial
     findings using homeopathically prepared pollens in hayfever. Br Homeopath J 1985;74:
     65–75.
[50] Reilly D, Taylor M, McSharry C, et al. Is homeopathy a placebo response? Controlled trial
     of homeopathic potency, with pollen in hayfever model. Lancet 1986;2:881–5.

[51] Reilly D, Taylor M, Beattie N, et al. Is evidence for homeopathy reproducible? Lancet 1994; 344:1601–6.
[52] Taylor M, Reilly D, Llewellyn-Jones R, et al. Randomised controlled trial of homeopathy versus placebo in perennial allergic rhinitis with overview of four trial series. Br Med J 2000;321:471–6.
[53] Kirby B. Safety of homeopathic products. J R Soc Med 2002;95:464–5.
[54] Chen E, Hanson M, Paterson L, et al. Socioeconomic status and inflammatory processes in childhood asthma: the role of psychological stress. J Allergy Clin Immunol 2006;117: 1014–20.
[55] Marshal G. Neuroendocrine mechanisms of immune dysregulation: applications to allergy and asthma. Ann Allergy Asthma Immunol 2004;93(2 Suppl 1):S11–7.
[56] Vazquez M, Buceta J. Psychological treatment of asthma: effectiveness of a self-management program with and without relaxation training. J Asthma 1993;30:171–83.
[57] Ewer T, Stewart D. Improvement in bronchial hyper-responsiveness in patients with moderate asthma after treatment with a hypnotic technique: a randomised controlled trial. BMJ 1986;293:1129–32.
[58] Kohen D, Wynne E. Applying hypnosis in a preschool family asthma education program: uses of storytelling, imagery and relaxation. Am J Clin Hypn 1997;39:169–81.
[59] Anbar R, Hummell K. Teamwork approach to clinical hypnosis at a pediatric pulmonary center. Am J Clin Hypn 2005;48:45–9.
[60] Bruton A, Lewith G. The Buteyko breathing technique for asthma: a review. Complement Ther Med 2005;13:41–6.
[61] Cooper S, Oborne J, Newton S, et al. Effect of two breathing exercises (Buteyko and pranayama) in asthma: a randomised controlled trial. Thorax 2003;58:649–50.
[62] Holloway E, Ram F. Breathing exercises for asthma. Cochrane Database Syst Rev 2004;1: CD001277.
[63] Slader C, Reddel H, Spencer L, et al. Double blind randomised controlled trial of two different breathing techniques in the management of asthma. Thorax 2006;61:643–5.
[64] Balon J, Aker P, Crowther E, et al. A comparison of active and simulated chiropractic manipulation as adjunctive treatment for childhood asthma. N Engl J Med 1998;339:1013–20.
[65] Bonfort G, Evans R, Kubic P, et al. Chronic pediatric asthma and chiropractic spinal manipulation: a prospective clinical series and randomized clinical pilot study. J Manipulative Physiol Ther 2001;24:369–77.
[66] Hondras M, Linde K, Jones A. Manual therapy for asthma. Cochrane Database Syst Rev 2005;2:CD001002.

ELSEVIER
SAUNDERS

PEDIATRIC CLINICS
OF NORTH AMERICA

Pediatr Clin N Am 54 (2007) 1025–1041

Pediatric Massage Therapy: An Overview for Clinicians

Shay Beider, MPH, LMT[a],*, Nicole E. Mahrer, BA[b],
Jeffrey I. Gold, PhD[c]

[a]Integrative Touch for Kids, 8306 Wilshire Boulevard, #530, Beverly Hills, CA 90211, USA
[b]Department of Anesthesiology Critical Care Medicine, Childrens Hospital Los Angeles,
4650 Sunset Boulevard, MS#12, Los Angeles, CA 90027, USA
[c]Department of Anesthesiology Critical Care Medicine, Keck School of Medicine,
University of Southern California, Childrens Hospital Los Angeles, Comfort,
Pain Management and Palliative Care Program, 4650 Sunset Boulevard,
MS#12, Los Angeles, CA 90027, USA

In humans, touch is the first sense to develop. Over the centuries, human touch has been shown to be emotionally and physically healing. Touch in the form of massage therapy (MT) was first described in China in the second century BC. Since being introduced to the United States in the 1850s, MT has been used for a wide variety of outcomes [1]. MT is part of a growing trend in complementary and alternative medicine (CAM) in the United States [2] and represents one of the most widely used CAM therapies by Americans [2]. A meta-analysis of massage therapy research in adults by Moyer and colleagues [3] found significant benefits of MT in reducing anxiety and depression. Given the current literature highlighting the benefits of MT in adults and the growing interest in the use of MT with children, examining the potential healing effects of MT in children who have various medical conditions has become critical.

This article provides clinicians with a broad overview of pediatric MT, including proven and promising effects of MT across disease-specific clinical applications, contraindications, safety, context and availability of services, and future directions. This evidence will support clinicians in reaching an informed decision about the usefulness of MT and acts as a guide for appropriate treatment recommendations.

---

* Corresponding author.
E-mail address: shay@integrativetouch.org (S. Beider).

0031-3955/07/$ - see front matter © 2007 Elsevier Inc. All rights reserved.
doi:10.1016/j.pcl.2007.10.001
pediatric.theclinics.com

Methods

Computerized databases, including PubMed, Medline, and PychInfo, were searched for relevant studies, including prior reviews, case studies, and randomized control trials of MT. Key terms included *pediatric massage* and *child massage*. Studies presented highlight qualitative and quantitative single-case and randomized control trials of pediatric MT. Clinical practice-based evidence was obtained through MT reference books and texts commonly referred to in the MT field. Studies were separated into two sections: proven effects and promising effects of MT. Studies presented in the "proven effects" section include meta-analyses and reviews of infant and pediatric MT that have shown positive outcomes, verifiable through effect size calculation. Research using less rigorous trials, case studies, and anecdotal clinical applications to show the benefits of MT are presented in the "promising effects" section of the paper.

Defining massage

Pediatric MT, defined as the manual manipulation of soft tissue intended to promote health and well-being in children and adolescents, can be applied with a wide range of variability in terms of pressure, pacing, and selected modality [4]. A skilled massage therapist will know how to go from light touch to deeper massage, as appropriate, and will be familiar with various modalities that can be incorporated into their practice. The pacing with which the treatment is applied can be substantially modified with the goal of increasing or decreasing stimulation through the use of faster or slower movements. Site restrictions may make one area of the body unavailable for MT, whereas other areas are safe to massage.

A wide variety of MT modalities exist, each providing suggested benefits. These include therapies such as cranial sacral, myofascial release, neuromuscular, trigger point, lymphatic drainage, and reflexology. Particular massage techniques and modalities have either stimulating or calming effects and a range of healing outcomes. One of the challenges in studying and defining MT is that it encompasses an increasing number of treatment modalities, each with distinct practice characteristics. As the field grows, individual modalities may be studied independently for effectiveness and treatment-related outcomes.

The type of pediatric MT appropriate for children who have chronic and acute illness may differ substantially from classic Swedish or circulatory massage. Often MT in a hospitalized or hospice setting can have significantly unique demands, and therefore the term *massage* can be confusing. New names are being used to describe these integrative MT treatments, such as Integrative Touch and Compassionate Touch. Integrative Touch is a gentle form of massage therapy that is sensitive to the medical needs of patients who are hospitalized or in hospice care [5]. Integrative Touch takes into consideration the whole patient, including mind, body, and spirit, and uses gentle, noncirculatory techniques as appropriate. Compassionate Touch describes a therapeutic modality created specifically for elderly and ill or dying individuals [6]. Compassionate Touch combines one-on-one focused attention, intentional touch, and sensitive massage with specialized communication skills to help enhance quality of life for those in later life stages.

This new language highlights the evolution of MT. In addition, differing notions exist about what constitutes therapeutic MT. At one end of the spectrum, MT is directed primarily at symptom management, while on the other, MT can be viewed as creating enhanced well-being through multisystem integration (MSI) and organization, which can lead to an optimal healing experience. MSI has similar goals to those expressed in acupuncture literature, emphasizing balance, homeostasis, healing, well-being, and a departure from symptom abatement alone. Western thinking has notoriously focused on symptom management, thus losing sight, at times, of the more global healing process. The authors propose that although the effectiveness of MT is often measured in terms of reduced symptom distress, holistically, MT may work through MSI, targeting the interactions among immune, muscular, cardiovascular, endocrine, and nervous system functions. The Samueli Institute is one medical research organization that has been exploring the scientific foundations of healing and applying that understanding in medicine and health care to create optimal healing environments.

Other theorists have posed plausible explanations for the effects of MT. For example, some studies have connected MT with weight gain in preterm/low–birth weight infants [7]. Field [8] theorizes that weight gain in preterm infants is caused by increased vagal activity after MT, resulting in the release of hormones in the gastrointestinal tract to promote more efficient food absorption. Vickers and colleagues [7] hypothesize that the weight gain could be caused by a combination of Field's theory and the possibility that MT may reduce adverse reactions to stress [9]. Nonetheless, these effects of MT have not been explained through reductionistic mechanisms, thus supporting an MSI approach.

The remainder of this article will emphasize the effects of MT across disease-specific states, as this is the common method used by the scientific and clinical communities to categorize research in MT. In this article, circulatory MT is generally the assumed therapeutic MT practice unless otherwise indicated. Gentle touch or light holding may be applied when circulatory MT is contraindicated. Following an overview of the clinical applications of pediatric MT, subdivided by proven and promising effects, the authors review contraindications, safety, context and availability of pediatric MT, and future directions in pediatric massage.

Clinical applications of pediatric massage therapy

Proven effects

Infant massage

An increasing amount of literature in MT for young children exists about preterm/low–birth weight infants. A meta-analysis conducted by Vickers and colleagues [7] examined the direct effects of MT to improve health and development in preterm/low–birth weight infants. These investigators report that preterm/low–birth weight infants who received daily massages showed improved weight gain (5g/d) and shorter hospital stays (4–5 days) in comparison to control groups who did not receive daily massages [7,8]; however, the authors were hesitant to connect these effects directly to the gentle-touch MT. Overall, the review concluded that researchers failed to reveal the underlying mechanisms of MT or provide proper information on data-gathering methodologies. More recently, Underdown and colleagues [10] looked at the effect of MT on infant physical and mental health. They found no effect on infant growth, but instead reported evidence of improved mother–infant interaction, sleep and relaxation, and reduced crying in infants receiving MT. No evidence of the benefit of MT on mental health outcomes was found.

Recent research examining caregiver-trained infant massage with fragile infants hospitalized in a neonatal intensive care unit showed feasibility/safety, as well as quantitative/qualitative improvements for infants and their caregivers [11]. Results indicated that caregivers randomized to administer infant touch/massage reported satisfaction with providing infant massage and declines in depressive symptoms. In addition, the study demonstrated the safety of infant massage based on physiologic stability and no change in agitation/pain scores in infants receiving MT. However, no evidence supported increased weight gain or shortened hospital stays. Livingston and colleagues [11] showed that caregiver-trained infant massage of fragile infants was feasible/safe and resulted in improved health and satisfaction outcomes compared with the control group. Although research on infant MT has targeted weight gain, shortened hospital stays, and other health/satisfaction outcomes, recent research on pediatric MT has focused more on general health-related outcomes (eg, psychologic or physiologic states).

Pediatric massage

Beider and Moyer [4] conducted a review of 24 randomized control trials of pediatric MT for children between the ages of 2 and 19 years. They differentiated between single-dose effects, or short-term effects, observed after a single session of MT versus multiple-dose effects or long-term effects, measured at various time points over the course of treatment [4]. A significant reduction of state anxiety was observed in the single-dose effects category. Other single-dose effects, purported to have potential benefit in other studies, such as the reduction of salivary cortisol, negative mood, and alteration in behavior, were not supported in this review. Multiple-dose effects, including improvements in trait anxiety, muscle tone, and arthritis pain, were found to be significant [4]. Table 1 [4] shows the effects of MT on various health outcomes from this review.

A recent review examining the effectiveness of MT for chronic, nonmalignant pain provided robust support for the analgesic effects of MT for nonspecific low back pain, moderate support for these effects on shoulder and headache pain, and preliminary support for MT in the treatment of fibromyalgia, mixed chronic pain conditions, neck pain, and carpal tunnel syndrome [12]. The review by Beider and Moyer [4,13] also found support for reduced pain in children who had juvenile rheumatoid arthritis.

Promising effects

Research using less-rigorous trials, case studies, and anecdotal clinical applications has provided findings indicative of promising effects of MT. These findings include decreased depression, negative mood, disruptive behavioral problems (eg, attention deficit hyperactive disorder), and increased airflow in those who have pulmonary disorders. Continued research using sound methodologies, standardized and measurable MT protocols, and multidimensional health outcomes to assess the effects of MT on children

Table 1
Mean effect sizes of massage therapy according to health outcome variable

Outcome variable	k^a	N	Effect size $(g)^b$	95% CI
Single-dose effects				
State anxiety, first session	4	81	0.59*	0.15–1.04
State anxiety, last session	4	81	1.10**	0.64–1.57
Negative mood	2	50	0.52	−0.05–1.10
Salivary cortisol	2	50	0.28	−0.27–0.84
Behavior	1	24	0.37	−0.43–1.35
Multiple-dose effects				
Depression	2	54	0.48	−0.06–1.02
Trait anxiety	1	30	0.94*	0.20–1.68
Arthritis pain	1	20	1.33**	0.37–2.29
Muscle tone	2	41	0.90**	0.23–1.57
Range of motion	1	20	0.31	−0.57–1.19
Immune measures	2	48	0.06	−0.52–0.63
Pulmonary function	1	20	0.47	−0.41–1.35
Developmental functioning	2	41	0.24	−0.38–0.86
Spasticity	1	20	0.26	−.0.62–1.14
Hostility	1	17	−0.85	−1.85–0.15
Classroom behavior	1	30	0.66	−0.07–1.39

[a] k indciates the nubmer of studies contributing to the effect size (g).
[b] A positive g indicates a reduction for any outcome variable.
* $P < .05$.
** $P < .01$.

and adolescents is needed. Although clinicians may espouse the benefits of MT with pediatric clinical samples, the empirical evidence still remains somewhat limited. However, clinical knowledge should not be dismissed in the absence of empirical data. Reference texts are available for massage therapists in the areas of pediatric massage therapy [14], pathology [15,16], and hospital massage [17] that provide valuable information for therapists working with children. The following information reports these promising effects of pediatric MT, organized according to system and disease-specific states.

Integumentary system conditions

There are a variety of integumentary system conditions that children may experience to which MT can be applied, so long as the lesion or compromised area is not directly touched. Children who have conditions such as eczema and psoriasis can benefit from MT if the skin has not been compromised such that it is vulnerable to infection. Benefits of MT have included reductions in skin redness, flakiness of the skin, and itching [18]. Infants and children who have thrush may receive MT if the thrush is not caused by a contraindicated disease [16]. Circulatory MT may be applied to very mild sunburns. More serious burns can be treated in the subacute stage to help with skin rehabilitation, scar status, and pruritus [19]. Perhaps of even greater benefit, MT may be useful for minimizing the stress, anxiety, and pain associated with skin debridement [20]. If burns have healed beyond the subacute stage, MT is appropriate, given a general sensitivity and inquisitiveness about any loss of sensation (eg, nerve damage) to the immediate area [15].

Through improving circulation, MT may also help prevent the development of pressure sores in children who spend prolonged periods in bed or a wheelchair [15]. Once a sore develops, MT is locally contraindicated because it may introduce infection. Children in wheelchairs with muscle atrophy may benefit from gentle and slow MT targeting increased blood circulation.

Musculoskeletal system conditions

The general rule for MT and musculoskeletal conditions is that the acute phase should be avoided, and that subacute and chronic injuries may be addressed. Investigators have shown that MT has promising effects for reducing pain in children who have juvenile rheumatoid arthritis, especially in the subacute phases with improved joint mobility [13]. Cherkin and colleagues [21] showed that MT has promising effects for decreasing back or neck pain of unknown origin when the areas are not acutely inflamed. Clinicians have indicated that children who have ankylosing spondylitis may benefit from MT to improve joint mobilization, muscle strength, and flexibility [16].

Physical therapists have shown that using MT for children who have undergone amputations or have limb length discrepancies due to birth defects can desensitize highly sensitive areas and minimize skin irritation resulting from prosthetics [16].

Duchenne muscular dystrophy (DMD) is marked by progressive weakness and degeneration of the skeletal muscles. Because scoliosis is common with DMD, MT is beneficial for relieving muscle soreness and tension in the back [22]. MT may also slow muscular atrophy associated with DMD. MT helps to provide release of muscular, tendinous, and ligamentous tension that is common with spinal changes (eg, postural deviations, including scoliosis and lumbar or thoracic curves). MT applied to the back and chest of patients who have DMD may also help minimize respiratory complications that are common after age 15 years. Because muscle function is impaired with DMD but sensation is intact, massage is indicated as long as the circulatory system is not compromised [15].

Any type of fracture or broken bone locally contraindicates MT, but collateral MT to surrounding areas can help with compensation patterns. MT applied proximally and distally to a fractured or broken bone can improve muscle tone and circulation, reducing the likelihood of developing edema. Dislocations, which can be fairly common in childhood, have specific MT indications during the subacute stage. Sprains, tendonitis, and shin splints also respond well to MT in the subacute stage [15]. MT can minimize swelling, reduce adhesions, support the healing process, and allow increased mobility in the joint. For a condition such as torticollis, local MT can promote muscle relaxation, loosen connective tissue, and reduce spasms [16].

Regular applications of MT, often practiced among rehabilitation specialists, have been shown to treat edema and contractures [23]. In addition to using circulatory MT for minimizing contractures, stretching, friction, and myofascial release techniques have also been suggested. Early treatment with regular MT may also reduce the development of severe contractures in young children who have cerebral palsy.

Nervous system conditions

MT has been shown to be helpful for nervous system conditions, specifically when peripheral nerves are impacted, and to be of clinical value in improving psychologically mediated neurologic outcomes, such as pain, anxiety, and depression [3]. Children who have complex regional pain syndrome (CRPS), formally known as *reflex sympathetic dystrophy* (RSD) *syndrome*, a chronic pathologic pain condition, will often not tolerate MT in the primarily identified area; however, clinical experience has shown that MT applied to other areas of the body may help to improve quality of life and reduce pain in the pain site. Furthermore, because of the high incidence of sleep disturbances in children who have CRPS, similar to other chronic pain conditions, MT has been used clinically to relax and initiate a parasympathetic state, which assists with sleep initiation.

Multiple sclerosis (MS) was long considered an adult disease; however, health care providers are now diagnosing MS in children and adolescents. MT can be beneficial during the subacute stage in children who have MS, and is often recommended as part of a stress management plan. Because symptoms can be aggravated by heat, MT must be provided in a cooler environment [24]. As indicated with other childhood conditions, MT can be useful for decreasing rigidity, contractures, and stiffness associated with MS [16].

Patients who have headaches can also respond favorably to MT, with treatment frequently preferred in the subacute stage. Generally, MT is indicated for tension-type headaches but contraindicated for headaches resulting from infection. The pattern and origin of the headache must be understood before proceeding with the therapy.

Children and adolescents with Erb's palsy and cerebral palsy (CP) can benefit from regular MT treatments [25]. Because of the variability in severity of CP and the symptoms expressed, MT treatments must be closely assessed and monitored on a case-by-case basis. Individuals who have hypertonic muscles will require a relaxing massage, whereas hypotonic muscles respond better to stimulating touch. MT can help maintain elasticity of the muscles and can provide comfort.

All three types of spina bifida, occulta, meningocele, and myelomeningocele can respond well to MT [15]. Children with spina bifida may have a shunt and full or partial paralysis, bladder and bowel control difficulties, depression, and latex allergy [15]. MT is particularly useful for stimulating blood circulation in the affected areas and increasing mobility, range of motion, and function/mobility.

Spinal cord injury can respond positively to MT in areas where sensation is present and underlying conditions are identified. Gentle touch or holding can also be applied to areas where sensation is absent due to injury. In general, when a child presents with paralysis, MT can be applied with specific precautionary guidelines. When sensation is limited, light pressure should be applied and joint mobilizations and stretches should be avoided [16].

Although strokes are rare in childhood, they do occur, especially as a consequence of other medical illnesses. MT can be used to augment other therapies, such as physical and occupational therapy. MT helps increase circulation and can counter unnecessary muscular degeneration sometimes caused by proprioceptive misinformation [15].

MT has been recommended for children and adolescents who have sleep disorders. In a study of adults who had fibromyalgia, results indicated that MT increased sleep, which led to decreased pain [26]. Researchers have shown that sleep is associated with decreases in substance P, a substance known to induce pain [26]. Researchers have also shown that MT is associated with increases in stage III and IV (N3) restorative sleep [27]. MT can improve the quality of sleep and may relieve some of the stressors that traditionally interfere with normal sleep architecture. Young infants and children who are hospitalized for prolonged periods may experience difficulty with sleep onset and maintenance and early awakening because their normal circadian rhythm is disrupted. MT, particularly applied in the evening, can help normalize this cycle.

MT has been shown to create a sense of calm and enhanced organization for children who have attention deficit hyperactivity disorder. The primary challenge for massage therapists working with this population is to apply MT in short doses and to be sensitive and flexible to the child's preferences and needs, which may quickly shift. Benefits of MT have been reported in terms of decreasing restlessness and increasing attention [28].

Anxiety disorders may be substantially improved through regular MT. Pediatric populations have shown strong effects resulting from MT in the area of anxiety reduction [4]. MT may be helpful for specific conditions, such as posttraumatic stress disorder and obsessive-compulsive disorder, and may also help minimize anxiety, worry, and general distress associated with treatments in hospitals or hospice settings. MT can also be a preventive measure for decreasing negative symptoms that may result from prolonged hospitalization.

Circulatory system conditions

Many of the conditions and diseases that contraindicate MT are contraindicated because of the specific functions of the circulatory system. Nonetheless, various circulatory system conditions have been shown to benefit from MT. MT for children who have Raynaud's syndrome may help stimulate vasodilation and increase blood flow to the desired area. MT can be applied as long as any serious underlying causes, such as lupus, have been ruled out. Children and adolescents experiencing heart failure may receive gentle holding and light touch only and no circulatory techniques. Similarly, MT has been shown to benefit children and adolescents during subacute stages of sickle cell disease. During acute pain episodes, very light touch and gentle holding may be provided to reduce pain and anxiety. In a recent study of children who have sickle cell disease, 54% of them used CAM therapies, with 5% reporting biomechanical therapy (ie, massage) [29].

Lymphatic and immune system conditions

Various immune system conditions, including chronic fatigue syndrome (CFS), HIV, and lupus, respond well to MT during the subacute stage. The section on "contraindications" discusses concerns about the clinical application of MT for various lymphatic and immune system conditions.

Respiratory system conditions

Pulmonary diseases, such as asthma, bronchiectasis, and chronic bronchitis, may benefit from MT in the subacute stage when infection is not present or during an ongoing asthma attack. Muscular relaxation in the back, chest, and neck may be particularly helpful for these conditions. Postural drainage may help clear the respiratory tract of excess mucus. Preliminary data on MT and pulmonary function have been promising and may be helpful for allergies that irritate respiratory function [4]. Some evidence suggests that children who have cystic fibrosis may experience improved pulmonary function with MT [30]. MT has also shown clinical benefit in improving pulmonary function for children who are experiencing difficulty breathing during end-of-life care.

Endocrine system conditions

There are endocrine system conditions for which MT may be indicated. MT may be indicated for children who have diabetes as long as they have healthy responsive tissue with good blood supply. Circulatory massage for children in advanced stages who have kidney failure or atherosclerosis is ill advised. MT in children who have diabetes should always be accompanied by careful glucose monitoring [31]. Hyper- and hypothyroidism, parathyroidism, and hyper- and hypopituitarism may benefit from MT as long as a careful treatment plan is established based on the child's symptoms and sensitivity [16].

Female reproductive system conditions

Endometriosis can affect girls as young as 9 years of age. This condition causes significant pain surrounding the abdomen, and therefore direct massage to this area is contraindicated. However, MT can help reduce stress, anxiety, and frustration that accompany the long-term consequences of the disease.

Premenstrual syndrome (PMS) strongly indicates massage. MT can reduce depression and anxiety, and can also alleviate some liquid retention that makes PMS physically uncomfortable [15].

Cancer

For most children who have cancer, MT can be safely applied with certain site and pressure restrictions. In a pilot study of 50 children undergoing hematopoeitic stem cell transplantation, participants were randomized to professional massage, parent massage, or standard care. Differences between groups emerged on the outcomes of number of days in the hospital and number of days to engraftment, suggesting potential cost or benefit for massage in this setting [32]. A 2001 randomized controlled trial conducted by Field and colleagues [33] reported that children who have leukemia who received daily massage from their parents for a month experienced an elevation in mood and a decrease in anxiety. The investigators also noted that MT might renew confidence and self-esteem. A study by Williams and colleagues assessed symptom monitoring by parents or caregivers of children who had cancer and strategies used to alleviate chemotherapy symptoms. MT was one of the methods that was found to be beneficial [34]. Children who have cancer must cope with many physical changes caused by the disease or treatment. These changes are accompanied by discomfort. A study of children with leukemia-related cancer pain found the most frequently used strategy for pain management was stressor modification, including MT [35]. Although children who undergo cancer treatment often experience many painful medical procedures and long-term health consequences, MT may serve to promote healing through providing comforting touch. Massage therapists can aid in the coping process by listening to the child express their sorrows and insecurities while aiding them through MT [36]. In terms of prevalence, alternative therapy use in families of children with cancer is comparable to use in families of well children [37].

Well children

Clinical experience suggests that gentle touch for well children, in the form of MT, can help promote optimal functioning across multiple systems. Parents and children receiving MT have expressed reductions in stress, muscular tension, and symptoms associated with sports-related injuries. Positive benefits include enhanced circulation and digestion, along with other benefits previously discussed. MT can help promote respectful and nonviolent communication between peers and family members. Parents have reported their children to be less aggressive after the family has received MT [38]. Another potential social impact of MT is the establishment of a sense of personal boundaries and awareness of appropriate and inappropriate touch. In general, MT for children can provide safe and loving touch that can both enhance relationships with others and develop a deep personal sense of connection with their bodies and themselves.

Pain management and palliative care

Massage therapists, biofeedback technicians, physician-acupuncturists, child-life specialists, psychologists, and physical and occupational therapists can all be used as allies to battle acute pain in children. Incorporating established and alternative forms of pain management, including education, relaxation techniques, hypnosis, guided imagery, biofeedback, and acupuncture into standard pediatric care may improve the management of acute, procedural, or chronic pain in children. Pain in children does not have to be managed with an "either/or" approach using traditional pharmacologic methods or the cognitive and alternative therapies discussed here. Current literature supports the use of adjunctive methods of pain management, which may complement traditional pharmacologic pain management, thereby providing optimal care for children experiencing pain.

MT as an integrative therapeutic intervention for pediatric palliative care is clinically important, even though empirical evidence is limited [39]. The palliative aspects of MT for children at end-of-life are critical. The therapeutic aspect of MT can provide children with a sense of comfort and safety, in addition to physiological improvement or symptom management. An National Institutes of Health pilot study of family-administered massage for children with cancer is currently being conducted [40]. This study seeks to examine the effectiveness of MT for controlling pain intensity and pain-related negative effects experienced by children who have cancer. Palliative care practice shows that MT can be useful for reducing pain and anxiety, and maximizing comfort, which is consistent with current findings in pediatric MT [4]. Perhaps the greatest strength of MT in a palliative care environment is that it allows children to feel comforted through touch. MT at end-of-life should always be gentle and applied with care and consideration for the patient's comfort.

Contraindications

Although MT may help treat a variety of pediatric medical conditions, MT is contraindicated in some circumstances. For example, although MT is clinically useful for various skin conditions, broken skin locally contraindicates the use of MT, as the lesion or compromised area should not be directly touched. Other locally contraindicated skin conditions include fungal infections, herpes, warts, contact dermatitis, hives, and psoriasis. Infections such as cellulitis and impetigo contraindicate the use of MT until the infection is resolved. Skin conditions that strictly contraindicate MT include lice, scabies, and mites. Circulatory MT is contraindicated for chickenpox and German measles until the child is completely recovered because of the systemic infection and communicability of the conditions. For musculoskeletal injury, the acute phase should be avoided, but subacute and chronic injuries may tolerate MT. Serious head injuries, concussions, and subdural hematomas contraindicate circulatory MT, but gentle holding and comforting touch techniques may be suitable. Because meningitis is a systemic infection, circulatory MT is contraindicated.

Disease affecting circulatory system functions largely contraindicate circulatory MT. However, MT theoretically provides less impact on the circulatory system than regular exercise, so it should not be ruled out for patients who can tolerate physical activity. For any condition that involves compromised blood vessels, circulatory MT is contraindicated. Massage therapists should only provide gentle holding or light touch for children with aneurysms, hypertension, or high blood pressure.

MT can cause fluid to be drawn into lymphatic capillaries and thereby increase lymphatic flow; therefore, massage therapists must be aware that MT can cause lymphedema in children who are at risk for this disease. Similarly, children who have edema should not receive circulatory MT, but rather light friction and gliding strokes with support and elevation to the edematous limb, which can promote lymphatic drainage. Proximal areas should be prioritized first, and then distal areas can receive therapy [16]. Although MT is contraindicated in children who have fever, acute inflammation, or acute kidney infection, very light touch could be provided without any circulatory enhancement [15].

Safety

Even though adverse events associated with MT are rare, safety remains an important concern. In a review study, Ernst [41] found 20 cases reporting adverse events as a result of MT. These events ranged from various pain syndromes and leg ulcers to more serious events, such as cerebrovascular accidents, hematoma, ruptured uterus, and strangulation of neck. In most of these cases, unconventional massage techniques other than circulatory massage were used and MT was not delivered by a trained massage therapist. Adverse outcomes by trained massage therapists following indication/contraindication guidelines are extremely rare.

Medical considerations

Knowledge of a child's medication use is important in constructing a MT treatment plan. This information assists in evaluating possible interactions between medications and MT. The following classes of medications are discussed as they relate to MT: anti-inflammatory and analgesics, muscle relaxants, clot management, antidepressants, anxiolytics, and diabetes management. Analgesics reduce the sensation of pain through either reducing inflammation or altering pain perception in the nervous system. This alteration changes tissue response, which then can alter the temperature, local blood flow, and muscle guarding of the child [42]. Therapists must be aware of this fact and extremely conservative with their treatment design. Muscle relaxants, which act on the brain, spinal cord, or muscle tissue to help diminish acute spasms or chronic plasticity from nervous system damage, can interfere with muscle reflexes. Therefore, deep tissue work, range of motion exercises, and excess stretching should be avoided. Typically, clot management medications come in two forms: anticoagulants to prevent the formation of new clots, and antiplatelets to prevent the clumping of platelets. All blood-clotting medications create risk for bruising, and therefore only gentle holding or light touch may be applied [43]. Antidepressant medications have common side effects, including dizziness, drowsiness, and lightheadedness, all of which can be exaggerated when combined with MT [44]. Anxiolytic medications that alter the sympathetic response in the central nervous system have side effects, including bleeding, poor reflexes, central nervous system depression, and exhaustion [45]. These side effects impact which type of MT should be performed, and patients and therapists must communicate about symptoms. Risks associated with diabetes management include systemic atherosclerosis, risk for stroke, diabetic ulcers, and peripheral neuritis [46]. MT should be conducted cautiously and with close communication with the medical team.

Context and availability of pediatric massage therapy

As CAM and integrative medicine increase in popularity, National Health Interview Survey data show that MT use is also rising. A 2005 survey of hospitals conducted by the Health Forum found that the growth in the number of hospitals offering CAM services has consistently increased each year from 1998 to 2004. A study of university-affiliated pain management centers (N = 43) in the United States and Canada found that 49% of centers offer MT [47]. The criteria used by a hospital to determine which CAM therapies to offer are a combination of patient demand (78.9%), evidence basis (64.5%), and practitioner availability (53.3%), as reported by the Health Forum Survey. Patients continue to pay for most services out-of-pocket, because insurance reimbursement is limited. According to the Health Forum Survey, patient satisfaction is currently the preferred metric in the evaluation of CAM services, and budgetary constraints and physician resistance are the major obstacles for implementing CAM programs.

A current challenge in offering pediatric MT to children who have serious medical conditions is that massage school graduates in the United States typically have little or no education in the area of pediatric MT, and few continuing education programs exist in this area [34,48]. Canadian programs tend to include education in the area of pediatric MT, but massage for children who have special health care needs is not necessarily covered. Several infant massage courses are taught nationally and internationally, although these courses tend to have a very limited amount of information on MT for infants who have special needs [37,49]. The development of high-quality training for massage therapists who wish to specialize in pediatric massage is needed. Additionally, collaborations between trained infant/pediatric licensed massage therapists and health care professionals is indicated.

Summary

For pediatricians and other clinicians considering the value of pediatric MT, many questions still remain. As family members and patients continue to be more educated about their health care and begin to request more holistic approaches for treatment (eg, alternative and complementary care), an increasing number of hospital and hospice settings are incorporating these modalities. Although MT has traditionally been considered a modality for symptom management, clinicians and researchers are beginning to view it as part of a larger holistic approach to health and healing involving multisystem integration and organization. Historically, pediatric MT has been provided by nurses and physical and occupational therapists in medical settings [17], but that is now beginning to change as more massage therapists are working as part of the health care team. An extensive body of clinical practice in this area shows benefit to children and, in some cases, their caregivers [14]. A substantial amount of qualitative data supports the physiologic and psychological benefits of MT for children [4]. Nevertheless, empirical studies that attain the gold standard remain limited by design and methodological considerations. The best empirical evidence shows reductions in anxiety and, to a lesser extent, reductions in pain. Improvements in pulmonary function and muscle tone seem promising, whereas the effects of MT on other health-related outcomes (eg, depression) require further investigation in children.

With the increased use of MT in medical and hospice settings, its demonstrated feasibility and safety, and the extreme rarity of negative outcomes, MT may be safely recommended for pediatric patients when provided by qualified and trained massage therapists who are working as part of the interdisciplinary medical team [41]. Significant reductions in anxiety alone are encouraging outcomes for children who have serious medical illness and may inevitably experience anxiety with their course of treatment. Cohen [50] argues that pediatricians are increasingly asked to advise pediatric patients and their caregivers on the integration of CAM into allopathic care and that including these therapies, as is the case with any medical subspecialty, is not itself "unethical," clinically inadvisable, or legally risky. He further states that pediatricians can help address potential malpractice liability issues by evaluating the level of clinical risk (which with MT seems minimal), engaging patients and their caregivers in shared decision making by obtaining parental permission and child assent, providing documentation in the medical record, continuing to monitor, not delaying medical treatment or substituting massage for conventional medical treatment, and being prepared to intervene conventionally when medically required. Given this overview, the stated considerations, the current evidence on pediatric MT, and the greater inclusion of CAM therapies into medical care, children and their caregivers may benefit from including MT in a comprehensive medical treatment plan.

References

[1] Onofrio J. The history of massage, bodywork and related modalities. Available at: http://www.thebodyworker.com/history.htm. Accessed August 1, 2007.

[2] Eisenberg DM, Davis RB, Ettner SL, et al. Trends in alternative medicine use in the United States, 1990–1997: results of a follow-up national survey. JAMA 1998;280:1569–75.

[3] Moyer CA, Rounds J, Hannum JW. A meta-analysis of massage therapy research. Psychol Bull 2004;130:3–18.

[4] Beider S, Moyer CA. Randomized control trials of pediatric massage: a review. eCAM 2007; 4:23–34.

[5] Integrative touch for kids. Available at: www.integrativetouch.org. Accessed September 16, 2007.

[6] The Center for compassionate touch. Available at: www.compassionate-touch.org. Accessed September 16, 2007.

[7] Vickers A, Ohlsson A, Lacy JB, et al. Massage for promoting growth and development of preterm/or low birth weight infants. Cochrane Review 2004;2(4):283–313.

[8] Field T. Massage therapy. Med Clin North Am 2002;86:163–71.

[9] Scafidi F, Field T. Massage therapy improves behavior in neonates born to HIV-positive mothers. J Pediatr Psychol 1996;21:889–97.

[10] Underdown A, Barlow J, Chung V, et al. Massage intervention for promoting mental and physical health in infants aged under six months. Cochrane Database Syst Rev 2006;4(3):1–28.

[11] Livingston, Beider S, Kant A, et al. Touch and massage for medically fragile infants. eCAM 2007.

[12] Tsao JC. Effectiveness of massage therapy for chronic, non-malignant pain: a review. Evid Based Complement Alternat Med 2007;4:165–79.

[13] Field T, Hernandez-Reif M, Seligman S, et al. Juvenile rheumatoid arthritis: benefits from massage therapy. J Pediatr Psychol 1997;22:607–17.

[14] Sinclair M. Pediatric massage therapy. 2nd edition. Philadelphia: Lippincott Williams & Wilkins; 2005.

[15] Werner R. A massage therapists' guide to pathology. 3rd edition. Philadelphia: Lippincott, Williams & Wilkins; 2005.

[16] Salvo S. Mosby's pathology for massage therapists. St. Louis (MO): Elsevier Mosby; 2004.

[17] MacDonald G. Massage for the hospital patient and medically frail client. Philadelphia: Lippincott Williams & Wilkins; 2005.

[18] Schachner L, Field T, Hernandez-Reif M, et al. Atopic dermatitis symptoms decreased in children following massage therapy. Pediatr Dermatol 1998;15:390–5.

[19] Roh YS, Cho H, Oh JO, et al. Effects of skin rehabilitation massage therapy on pruritus, skin status, and depression in burn survivors. Taehan Kanho Hakhoe Chi 2007;37:221–6.

[20] Field T. Massage therapy for skin conditions in young children. Dermatol Clin 2005;23: 717–21.

[21] Cherkin DC, Eisenberg D, Sherman KJ, et al. Randomized trial comparing traditional Chinese medical acupuncture, therapeutic massage, and self-care education for chronic low back pain. Arch Intern Med 2001;161:1081–8.

[22] Hawes MC, Brooks WJ. Reversal of the signs and symptoms of moderately severe idiopathic scoliosis in response to physical methods. Stud Health Technol Inform 2002;91:365–8.

[23] Vasudevan SV, Melvin JL. Upper extremity edema control: rationale of the techniques. Am J Occup Ther 1979;33:520–3.

[24] Meyer-Heim A, Rothmaier M, Weder M, et al. Advanced lightweight cooling-garment technology: functional improvements in thermosensitive patients with multiple sclerosis. Mult Scler 2007;13:232–7.

[25] Powell L, Barlow J, Cheshire A. The training and support programme for parents of children with cerebral palsy: a process evaluation. Complement Ther Clin Pract 2006;12:192–9.

[26] Field T, Diego M, Cullen C, et al. Fibromyalgia pain and substance P decrease and sleep improves after massage therapy. J Clin Rheumatol 2002;8:72–6.

[27] Field T. Touch therapy. London: Churchill Livingston Press; 2007.

[28] Field T, Quintino O, Hernandez-Reif M, et al. Adolescents with attention deficit hyperactivity disorder benefit from massage therapy. Adolescence 1998;33:103–8.

[29] Sibinga EM, Shindell DL, Casella JF, et al. Pediatric patients with sickle cell disease: use of complementary and alternative therapies. J Altern Complement Med 2006;12:291–8.

[30] Hernandez-Reif M, Field T, Krasnegor J, et al. Children with cystic fibrosis benefit from massage therapy. J Pediatr Psychol 1999;24:175–81.

[31] Guthrie DW, Gamble M. Energy therapies and diabetes mellitus. Diabetes Spectrum 2001; 14:149–53.

[32] Phipps S, Dunavant M, Gray E, et al. Massage therapy in children undergoing hematopoeitic stem cell transplantation: Results of a pilot trial. J Cancer Integrative Medicine 2005;3:62–70.

[33] Field T, Cullen C, Diego M, et al. Leukemia immune changes following massage therapy. Journal of Bodywork and Movement Therapies 2001;5:271–4.

[34] Williams PD, Schmideskamp J, Ridder EL, et al. Symptom monitoring and dependent care during cancer treatment in children: Pilot study. Cancer Nurs 2006;29:188–97.

[35] Van Cleve L, Bossert E, Beecroft P, et al. The pain experience of children with leukemia during the first year after diagnosis. Nurs Res 2004;53:1–10.

[36] Gentle massage for children. Available at: www.massageforchildren.com. Accessed July 24, 2007.

[37] Friedman T, Slayton WB, Allen LS, et al. Use of alternative therapies for children with cancer. Pediatrics 1997;100:E1.

[38] Beider S. Gentle massage for children. Massage Magazine 2006;126:60–70.

[39] Lafferty WE, Downey L, McCarty RL, et al. Evaluating CAM treatment at the end of life: a review of clinical trials for massage and meditation. Complement Ther Med 2006;14: 100–12.

[40] International association of infant massage. Available at: www.iaim.net. Accessed August 1, 2007.

[41] Ernst E. The safety of massage therapy. Rheumatology 2003;42:1101–6.

[42] Uretsky S. Analgesics. In: Jeryan C, Boyden K, editors. Gale Encyclopedia of Medicine. Gale Group; 2006.

[43] Ross-Flanigan N. Antidepressant medications. Available at: www.healthatoz.com. Accessed July 24, 2007.

[44] Health A to Z. Antidepressant medications. Available at: www.healthatoz.com. Accessed July 24, 2007.

[45] Health A to Z. Anti-anxiety medications. Available at: www.healthatoz.com. Accessed July 24, 2007.

[46] American Diabetes Association. Type 2 diabetes in children and adolescents. Diabetes Care 2000;23:381–9.

[47] Lin Y, Lee AC. Acupuncture for the management of pediatric pain. Annual Meeting of the Pediatric Academic Societies. San Francisco (CA), May 1999.

[48] A foundation for healthy family living. Available at: www.healthyfamily.org. Accessed August 1, 2007.

[49] Infant massage USA. Available at: www.infantmassageusa.org. Accessed August 1, 2007.

[50] Cohen MH. Legal and ethical issues relating to use of complementary therapies in pediatric hematology/oncology. J Pediatr Hematol Oncol 2006;28:190–3.

ELSEVIER
SAUNDERS

PEDIATRIC CLINICS
OF NORTH AMERICA

Pediatr Clin N Am 54 (2007) 1043–1060

Complementary and Alternative Therapies in Pediatric Oncology

Susan F. Sencer, MD[a],*, Kara M. Kelly, MD[b]

[a]Department of Pediatric Oncology, Children's Hospitals and Clinics of Minnesota,
2525 Chicago Avenue S., Minneapolis, MN 55404, USA
[b]Columbia University Medical Center, Division of Pediatric Oncology,
161 Fort Washington Avenue, IP-7, New York, NY 10032, USA

Complementary and alternative medicine (CAM) therapies, defined as "a group of diverse medical and health care systems, practices, and products that are not presently considered to be part of conventional medicine" [1], are often sought by cancer patients or, in the case of pediatric oncology, by their parents. Such therapies are chosen in part because they provide the opportunity to maintain a degree of control over care and offer hope for symptom management and even cure [2]. By definition, however, such therapies have not undergone the research scrutiny of those labeled "conventional," and therefore are often a significant source of concern for oncologists. Historically, many of the most notorious and high profile alternative therapies have been touted as a cure for cancer, contributing to the public and professional skepticism toward CAM in general. In addition, most CAM use among children with cancer is parent rather than provider driven, with the information obtained from friends, family or the Internet. Physicians often feel they are playing "catch-up" in trying to remain knowledgeable about the agents their patients are using.

The purpose of this article is to provide a practitioner working with pediatric oncology patients with an overview of the scope of CAM use in that population, including the types of therapies most commonly chosen. The authors discuss the research issues unique to CAM and pediatric oncology and hope to provide the reader with a knowledge base to begin discussions about CAM with patients and their parents, and the tools to further find reputable information about these therapies.

---

* Corresponding author.
  E-mail address: susan.sencer@childrensmn.org (S.F. Sencer).

0031-3955/07/$ - see front matter © 2007 Elsevier Inc. All rights reserved.
doi:10.1016/j.pcl.2007.10.007

Incidence and history

Recent surveys have demonstrated that between 31% and 84% of pediatric oncology patients world-wide use some type of CAM [2–11]. Children with cancer and chronic illness report more CAM use than children seen in general pediatric clinics. Most parents say they choose CAM for their child to help manage side effects and to do everything they can for their child. Families are more likely to use CAM for their child if a parent uses CAM, the child has a poor prognosis, or the parents are of an older age and are more educated. Children with cancer most commonly use prayer and spiritual healing [6], although the inclusion of prayer in CAM surveys is controversial and is felt by some researchers to unfairly inflate estimates of CAM use. Children with cancer also frequently use mind-body therapies, nutritional and herbal supplements, vitamins, and massage [5,9–11]. Hypnosis, guided imagery, and biofeedback are standard approaches in pediatric pain centers, with acupuncture increasingly being used for sickle cell disease [12] and other pain conditions. The authors have noticed an increase, especially among adolescents, in the use of biologically based supplements.

Of concern to pediatric oncologists is that only about half of parents, and even fewer adolescents, disclose their use of CAM to their providers [5]. The primary reason given, however, for not disclosing CAM use is that providers rarely ask. Many children with cancer are enrolled on cooperative group trials, adding a potentially confounding factor to already complex trial designs. Asking and documenting CAM use are critical steps in providing comprehensive care.

The International Society for Pediatric Oncology recently published guidelines that called for the health care team to be attentive to complementary therapies that may be physically or psychologically harmful to children and their parents, but also concur that the health care team should not automatically and dismissively discourage the use of nonharmful complementary therapies [13].

Integrative oncology

"Integrative oncology" is the term now preferred by many oncologists who choose to combine "high tech" conventional oncology treatment with "high touch" supportive care therapies. Integrative oncology is the evolving evidence-based specialty that uses complementary therapies in concert with medical treatment to enhance efficacy, improve symptom control, alleviate patient distress, and reduce suffering. Many hospitals or cancer programs are developing integrative medicine programs that provide services such as massage, mind-body techniques, and counseling on herbs and supplements. Most of these arise originally in adult centers; pediatricians should ensure that practitioners who offer services to children have been trained in the unique developmental needs of children and their families.

The integration of CAM therapies with conventional treatment for childhood cancer at a pediatric hospital or larger medical center offers several opportunities, especially the ability to provide truly multidisciplinary care. Programs such as these can provide not only access to CAM services, but also the ability to counsel patients on the risks and benefits of CAM therapies in the care of a child with cancer. CAM programs may also enhance the development of a research platform to facilitate access to patients for research studies, enhance collaborations with CAM practitioners for research, provide opportunities for feedback on CAM therapies from patients and their families, and also allow investigation of therapies via small pilot approaches that can subsequently be evaluated in a larger cooperative research group setting.

Increasingly, integrative oncology programs are stressing the concept of "wellness" for their cancer patients. Although "wellness" may seem a peculiar term to use when discussing a child with a life-threatening disease, the authors are more and more coming to realize that general tenets of good health, such as appropriate nutrition, adequate restful sleep, and especially exercise, are essential. Pediatric oncologists have historically thought of nutrition as hyperalimention, but nutritionists working with this population have been forceful in retraining pediatric oncologists to consider not only the importance of enteral feeding, but also of nutritional supplements, such as glutathione [14] and essential fatty acids [15,16]. A cooperative group trial of a whey protein-based glutathione supplement for children with cancer is in the final stages of development [17].

Multiple meta-analysis and systemic reviews in adults with cancer have found exercise to be a safe and effective intervention for treating fatigue and other symptoms during cancer treatment [18]. Research is just beginning in children with cancer; in children with acute lymphoblastic leukemia, exercise programs have been found to be safe and effective in improving aerobic fitness, strength, and functional mobility [19,20]. Research has found that children frequently experience physical performance changes during cancer treatment [21,22]; cancer survivors report in questionnaires that they have lower levels of physical activity when compared with healthy controls [23]. Exercise has the potential for improving fatigue, pain, nausea, sleep, and mood.

Complementary and alternative medicine therapies used in pediatric oncology

Most parents of children with cancer want their children to receive state-of-the-art therapy, which generally includes chemotherapy, radiation, and surgery. Increasingly, they also want the concomitant use of CAM therapies to help effect a cure or to alleviate symptoms. CAM therapies cover a wide spectrum, and include spiritual and psychologic approaches, energy systems approaches, chiropractic, massage, and the use of herbs or nutritional supplements. Specific CAM therapies used by children with cancer have geographic variability and go through waves of popularity.

Mind-body interventions

Many of the mind-body techniques, considered alternative in adult practice, are mainstream in pediatrics. Some of the earliest work with children and self-hypnosis was done with pediatric cancer patients [24,25]. These and later studies demonstrated that self-hypnosis, imagery, and distraction all can effectively decrease nausea and vomiting [26], as well as pain and anxiety related to procedures such as spinal taps and bone marrows [27]. The authors recommend that all children with malignancies be offered the opportunity to learn a self-regulatory skill early in their therapy. Child-life practitioners, available in all pediatric hospitals, are trained in guided imagery and other self-regulatory techniques, as are many developmental pediatricians. Therefore, even if a pediatric integrative medicine program is not directly available, these techniques should still be available to any child with cancer. Music therapy, also available in most pediatric hospitals, has been shown to affect a child's emotional state [28] as well as immune function [29]. There is currently an ongoing Children's Oncology Group (COG) limited institution study examining the role of music therapy in promoting resilience and coping in oncology patients.

Energy field therapies

Any article about CAM reflects the current state-of-the-art and the science, but is outdated rapidly as therapies once considered alternative or complementary are validated and move into the mainstream. Acupuncture, for instance, was previously considered CAM, but has been proven to be effective in adults for the nausea and vomiting related to chemotherapy and for certain types of pain. It has therefore moved into the realm of conventional therapies and is available in both integrative medicine programs and anesthesia departments. There have been few trials documenting the effectiveness of acupuncture in children for nausea and vomiting [30], although both acupressure bands and acupressure has been shown to be helpful in small studies [31,32]. Acupuncture is acceptable to even very young children, and bleeding or infectious complications have not been observed in the preliminary studies in children with cancer [33]. Currently, there is a cooperative group trial through the National Cancer Institute and COG to further define acupuncture's role in nausea and vomiting associated with chemotherapy for adolescents who have solid tumors.

Bodywork

Body-based therapies, such as massage, are associated with improvements in mood and anxiety [34]. In a recently published review of 24 randomized pediatric massage studies for various conditions, anxiety was consistently reduced after just one massage session [35]. The authors found similar effects in two pilot studies of massage in children with cancer, conducted at Children's Hospitals and Clinics in Minneapolis and St. Paul.

Biologically based complementary and alternative medicine therapies

While the integrative oncologist may feel that his or her primary role is to stress nonpharmacologic adjuncts to therapy for supportive care, the reality is that patients are increasingly using biologically based therapies, either as adjuncts to or substitutes for conventional therapics. A major concern among pediatric oncologists is the potential for interactions among biologic therapies with chemotherapy and radiation therapy. St. John's Wort was observed to interfere with irinotecan, which is metabolized through the cytochrome P450 CYP3A4 pathway [36], raising concerns that other herbal therapies may have similar interactions. Although there are few reports of clinically significant adverse interactions at the doses used, all biologic agents intended for use in cancer should be tested for pharmacokinetic interactions with standard chemotherapy drugs, particularly those metabolized by the CYP3A4 enzyme pathways. Of those tested, melatonin, whey protein, and St. John's Wort are inducers of the CYP pathway, and curcumin is an inhibitor. Agents tested and found to have no effect include milk thistle, echinacea, saw palmetto, ginkgo biloba, valerian, and green tea [37]. Table 1 lists interactions which are theoretically possible between herbs and drugs commonly used by children with cancer.

Adverse events have been reported with CAM therapies [38], especially from contamination of herbal products [2]. Despite these caveats, however, no actual herb-drug interactions resulting in adverse outcomes have been reported in human beings undergoing cancer treatment. Nonetheless, caution should be employed in recommending biologically active agents. Tremendous strides have been made in the care of children with cancer; we should not allow potentially life-saving therapies to be shortchanged in an effort to provide a less toxic, or more natural therapy.

Antioxidants

Antioxidant supplementation by patients during conventional cancer treatment is especially controversial. Antioxidants have gained increasing popularity for their role in reducing free radicals that are a cause of tissue damage, of the type seen in chemotherapy and radiation toxicities. Few studies have evaluated the use of antioxidant supplements specifically among children with cancer [5], and estimates of antioxidant use by adults with cancer vary widely depending on the survey, cancer type, and a variety of other individual and demographic factors [39–45]. Typically, antioxidants are used in conjunction with conventional cancer therapies.

Data from preclinical studies often support the potential role of antioxidants in preventing and treating disease in that oxidative stress and an antioxidant-depleted diet have been identified to correlate with the

Table 1
Drug herb interactions

Drug	Agent and potential interaction
Anticoagulation	**Agents which may increase bleeding potential**: Angelica root, anise, arnica flower, Asa foetida, black cohosh, capsicum, celery, chamomiles, clove, Denshen, Devils Claw, dong quai, Evening Primrose, fenugreek, feverfew, garlic, ginkgo biloba, guarana, Horse chestnut, licorice, onion, papain, parsley, Passion flower, Quassia, quinine, red clover, sweet clover, sunflower seeds (vitamin E)
	Agents which may increase effectiveness of anticoagulation leading to increased risk of bleeding: Broccoli, ginseng, green tea, plantain, Saint John's Wort, alfalfa (vitamin K), turmeric, inositol hexaphosphate (IP-6)
Corticosteroids, cyclosporine (immunosuppressive agents)	**Agents that may block the effectiveness of immunosuppressive agents**: Alfalfa sprouts, echinacea, licorice, Saint John's wort, vitamin E, zinc
	Agents that increase cyclosporine toxicity (increase levels): Grapefruit juice.
	Agents that may reduce immunosuppression: Cordyceps (with prenisolone), country mallow, ephedra, marshmallow (with dexamethasone)
Methotrexate	**Agents that may increase hepatotoxicity**: Echinacea, black cohosh, salicylate-containing herbs such as bilberry, cramp bark, meadowsweet, poplars, red clover, uva ursi, white willow, wintergreen
Tamoxifen	**Agents that may decrease effectiveness**: Black cohosh, soy
Cisplatin	**Agents that may increase toxicity**: Selenium
Itraconazole	**Agents that may decrease effectiveness**: Grapefruit juice
Penicillin	**Agents that may decrease effectiveness**: Khat
Etoposide	**Agents that may increase toxicity**: Saint John's Wort

Herbs that over time cause liver damage and can also interfere with chemotherapy

Herb	Reported hepatic adverse reactions
Gerimandu	Hepatic necrosis
Comfrey (pyrrolizidine alkaloids)	Veno-occlusive disease of the liver (VOD)
Chaparral	Hepatocellular damage
Konbacha tea	Hepatocellular damage

This list is not to suggest that these agents should be avoided altogether, but to suggest caution as with any possible drug interactions.

development of cancer [46]. Although some epidemiologic studies have observed an association between an increased intake of dietary antioxidants and a decreased risk of developing various adult cancers, these same correlations have not been seen with childhood cancer. Recent reports of decreased cancers with the supplemental use of vitamin D are intriguing [47], and may have a role in the recommendations the authors give to long-term follow up patients. Proponents claim that antioxidant supplementation may also protect normal tissues and allow for higher doses of chemotherapy to be administered. For instance, in a small study, the authors have demonstrated a hepatoprotectant effect of milk thistle during maintenance therapy for acute lymphoblastic leukemia [48]. Additionally, at certain concentrations, antioxidants might also be able to directly affect cancer cells through pro-oxidant effects.

Certain chemotherapy agents (especially anthracyclines, platinum-containing complexes, and alkylating agents) and radiation therapy both gain at least part of their anticancer effects by generating reactive oxygen species, or free radicals [49]. Much of the controversy surrounding antioxidants and cancer therapy is that, theoretically at least, these actions may be inhibited by the use of antioxidant supplements. However, chemotherapy agents often have multiple mechanisms of action beyond just free radical generation.

Few clinical trials have investigated antioxidant supplementation for the treatment of specific cancers, or for the reduction in or prevention of common adverse effects associated with anticancer therapy [50–55]. Most clinical trials have been limited by inadequate sample sizes, heterogeneous patient populations, variation in the routes of antioxidant administration, or study designs that lacked appropriate blinding to randomization [50]. Although the data on antioxidant use during chemotherapy has not been associated with an attenuation of the effects of the particular anticancer treatment on tumor control, the studies have not yet thoroughly investigated this issue to allow for the routine recommendation of antioxidant supplementation. More research is needed to determine the biologic mechanisms, appropriate antioxidant mixtures, and dosing for each clinical setting.

Because the clinical research on antioxidant supplementation has not yet adequately demonstrated that the benefits of supplementation clearly outweigh the risks, patients should be counseled to avoid dietary antioxidant supplements above the basic nutritional requirements during radiation therapy. Patients should exert caution in supplementing with antioxidants, while receiving treatment with chemotherapy agents, until their combined use is found to be safe and does not compromise the efficacy of chemotherapy agents.

Immune modulators

Immune modulators are another broad category of CAM therapies that are often used by cancer patients. It is understandable that patients assume that their immune systems, dampened by both malignancy and chemotherapy, need "boosting" to fight infection and the return of cancer. Many agents, including Asian mushrooms [56] and mistletoe [57], have been shown to increase cytotoxic T lymphocytes, natural killer cells, or endogenous production of cytokines. Whether these actions have in vivo efficacy to fight cancer is not yet well defined. Other agents, such as blue-green algae, (*spirulina* sp), have been shown in vitro to produce some immune stimulation, but not with validity in human studies [58]. In addition, blue-green algae may be contaminated with either heavy metals or toxic algae strains (eg, microcystin species), which can cause hepatotoxicity [59]. For this reason, blue-green algae products are not recommended for use in children with cancer.

The potential interactions of immune modulators with chemotherapy requires further study, along with phase I trials of dose, toxicities, and length of treatment. Until there is more evidence, children with leukemia or lymphoma, or having a stem cell transplant, should be discouraged from taking immune modulators.

Symptom control

The push toward integrative medicine has primarily come from patients and parents who perceive CAM as being more patient-friendly and more natural than more conventional therapies. This "natural" approach is appealing because of the often debilitating side effects of chemotherapy and radiation. However, because most pediatric cancers are curable with conventional treatment, the health care team must continue to stress to parents that conventional therapies are in general the best treatment for their children and that CAM therapies may be positive adjuncts. There is currently no systematic cure for any type of cancer in complementary therapies, and there is little scientific evidence yet as to whether CAM therapies increase survival, extend life, or improve quality of life. Nonetheless, preliminary and anecdotal evidence suggests that some therapies offer relief of symptoms associated with cancer treatment. A recent review summarized the CAM therapies that have some evidence of efficacy in children and adults for cancer symptom management [17]. Small clinical trials document effectiveness for acupuncture or ginger for nausea and vomiting, and hypnosis and imagery for pain and anxiety. Some supplements or herbs have shown effectiveness in adults for anxiety or fatigue, but few studies have been conducted in children. Although preliminary evidence supports the safety and effectiveness of acupuncture, hypnosis, imagery, and massage in cancer, more studies are needed to test the role of herbs, supplements, and homeopathic remedies in preventing and managing symptoms.

Chemotherapy induced mucositis is particularly troubling in the pediatric population; a homeopathic mouth rinse preparation was reported in a pilot study to be effective in both preventing and treating mucositis in children undergoing stem cell transplant [60], leading to a large COG group-wide trial. Patient accrual is complete for this and data analysis is underway. Adult clinical trials of glutamine, that uses a novel delivery system, has shown efficacy in reducing the incidence of mucositis following anthracycline therapy [61]; a clinical trial evaluating this agent in children is being developed.

Table 2 outlines both pharmacologic and nonpharmacologic CAM therapies for many of the most distressing symptoms of cancer and its therapies.

Table 2
Complementary and alternative medicine therapies for children with cancer

Symptom	Pharmacologic therapies	Nonpharmacologic therapies
Mucositis	Glutamine Homeopathic mouth rinses	
Pain		Heat Acupuncture Massage Exercise
Procedural pain		Hypnosis or imagery Massage Music Peppermint oil Healing Touch
Fatigue	Levocarnitine	Massage Acupuncture Relaxation or imagery Exercise
Loss of appetite	Essential fatty acids Cannabinoids Whey protein	
Anxiety and insomnia	Valerian Melatonin Chamomile tea	Aromatherapy Acupuncture Massage Hypnosis Exercise Music Therapy Yoga
Diarrhea	Colostrum Probiotics	
Constipation	Senna	Biofeedback Massage
Neuropathy and deconditioning	Glutamine Vitamin E	Exercise
Nausea	Ginger	Aromatherapy Acupressure Acupuncture Hypnosis Massage Yoga

The long term follow-up patient

Childhood cancer survivors are a growing population that faces unique challenges, such as obesity, infertility, osteopenia, reduced cardiac function, chronic fatigue, and a higher risk of second malignancies. They have been shown to have higher death rates than the general population because of recurrence of the original cancer or late effects of treatment, such as a second malignancy, cardiac abnormalities, or pulmonary complications [62]. A 2005 analysis of the Childhood Cancer Survivors Study (CCSS) reported that of over 14,000 adults who survived childhood cancer, 57% of survivors had a moderate health problem by age 45, compared with 18% of their siblings, and 37% had a severe health problem, compared with less than 5% of their siblings. It has also been shown that survivors think about their health differently than the general public, exhibited by lower rates of smoking and alcohol use in survivors [62,63]. Although the authors hypothesized that survivors may turn to CAM therapies to decrease their risk of cancer recurrence, or to treat their late effects, a recent survey of close to 10,000 survivors followed by CCSS revealed that survivors were no more likely than their siblings to use CAM, suggesting that survivors may be using other means to cope with stressors than using complementary modalities [64].

Research

The treatment of children with cancer is one of the great medical success stories of the last half-century. More than three-quarters of all children diagnosed with cancer will now be cured [65,66]. This is in distinction from many adult cancers, which are increasingly being treated as chronic conditions, rather than curable diseases. These remarkable gains in pediatric oncology have all been through careful, cumulative research, primarily under the umbrella of cooperative trial groups, such as the Children's Oncology Group and others throughout the world. All health care providers know now about treating childhood cancers was learned through research, with clinical trials as a final common pathway applying basic and clinical science discoveries. The rationale has been that the numbers of children with cancer are relatively low, and that few single institutions will have sufficient numbers to answer important questions. A similar approach is necessary as health care providers seek to answer questions about CAM use in children.

The Complementary and Alternative Medicine Subcommittee of COG (of which the authors are co-chairs) has as its charge to promote scientific investigation of complementary therapies as they relate to childhood cancer, and to provide reputable information on these therapies to health care providers and patients. The CAM Subcommittee's primary goal, however, is to design and execute intervention-based clinical trials to evaluate the efficacy of specific complementary therapies in use by children with cancer. To date, two large scale clinical trials have been undertaken; besides the aforementioned acupuncture trial, another study of the use of a homeopathic agent in the prevention and treatment of the mucositis associated with stem cell transplant has completed patient accrual and is in the final stages of analysis. Through the subcommittee's individual members, many smaller pilot studies have been done, as well as many surveys about CAM use in this population.

Most of the initial research on CAM in pediatric cancer relied upon surveys to determine prevalence of CAM use. Surveys are useful to identify areas for further research, but the current emphasis among researchers is to move away from descriptive studies and toward interventional studies.

The majority of studies to date, investigating CAM in children with cancer, have focused on CAM as supportive care agents and have been limited institution projects, with plans to move promising agents or modalities to group-wide trials. Investigators are also looking at developing new agents, such as curcumin, that have direct anticancer properties, with the hope of being able to bring them into phase I trials as well.

There are, however, barriers to mounting large-scale research studies of complementary therapies in children with cancer. There are many different types of CAM therapies in use by children with cancer, and very few have been evaluated for safety and efficacy. There is often little pre-existing literature, even in adults with cancer, to guide the prioritization of research studies. In addition, firmly held preconceptions by physicians, patients, and complementary or alternative medical practitioners about individual therapies have made the design and execution of studies difficult. Institutional review boards at individual institutions have been reluctant to take on potentially controversial complementary modalities. As CAM has become more accepted throughout the medical community, these issues have become less problematic. Many academic institutions, for instance, now have departments of integrative medicine. Nonetheless, the obstacles to designing and implementing CAM studies on a large scale are instructive.

However, it bears repeating that the bottom line is that CAM therapies offer no systematic cure for any type of cancer and there is little scientific evidence available as to whether these therapies result in survival advantage, life extension, or improved quality of life. Lack of evidence does not mean there is absence of effect. The small clinical studies, lack of standardization of the interventions, and lack of control over the many factors influencing responses, all reduce the quality of the trials that have been conducted to date. Finally, pediatric-specific research studies are particularly important, as results from studies in adults cannot always be extrapolated to a pediatric population because of children's unique developmental, social, and metabolic aspects.

Challenges in conducting research in CAM and pediatric oncology have been previously discussed; however, one of the foremost challenges in conducting CAM research remains effectively investigating fundamentally different medical systems within a western medical model. Medical models, such as traditional Chinese medicine, Ayurvedic medicine, and homeopathy employ diagnostic features not readily recognized in a western medical model. In traditional Chinese medicine, individuals with the same diagnosis may be treated with immensely different protocols dependent upon the individual's "chi" or energy. Within the western medical model, these patients with similar diagnosis would generally be treated in a similar fashion. However, individual-based therapies, a burgeoning new field in cancer research, reflects the understanding that every individual reacts to disease and therapeutic approaches in a unique fashion. Health care providers may in the future see new ways to study cancer therapies within alternative medical models.

Leading the way for families

The diagnosis of cancer in a child leaves parents and families devastated and vulnerable. Parents feel tremendous responsibility to ensure that they have researched the best therapies to treat their child's cancer. Although most families choose conventional treatment under the care of a pediatric oncologist, many also choose supplemental therapies from the complementary and alternative realm to support their children through treatment. Rarely, parents may choose alternative treatment instead of conventional therapies for their children with cancer. Western trained medical providers have often been hesitant to embrace complementary and alternative therapies because they have seen the negative consequences for patients who have foregone conventional therapy in hopes that a more "natural" therapy will be as effective with less toxicity. Pediatric oncologists in particular can point to the tremendous successes over the last 30 years in treating children with cancer, and are understandably reluctant to diverge from this path. This hesitancy to consider less proven therapies has often created animosity or tension between provider and patients or their parents, as well as with CAM providers themselves.

This tension is further increased because the oncologist is no longer the sole, or perhaps even primary, source of information, about their disease and its treatment, for most cancer patients and their families. The Internet, in particular, has become a powerful tool, allowing individuals to exchange information about therapies, both conventional and alternative. This rapid exchange of information has contributed to the increased use of unproven therapies, because anecdotal tributes and commercial Web sites are often more readily accessible and understandable to the Internet user than are results of scientific studies.

It is easy to understand the desire to try new approaches, to offer any possibility of cure or relief of pain. Parents of children with life-threatening diseases have a strong desire to alleviate pain and suffering for their children, and will search for every available means to this end. Pediatric oncologists are well-experienced in holding difficult discussions about painful subjects, but are not generally comfortable with families who may suggest alternatives to the treatment plan. Oncologists may find themselves in the perplexing position of trying to support these families in distress, while objectively researching new approaches the parents yearn to offer their children. The Appendix lists resources the authors find to be helpful in researching CAM therapies.

The decision to use CAM involves weighing the potential risks and benefits, along with preferences of families and developmental age and interest of the patient. Some therapies, such as mind-body therapies, carry little to no risk and, although they consume resources, are often justified by the rationale that they might provide some benefit. A trial approach is often used to determine which therapies are most appropriate for individual patients.

CAM therapies can increase a patient's feeling of control, which can increase compliance and have a therapeutic benefit. Patients and parents who seek additional therapies for their cancer are seeking to become partners in the healing process. Adult studies show a survival advantage to those individuals who take an active part in their own health care. We should no longer be threatened when patients are interested in taking a more active role in their health care, which includes CAM. However, it is important to assess and document the child's use of CAM, critically evaluate the evidence or lack of evidence, balance the potential risks with possible benefits, and assist the family in their choices and decisions regarding use of CAM for their child. All therapies should be monitored for ongoing safety, effectiveness, and clinical relevance.

Summary

Evidence on the science of CAM in children with cancer is slowly evolving. The ideal model of integrative pediatric oncology would offer CAM therapies that are deemed safe and effective, in conjunction with effective standard medical treatment. Because of potential interactions, herbs and supplements should be used with caution while on treatment. Health and wellness should be the emphasis, with CAM therapies supporting health promotion and key disease prevention strategies for childhood cancer survivors. All uses, responses, and effects of CAM therapies should be carefully documented. A desire to use CAM therapies may be an effort to become an active participant in the healing process. Health care providers should encourage, not discourage this partnership.

Acknowlegement

Our thanks to Elena Ladas, Janice Post-White, Casey Hooke, Kelly Finstrom, and Jan Watterson Schaeffers for their help in the preparation of this, and other manuscripts.

Appendix: Resources on complementary and alternative medicine

Book references

Physicians Desk Reference for Herbal Products. Published by Medical Economics Company, Inc., Montvale, New Jersey

Physicians Desk Reference for Nutritional Supplements. Published by Medical Economics Company, Inc., Montvale, New Jersey

Centers and institutions

National Center for Complementary and Alternative Medicine (http://nccam.nih.gov/)

National Cancer Institute PDQ (http://www.cancer.gov/cancertopics/pdq/cam)

Children's Oncology Group (www.childrensoncologygroup.org)

Integrative Therapies Program for Children with Cancer, Columbia University (www.integrativetherapiesprogram.org)

Memorial Sloan Kettering (http://www.mskcc.org/mskcc/html/11,570.cfm)

Children's Hospitals and Clinics of Minnesota (www.childrensmn.org/Communities/IntegrativeMed.asp)

Curriculum and conferences

CancerGuides, sponsored by the Center for Mind Body Medicine, an annual conference which explores CAM therapies for patients with cancer

Databases

National Library of Medicine (MEDLINE) (www.ncbi.nlm.nih.gov/)

The Natural Medicines Comprehensive Database (www.naturaldatabase.com)

The Cochrane Library (http://www3.interscience.wiley.com/cgi-bin/mrwhome/106,568,753/HOME)

Journals

Alternative Therapies in Health and Medicine (InnerDoorway Health Media, Inc.)

Integrative Cancer Therapies (Sage Publications)

Journal Complementary/Alternative Medicine (Mary Ann Lierbert, Inc. Publishers)

Product information

Consumer Lab (www.consumerlab.com)

Reviews

Sencer SF; Kelly KM. Bringing Evidence to Complementary and Alternative Medicine for Children With Cancer. Journal of Pediatric Hematology/Oncology. 28(3):186–9, 2006.

Cohen MH. Legal and Ethical Issues Relating to Use of Complementary Therapies in Pediatric Hematology/Oncology. Journal of Pediatric Hematology/Oncology. 28(3):190–3, 2006.

Sung L, Feldman BM. N-of-1 Trials: Innovative Methods to Evaluate Complementary and Alternative Medicines in Pediatric Cancer. Journal of Pediatric Hematology/Oncology. 28(4):263–6, 2006.

Melnick SJ. Developmental Therapeutics: Review of Biologically Based CAM therapies for Potential Application in Children With Cancer: Part I. Journal of Pediatric Hematology/Oncology. 28(4):221–30, 2006. (Part II, 2006;28(5):271–85.)

References

[1] National Institutes of Health National Center for Complementary and Alternative Medicine. Classification of complementary and alternative medical practices. NCCAM Publication No. D156, May 2002. Available at: http://nccam.nih.gov/health/whatiscam/#sup2. Accessed October 22, 2007.

[2] Kelly KM. Complementary and alternative medical therapies for children with cancer. Eur J Cancer 2004;40:2041–6.

[3] Sawyer MG, Gannoni AF, Toogood IR, et al. The use of alternative therapies by children with cancer. Med J Aust 1994;160:320–4.

[4] Friedman T, Slayton WB, Allen LS, et al. Use of alternative therapies for children with cancer. Pediatrics 1997;100:e1–6.

[5] Kelly KM, Jacobson JS, Kennedy DD, et al. Use of unconventional therapies by children with cancer at an urban medical center. J Pediatr Hematol Oncol 2000;22:412–6.

[6] McCurdy EA, Spangler JG, Wofford MM, et al. Religiosity is associated with the use of complementary medical therapies by pediatric oncology patients. J Pediatr Hematol Oncol 2003; 25:125–9.

[7] Copeland DR, Silberberg Y, Pfefferbaum B. Attitudes and practices of families of children in treatment for cancer: a cross-cultural study. Am J Pediatr Hematol Oncol 1983;5:65–71.

[8] Post-White J, Sencer S, Fitzgerald M. Complementary therapy use in pediatric cancer. Oncol Nurs Forum 2000;27(2):342–3.

[9] Mottonen M, Uhari M. Use of micronutrients and alternative drugs by children with acute lymphoblastic leukemia. Med Pediatr Oncol 1997;28:205–8.

[10] Fernandez CV, Stutzer CA, MacWilliam L, et al. Alternative and complementary therapy use in pediatric oncology patients in British Columbia: prevalence and reasons for use and nonuse. J Clin Oncol 1998;16:1279–86.

[11] Grootenhuis MA, Last BF, deGraaf-Nijkerk JH, et al. Use of alternative treatment in pediatric oncology. Can Nurs 1998;21:282–8.

[12] Hennessey J, Post-White J, Sencer S, et al. Complementary and alternative medicine use in pediatric patients with sickle cell disease. Presented at the 25th Annual Meeting of National Sickle Cell Disease Programs. New York, April 13–17, 2001.

[13] Jankovic M, Spinetta JJ, Martins AG, et al. Non-conventional therapies in childhood cancer: guidelines for distinguishing non-harmful from harmful therapies: a report of the SIOP working committee on psychosocial issues in pediatric oncology. Pediatr Blood Cancer 2004;42:106–8.

[14] Melnick SJ, Rogers P, Sacks N, et al. A pilot limited institutional study to evaluate the safety and tolerability of immunocal®, a nutraceutical cysteine delivery agent in the management of wasting in high-risk childhood cancer patients. Presented at the 1st Annual Chicago Supportive Oncology Conference. Chicago, October 6–8, 2005.

[15] Bruera E, Strasser F, Palmer JL, et al. Effect of fish oil on appetite and other symptoms in patients with advanced cancer and anorexia/cachexia: a double-blind, placebo-controlled study. J Clin Oncol 2003;21:129–34.

[16] Gogos CA, Ginopoulos P, Salsa B, et al. Dietary omega-3 polyunsaturated fatty acids plus vitamin E restore immunodeficiency and prolong survival for severely ill patients with generalized malignancy: a randomized control trial. Cancer 1998;82:395–402.

[17] Ladas EJ, Post-White J, Hawks R, et al. Evidence for symptom management in the child with cancer. J Pediatr Hematol Oncol 2006;28(9):601–15.

[18] Mitchell S, Beck S, Hood L, et al. 2005. What interventions are effective in preventing and treating fatigue during and following cancer and its treatment? ONS putting evidence into practice. Available at: http://www.ons.org/outcomes/resources/fatigue.shtml. Accessed April 27, 2007.

[19] San Juan AF, Fleck SJ, Chamorro-Viña C, et al. Effects of an intrahospital exercise program intervention for children with leukemia. Med Sci Sports Exerc 2007;39(1):13–21.

[20] Marinovic D, Dorgeret S, Lescoeur B, et al. Improvement in bone mineral density and body composition in survivors of childhood acute lymphoblastic leukemia: a 1-year prospective study. Pediatrics 2005;116(1):e102–8.

[21] Tillmann V, Darlington AS, Eiser C, et al. Male sex and low physical activity are associated with reduced spine bone mineral density in survivors of childhood acute lymphoblastic leukemia. J Bone Miner Res 2002;17(6):1073–80.

[22] Hockenberry M, Hooke MC. Symptom clusters in children with cancer. Semin Oncol Nurs 2007;23(2):152–7.

[23] Demark-Wahnefried W, Werner C, Clipp EC, et al. Survivors of childhood cancer and their guardians. Cancer 2005;103(10):2171–80.

[24] Lansky S. Imagery (self-hypnosis) as adjunct therapy in childhood cancer. Am J Pediatr Hematol Oncol 1981;3:313–21.

[25] Olness K. Imagery (self-hypnosis) as an adjunct therapy in childhood cancer: clinical experience with 25 patients. Am J Pediatr Hematol Oncol 1981;3:313–21.

[26] Zeltzer L, LeBaron S, Zeltzer P. The effectiveness of behavioral intervention for reduction of nausea and vomiting in children and adolescents receiving chemotherapy. J Clin Oncol 1984; 2:683–90.

[27] Zeltzer L, LeBaron S. Hypnosis and nonhypnotic techniques for reduction of pain and anxiety during painful procedures in children and adolescents with cancer. J Pediatr 1982; 101:1032–5.

[28] Barrera EM, Rykov MH, Doyle SL. The effects of interactive music therapy on hospitalized children with cancer: a pilot study. Psychooncology 2002;11:379–88.

[29] Marwick C. Leaving concert hall for clinic, therapists now test music's charms. JAMA 1996; 275:267–8.

[30] Reindl TK, Geilen W, Hartmann R, et al. Acupuncture against chemotherapy-induced nausea and vomiting in pediatric oncology interim results of a multicenter crossover study. Support Care Cancer 2006;14:172–6.

[31] Roscoe JA, Morrow GR, Hickok JT, et al. The efficacy of acupressure and acustimulation wrist bands for the relief of chemotherapy-induced nausea and vomiting. A University of Rochester Cancer Center Community Clinical Oncology Program multicenter study. J Pain Symptom Manage 2003;26:731–42.

[32] Treish I, Shord S, Valgus J, et al. Randomized double-blind study of the relief band as an adjunct to standard antiemetics in patients receiving moderately-high to highly emetogenic chemotherapy. Support Care Cancer 2003;11:516–21.

[33] Zeltzer LK, Tsao JC, Stelling C, et al. A phase I study on the feasibility and acceptability of an acupuncture/hypnosis intervention for chronic pediatric pain. J Pain Symptom Manage 2002;24:437–46.

[34] Field T, Cullen C, Diego M, et al. Leukemia immune changes following massage therapy. Journal of Bodywork and Movement Therapies 2001;5:271–4.

[35] Beider S, Moyer CA. Randomized controlled trials of pediatric massage: a review. Evid Based Complement Alternat Med 2007;4(1):23–34, Epub 2006 Nov.

[36] Mathijssen RH, Verweij J, de Bruijn P, et al. Effects of St. John's wort on irinotecan metabolism. J Natl Cancer Inst 2002;94:1247–9.

[37] Sencer SF, Reaman GH, Kelly KM. Complementary and alternative medicine utilization in childhood cancer: truth or consequences. American Society of Clinical Oncology Education Book; 2007. p. 617–21.

[38] Ernst E. Serious adverse effects of unconventional therapies for children and adolescents: a systematic review of recent evidence. Eur J Pediatr 2003;162:72–80.

[39] Lesperance ML, Olivotto IA, Forde N, et al. Mega-dose vitamins and minerals in the treatment of non-metastatic breast cancer: an historical cohort study. Breast Cancer Res Treat 2002;76:137–43.

[40] Legha SS, Wang YM, Mackay B, et al. Clinical and pharmacologic investigation of the effects of alpha-tocopherol on adriamycin cardiotoxicity. Ann N Y Acad Sci 1982;393:411–8.

[41] Clemens MR, Waladkhani AR, Bublitz K, et al. Supplementation with antioxidants prior to bone marrow transplantation. Wien Klin Wochenschr 1997;109:771–6.

[42] Burstein HJ, Gelber S, Guadagnoli E, et al. Use of alternative medicine by women with early-stage breast cancer. N Engl J Med 1999;340:1733–9.

[43] Branda RF, Naud SJ, Brooks EM, et al. Effect of vitamin B12, folate, and dietary supplements on breast carcinoma chemotherapy—induced mucositis and neutropenia. Cancer 2004;101:1058–64.

[44] Block KI, Koch AC, Mead MN, et al. Impact of antioxidant supplementation on chemotherapeutic efficacy: a systematic review of the evidence from randomized controlled trials. Cancer Treat Rev 2007;33:407–18.

[45] Mills EE. The modifying effect of beta-carotene on radiation and chemotherapy induced oral mucositis. Br J Cancer 1988;57:416–7.

[46] Salganik RI, Albright CD, Rodgers J, et al. Dietary antioxidant depletion: enhancement of tumor apoptosis and inhibition of brain tumor growth in transgenic mice. Carcinogenesis 2000;21(5):909–14.

[47] Lappe JM, Travers-Gustafson D, Davies KM, et al. Vitamin D and calcium supplementation reduces cancer risk: results of a randomized trial. Clin Nutr 2007;85(6):1586–91.

[48] Post-White J, Ladas EJ, Kelly KM. Advances in the use of milk thistle (Silybum marianum). Integr Cancer Ther 2007;6(2):104–9.

[49] Moss RW. Should patients undergoing chemotherapy and radiotherapy be prescribed antioxidants? Integr Cancer Ther 2006;5:63–82.

[50] Ladas EJ, Jacobson JS, Kennedy DD, et al. Antioxidants and cancer therapy: a systematic review. J Clin Oncol 2004;22:517–28.

[51] Bairati I, Meyer F, Gelinas M, et al. Randomized trial of antioxidant vitamins to prevent acute adverse effects of radiation therapy in head and neck cancer patients. J Clin Oncol 2005;23:5805–13.

[52] Drisko JA, Chapman J, Hunter VJ. The use of antioxidant therapies during chemotherapy. Gynecol Oncol 2003;88:434–9.

[53] Drisko JA, Chapman J, Hunter VJ. The use of antioxidants with first-line chemotherapy in two cases of ovarian cancer. J Am Coll Nutr 2003;22:118–23.

[54] Hoenjet KM, Dagnelie PC, Delaere KP, et al. Effect of a nutritional supplement containing vitamin E, selenium, vitamin C and coenzyme Q10 on serum PSA in patients with hormonally untreated carcinoma of the prostate: a randomised placebo-controlled study. Eur Urol 2005;47:433–9.

[55] Pathak AK, Bhutani M, Guleria R, et al. Chemotherapy alone vs. chemotherapy plus high dose multiple antioxidants in patients with advanced non small cell lung cancer. J Am Coll Nutr 2005;24:16–21.

[56] Borchers AT, Stern JS, Hackman RM, et al. Mushrooms, tumors, and immunity. Exp Biol Med 1999;221:281–93.

[57] Ernst E, Schmidt K, Steuer-Vogt MK. Mistletoe for cancer? A systematic review of randomized clinical trials. Int J Cancer 2003;107(2):262–7.

[58] Jensen GS, Ginsberg DI, Drapeau C. Blue-green algae as an immuno-enhancer and biomodulator. J Amer Nutraceut Assoc 2001;3(4):24–30.

[59] Wasa M, Yamamoto M, Tanaka Y, et al. Spirulina-associated hepatotoxicity. Am J Gastroenterol 2002;97(12):3212–3.

[60] Oberbaum M, Yaniv I, Ben-Gal Y, et al. A randomized, controlled clinical trial of the homeopathic medicine TRAUMEEL S™ in the treatment of chemotherapy-induced stomatitis in children undergoing stem cell transplantation. Cancer 2001;92:684–90.

[61] Peterson DE, Jones JB, Petit RG. Randomized, placebo-controlled trial of Saforis for prevention and treatment of oral mucositis in breast cancer patients receiving anthracycline-based chemotherapy. Cancer 2007;109(2):322–31.

[62] Mertens AC, Yasui Y, Neglia J, et al. Late mortality experience in five-year survivors of childhood and adolescent cancer: the childhood cancer survivor study. J Clin Oncol 2001; 19:3163–72.

[63] Emmons K, Li F, Whitton J, et al. Predictors of smoking initiation and cessation among childhood cancer survivors. J Clin Oncol 2002;20:1608–16.

[64] Mulhern RK, Tyc VL, Phipps S, et al. Health-related behaviors of survivors of childhood cancer. Med Pediatr Oncol 1995;25:159–65.

[65] Mertens AC, Sencer S, Myers CD, et al. Complementary and alternative therapy use in adult survivors of childhood cancer: a report from the childhood cancer survivor study. Pediatr Blood Cancer 2007, [e-pub ahead of print].

[66] Ries LAG, Smith MA, Gurney JG, et al, editors. Cancer incidence and survival among children and adolescents: United States SEER Program 1975–1995, National Cancer Institute, SEER Program. NIH Pub. No. 99–4649. Bethesda (MD); 1999.

PEDIATRIC CLINICS

OF NORTH AMERICA

ELSEVIER
SAUNDERS   Pediatr Clin N Am 54 (2007) 1061–1070

Index

Note: Page numbers of article titles are in **boldface** type.

Moving?

Make sure your subscription moves with you!

To notify us of your new address, find your **Clinics Account Number** (located on your mailing label above your name), and contact customer service at:

E-mail: elspcs@elsevier.com

800-654-2452 (subscribers in the U.S. & Canada)
407-345-4000 (subscribers outside of the U.S. & Canada)

Fax number: 407-363-9661

Elsevier Periodicals Customer Service
6277 Sea Harbor Drive
Orlando, FL 32887-4800

*To ensure uninterrupted delivery of your subscription, please notify us at least 4 weeks in advance of move.